T0259609

Flow Cytometry

Editor

DAVID M. DORFMAN

CLINICS IN LABORATORY MEDICINE

www.labmed.theclinics.com

Editor-in-Chief
MILENKO JOVAN TANASIJEVIC

December 2017 • Volume 37 • Number 4

ELSEVIER

1600 John F. Kennedy Boulevard • Suite 1800 • Philadelphia, Pennsylvania, 19103-2899

http://www.theclinics.com

CLINICS IN LABORATORY MEDICINE Volume 37, Number 4
December 2017 ISSN 0272-2712, ISBN-13: 978-0-323-55282-0

Editor: Stacy Eastman
Developmental Editor: Laura Fisher

© **2017 Elsevier Inc. All rights reserved.**

This periodical and the individual contributions contained in it are protected under copyright by Elsevier, and the following terms and conditions apply to their use:

Photocopying

Single photocopies of single articles may be made for personal use as allowed by national copyright laws. Permission of the Publisher and payment of a fee is required for all other photocopying, including multiple or systematic copying, copying for advertising or promotional purposes, resale, and all forms of document delivery. Special rates are available for educational institutions that wish to make photocopies for non-profit educational classroom use. For information on how to seek permission visit www.elsevier.com/permissions or call: (+44) 1865 843830 (UK)/(+1) 215 239 3804 (USA).

Derivative Works

Subscribers may reproduce tables of contents or prepare lists of articles including abstracts for internal circulation within their institutions. Permission of the Publisher is required for resale or distribution outside the institution. Permission of the Publisher is required for all other derivative works, including compilations and translations (please consult www.elsevier.com/permissions).

Electronic Storage or Usage

Permission of the Publisher is required to store or use electronically any material contained in this periodical, including any article or part of an article (please consult www.elsevier.com/permissions). Except as outlined above, no part of this publication may be reproduced, stored in a retrieval system or transmitted in any form or by any means, electronic, mechanical, photocopying, recording or otherwise, without prior written permission of the Publisher.

Notice

No responsibility is assumed by the Publisher for any injury and/or damage to persons or property as a matter of products liability, negligence or otherwise, or from any use or operation of any methods, products, instructions or ideas contained in the material herein. Because of rapid advances in the medical sciences, in particular, independent verification of diagnoses and drug dosages should be made.

Although all advertising material is expected to conform to ethical (medical) standards, inclusion in this publication does not constitute a guarantee or endorsement of the quality or value of such product or of the claims made of it by its manufacturer.

Reprints. For copies of 100 or more, of articles in this publication, please contact the Commercial Reprints Department, Elsevier Inc., 360 Park Avenue South, New York, New York 10010-1710. Tel. 212-633-3874, Fax: 212-633-3820, E-mail: reprints@elsevier.com.

Clinics in Laboratory Medicine (ISSN 0272-2712) is published quarterly by Elsevier Inc., 360 Park Avenue South, New York, NY 10010-1710. Months of issue are March, June, September, and December. Business and Editorial offices: 1600 John F. Kennedy Blvd., Suite 1800, Philadelphia, PA 19103-2899. Periodicals postage paid at New York, NY and additional mailing offices. Subscription prices are $258.00 per year (US individuals), $488.00 per year (US institutions), $100.00 per year (US students), $314.00 per year (Canadian individuals), $593.00 per year (Canadian institutions), $185.00 per year (Canadian students), $402.00 per year (international individuals), $593.00 per year (international institutions), $185.00 (international students). Foreign air speed delivery is included in all Clinics subscription prices. All prices are subject to change without notice. POSTMASTER: Send address changes to *Clinics in Laboratory Medicine*, Elsevier Health Sciences Division, Subscription Customer Service, 3251 Riverport Lane, Maryland Heights, MO 63043. **Customer Service: 1-800-654-2452 (US). From outside of the US and Canada, call 1-314-447-8871. Fax: 1-314-447-8029. E-mail: journalscustomerservice-usa@elsevier.com (for print support) or journalsonlinesupport-usa@elsevier.com (for online support).**

Clinics in Laboratory Medicine is covered in *EMBASE/Exerpta Medica, MEDLINE/PubMed (Index Medicus), Cinahl, Current Contents/Clinical Medicine, BIOSIS and ISI/BIOMED.*

Contributors

CONSULTING EDITOR

MILENKO JOVAN TANASIJEVIC, MD, MBA
Vice Chair for Clinical Pathology and Quality, Department of Pathology, Director of Clinical Laboratories, Brigham and Women's Hospital and Dana Farber Cancer Institute, Associate Professor of Pathology, Harvard Medical School, Boston, Massachusetts, USA

EDITOR

DAVID M. DORFMAN, MD, PhD
Department of Pathology, Brigham and Women's Hospital, Harvard Medical School, Boston, Massachusetts, USA

AUTHORS

GREGORY K. BEHBEHANI, MD, PhD
Assistant Professor of Internal Medicine, Division of Hematology, The Ohio State University, Arthur G. James Cancer Hospital, Columbus, Ohio, USA

MICHAEL BITAR, MSc
Medical Faculty, Department of Diagnostics, Institute of Clinical Immunology, University of Leipzig, Leipzig, Germany

ANDREAS BOLDT, PhD
Medical Faculty, Department of Diagnostics, Institute of Clinical Immunology, University of Leipzig, Leipzig, Germany

JACK BUI, MD, PhD
Associate Professor, Department of Pathology, UC San Diego, La Jolla, California, USA

XUEYAN CHEN, MD, PhD
Assistant Professor, Department of Laboratory Medicine, University of Washington, Seattle, Washington, USA

SINDHU CHERIAN, MD
Associate Professor, Department of Laboratory Medicine, University of Washington, Seattle, Washington, USA

JACQUELINE M. CORTAZAR, MD
Department of Pathology, Brigham and Women's Hospital, Harvard Medical School, Boston, Massachusetts, USA

JEFFREY W. CRAIG, MD, PhD
Department of Pathology, Brigham and Women's Hospital, Harvard Medical School, Boston, Massachusetts, USA

DAVID M. DORFMAN, MD, PhD
Department of Pathology, Brigham and Women's Hospital, Harvard Medical School, Boston, Massachusetts, USA

ALEXANDRA M. HARRINGTON, MD
Associate Professor, Department of Pathology, Medical College of Wisconsin, Milwaukee, Wisconsin, USA

ANDREA ILLINGWORTH, MS, H(ASCP), SCYM
Dahl Chase Diagnostic Services, Bangor, Maine, USA

DRAGAN JEVREMOVIC, MD, PhD
Assistant Professor of Pathology, Division of Hematopathology, Mayo Clinic, Rochester, Minnesota, USA

JEFFREY L. JORGENSEN, MD, PhD
Professor, Department of Hematopathology, The University of Texas MD Anderson Cancer Center, Houston, Texas, USA

MIKE KEENEY, ART, FCSMLS(D)
Associate Scientist, Pathology and Laboratory Medicine, London Health Sciences Centre, Ontario, Canada

STEVEN H. KROFT, MD
Professor and Executive Vice Chair of Pathology, Director of Clinical Pathology and Hematopathology, Department of Pathology, Medical College of Wisconsin, Milwaukee, Wisconsin, USA

CATHERINE P. LEITH, MB BChir
Professor, Department of Pathology and Laboratory Medicine, University of Wisconsin–Madison School of Medicine and Public Health, Madison, Wisconsin, USA

JIE LI, MD
Department of Pathology and Laboratory Medicine, Division of Hematopathology, The Children's Hospital of Philadelphia, Hospital of University of Pennsylvania, Perelman School of Medicine, University of Pennsylvania, Philadelphia, Pennsylvania, USA

PHUONG NGUYEN, MD
Associate Professor of Pathology, Division of Hematopathology, Mayo Clinic, Rochester, Minnesota, USA

MICHELE PAESSLER, DO
Associate Professor, Department of Pathology and Laboratory Medicine, Division of Hematopathology, The Children's Hospital of Philadelphia, Philadelphia, Pennsylvania, USA

VINODH PILLAI, MD, PhD
Assistant Professor, Department of Pathology and Laboratory Medicine, Division of Hematopathology, The Children's Hospital of Philadelphia, Hospital of University of Pennsylvania, Perelman School of Medicine, University of Pennsylvania, Philadelphia, Pennsylvania, USA

YU QIAN, PhD
Assistant Professor, Department of Informatics, J. Craig Venter Institute, La Jolla, California, USA

ULRICH SACK, MD
Professor, Department of Diagnostics, Institute of Clinical Immunology, University of Leipzig, Leipzig, Germany

RICHARD H. SCHEUERMANN, PhD
Professor and Campus Director, Department of Informatics, J. Craig Venter Institute, Adjunct Professor, Department of Pathology, UC San Diego, La Jolla, California, USA

ADAM C. SEEGMILLER, MD, PhD
Associate Professor, Department of Pathology, Microbiology, and Immunology, Vanderbilt University Medical Center, Nashville, Tennessee, USA

AARON C. SHAVER, MD, PhD
Assistant Professor, Department of Pathology, Microbiology, and Immunology, Vanderbilt University Medical Center, Nashville, Tennessee, USA

MIN SHI, MD, PhD
Assistant Professor of Pathology, Division of Hematopathology, Mayo Clinic, Rochester, Minnesota, USA

KAH TEONG SOH, MS
Department of Flow and Image Cytometry, Roswell Park Cancer Institute, Buffalo, New York, USA

D. ROBERT SUTHERLAND, MS
Professor of Medicine, Laboratory Medicine Program, Toronto General Hospital, University Health Network, Toronto, Ontario, Canada

JOSEPH D. TARIO Jr, PhD
Department of Flow and Image Cytometry, Roswell Park Cancer Institute, Buffalo, New York, USA

PAUL K. WALLACE, PhD
Professor, Department of Flow and Image Cytometry, Roswell Park Cancer Institute, Buffalo, New York, USA

HUAN-YOU WANG, MD, PhD
Professor, Department of Pathology, UC San Diego School of Medicine, La Jolla, California, USA

SA A. WANG, MD
Professor, Department of Hematopathology, The University of Texas MD Anderson Cancer Center, Houston, Texas, USA

GERALD WERTHEIM, MD, PhD
Assistant Professor, Department of Pathology and Laboratory Medicine, Division of Hematopathology, The Children's Hospital of Philadelphia, Hospital of University of Pennsylvania, Perelman School of Medicine, University of Pennsylvania, Philadelphia, Pennsylvania, USA

JIE XU, MD, PhD
Assistant Professor, Department of Hematopathology, The University of Texas MD Anderson Cancer Center, Houston, Texas, USA

Contents

of hematogones, the normal counterpart of leukemic B lymphoblasts. Assessment of multiple flow cytometry markers, in concert with each other in multidimensional histograms, is necessary to distinguish hematogones from malignant blasts. Emerging therapies targeting CD19 and other B-cell markers can disrupt the most frequently used MRD assessment, requiring a revised approach as the use of targeted therapies becomes widespread.

Multicolor flow cytometry (MFC), combined with molecular and cytogenetic studies, is the most common method for detecting minimal residual disease (MRD) in acute myeloid leukemia (AML). Studies have shown that a positive MFC MRD study after induction and/or consolidation, or before allogeneic hematopoietic stem cell transplantation, correlates with risk of relapse and inferior survival. However, there is little information on technical and analytical details. This article shares the authors' experience using MFC for AML MRD detection, including antibody panel design, data analysis, and interpretation. It summarizes diagnostic pearls and pitfalls and provides practical information for pathologists or hematologists.

Flow cytometry immunophenotyping of the hematopoietic cells from the bone marrow can help with diagnosis, prognosis, and therapy of chronic myeloid neoplasms. Unlike with B-cell neoplasms, there is no simple phenotypic test to substitute for clonality. Therefore, antigen panels to evaluate myeloid neoplasms are larger and the gating strategies more complex than for lymphoid neoplasms. The number of phenotypic abnormalities in hematopoietic cells correlates with disease severity and cytogenetic complexity and can be integrated into a scoring system for diagnostic and prognostic purposes. However, flow cytometry remains only an adjunct diagnostic modality.

Plasma cell dyscrasia (PCD) is a heterogeneous disease that has seen a tremendous change in outcomes as a result of improved therapies. Over the past few decades, multiparametric flow cytometry has played an important role in the detection and monitoring of PCDs. Flow cytometry is a high-sensitivity assay for early detection of minimal residual disease (MRD) that correlates well with progression-free survival and overall survival. Before flow cytometry can be effectively implemented in the clinical setting, sample preparation, panel configuration, analysis, and gating strategies must be optimized to ensure accurate results. Current consensus methods and reporting guidelines for MRD testing are discussed.

to identify rare diseases that need additional FC testing. Strategies to limit FC testing include the use of algorithms to predict disease probability, with limited FC performed if disease is unlikely. Successful algorithms use easily available parameters, have well-defined rules for use, and are periodically reviewed and updated to maximize efficiency while containing costs.

Richard H. Scheuermann, Jack Bui, Huan-You Wang, and Yu Qian

Flow cytometry is used in cell-based diagnostic evaluation for blood-borne malignancies, including leukemia and lymphoma. The current practice for cytometry data analysis relies on manual gating to identify cell subsets in complex mixtures, which is subjective, labor intensive, and poorly reproducible. This article reviews recent efforts to develop, validate, and disseminate automated computational methods and pipelines for cytometry data analysis that could help overcome the limitations of manual analysis and provide for efficient and data-driven diagnostic applications. It demonstrates the performance of an optimized computational pipeline in a pilot study of chronic lymphocytic leukemia data from the authors' clinical diagnostic laboratory.

Gregory K. Behbehani

Mass cytometry is a novel technology similar to flow cytometry in which antibodies are tagged with heavy metal molecules rather than fluorophores and then detected with time-of-flight mass spectrometry. This method enables the measurement of up to 50 simultaneous parameters with no autofluorescent background and little or no spillover or required compensation. Mass cytometry has tremendous potential for the analysis of highly complex clinical samples for the diagnosis and monitoring of malignant and autoimmune disorders. The technology also presents several unique challenges for clinical use and will require new approaches to analyze the large amounts of data generated.

CLINICS IN LABORATORY MEDICINE

THE CLINICS ARE NOW AVAILABLE ONLINE!
Access your subscription at:
www.theclinics.com

Preface

Clinical Flow Cytometry: State-of-the-Art and New Approaches

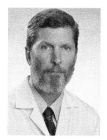

David M. Dorfman, MD, PhD
Editor

Flow cytometric immunophenotypic analysis is critical for diagnosing and subtyping a number of hematopoietic neoplasms. In recent years, significant advances in clinical flow cytometry have included the development of robust commercial flow cytometers suitable for the multiparametric assessment of clinical samples, a wide range of fluorochrome-conjugated antibodies directed at antigens that are useful for the identification of hematopoietic cells at various stages of development and differentiation, as well as sophisticated data analysis software.

This 2017 issue of *Clinics in Laboratory Medicine* summarizes the current state of the field. It reviews the flow cytometric analysis of B-cell and T-cell neoplasms and acute leukemias and discusses the rationale for flow cytometric testing, gating strategies, antibody panels for diagnosis and disease subtyping, and specific immunophenotypic patterns important for differential diagnosis. It discusses flow cytometric testing of systemic mastocytosis and paroxysmal nocturnal hemoglobinuria, two rare diseases well suited to assessment by flow cytometric analysis, particularly with new immunophenotypic markers and approaches. It reviews flow cytometric analysis of minimal residual disease in patients with acute lymphoblastic leukemia, which has become a standard clinical practice. In addition, Dr Sa A. Wang and colleagues at MD Anderson Cancer Center describe here their approach for the flow cytometric assessment of minimal residual disease in patients with acute myeloid leukemia, an application of clinical flow cytometry that is not yet widely employed.

This issue also discusses the flow cytometric analysis of hematopoietic neoplasms in pediatric patients and in patients with primary immunodeficiencies. Several articles discuss timely and emerging topics, such as algorithms and strategies for cost-effective flow cytometric testing of clinical samples and sophisticated approaches and scoring systems to assess chronic myeloid neoplasms, another area of clinical flow cytometry that is still in development. Dr Richard H. Scheuermann, one of the pioneers of

Clin Lab Med 37 (2017) xiii–xiv
http://dx.doi.org/10.1016/j.cll.2017.09.001
0272-2712/17/© 2017 Published by Elsevier Inc.

the field, discusses automated analysis of clinical flow cytometry data using computer algorithms. This approach has been employed for the assessment of a number of hematopoietic neoplasms and holds great promise for identifying important patterns in complex multiparametric data generated by contemporary flow cytometers. In the future, clinical flow cytometry and related technology will likely permit increasingly multiparametric immunophenotyping approaches to be employed in routine clinical practice. Dr Gregory K. Behbehani discusses the potential clinical application of mast cytometry, a novel technology that has the potential to significantly expand the ability to perform immunophenotyping with up to 50 simultaneous parameters, as well as a number of highly sophisticated data analysis approaches developed to analyze mass cytometry data.

I wish to express my gratitude to the authors of these articles for their contributions, which I hope will enlighten students and practitioners of clinical flow cytometry and hematopathology.

David M. Dorfman, MD, PhD
Department of Pathology
Brigham and Women's Hospital
and Harvard Medical School
75 Francis Street
Boston, MA 02115, USA

E-mail address:
ddorfman@bwh.harvard.edu

Flow Cytometry of B-Cell Neoplasms

Steven H. Kroft, MD*, Alexandra M. Harrington, MD

KEYWORDS

- Flow cytometry • Immunophenotypic aberrancy • Light chains/clonality
- Chronic lymphoproliferative disorders • Small B-cell lymphomas
- Aggressive B-cell lymphomas

KEY POINTS

- Light chain restriction or absence of light chain expression is evidence of clonality for most mature B-cell neoplasms; however, assessment of light chains by flow cytometry has technical, specimen source, and disease-specific challenges.
- Most B-cell neoplasms show immunophenotypic aberrancy, when compared with their normal cell counterparts.
- Chronic lymphocytic leukemia/small lymphocytic lymphoma is defined by its immunophenotype: CD5(+), CD10(−), CD20 dim(+), CD23(+), FMC7(−), CD79b(−), CD200(+), surface immunoglobulin(dim+).
- Hairy cell leukemia can be distinguished from its morphologic mimickers with CD25, CD103, and CD123.
- Double-hit lymphomas have a characteristic immunophenotype, showing diminished CD19, CD20, and light chain expression and positivity for CD10 and CD38 (bright).

INTRODUCTION

The role of flow cytometry in the evaluation of B-cell neoplasia has been well established for several decades. It has expanded, however, from an early focus on classification of leukemic disorders in blood or bone marrow to far broader applications in the identification, classification, prognostication, and follow-up of many different disorders in virtually any body site. Consequently, the literature pertaining to this topic is voluminous and complex; therefore, this review focuses mainly on the general approach to and major issues in the flow cytometric evaluation of this group of disorders.

The authors have nothing to disclose.
Department of Pathology, Medical College of Wisconsin, 8701 Watertown Plank Road, Milwaukee, WI 53226, USA
* Corresponding author.
E-mail address: skroft@mcw.edu

GENERAL APPROACH AND TECHNICAL ISSUES

The diagnosis of neoplasia by immunophenotypic methods can be divided into 2 general categories: demonstration of clonality and demonstration of antigenic differences from normal counterparts (aberrancy). The former, accomplished through analysis of surface light chain expression, is most often emphasized in the assessment for mature B-cell malignancies. This approach is not applicable, however, to most B-lymphoblastic processes and the small proportion of mature B-cell malignancies that lack surface light chain expression. In these scenarios, the demonstration of deviations from normal patterns forms the primary basis of flow cytometric diagnosis.

Light Chain Analysis

The classic approach to light chain analysis involves gross gating on lymphocytes or B cells, enumerating the percentage of cells expressing either kappa or lambda, often by quadrant analysis, and calculating a kappa to lambda ratio. If the ratio is within normal limits, a B-cell clone is presumed to be absent. If the ratio exceeds the normal range, a clonal process is assumed to be present. The normal range for kappa to lambda ratios given for gross B-cell populations is variable, but a typical range is 0.5 to 3.0.[1–5] From a technical standpoint, a few issues are worth mentioning. First, it is essential that kappa and lambda be assessed in the same tube and visualized in a bivariate plot. Light chains often demonstrate significant nonspecific fluorescence, and bivariate plots of these mutually exclusive antigens allow more precise discrimination of kappa and lambda expressing cells. Second, B cells should be gated as precisely as possible, preferably with more than one pan-B-cell antigen, to avoid noise in the light chain analysis. Finally, the kappa and lambda clusters should be defined as precisely as possible; gross quadrant analysis may not be sufficient. When this more rigorous approach is applied, the normal kappa to lambda ratio in most tissues shrinks to approximately 1.0 to 2.0.[3]

Even with precise gating on B cells, this approach can lack sensitivity. Clonal B-cell populations may be outnumbered by reactive, polyclonal B cells (in many extranodal marginal zone lymphomas, for example) (**Fig. 1**), and the kappa to lambda ratio may be normal despite the presence of a clone. Fortunately, lymphoma cells in most cases are not only light chain restricted but also deviate from normal B cells by expression of or intensity of expression of one or more antigens.[6–9] These deviations create variably distinct populations in virtual high dimensional space; precise analysis of these populations demonstrates true light chain restriction (as opposed to light chain skew) and, therefore, confident diagnosis of neoplasia (by both clonality and aberrancy) (see **Fig. 1**). Kappa to lambda ratios become almost beside the point, other than as a trigger to perform more detailed analysis when skewed. Implicit in this concept is the fact that the more antigens assessed per tube (ie, the higher the dimensionality of the data), the easier it will be to discriminate populations. However, sufficiently robust analysis techniques are required for these discriminations; gross gating is not sufficient. Ideally, an iterative approach that maximally uses the multidimensional data available should be applied. One such approach (sometimes termed *cluster analysis*) has been repeatedly demonstrated to effectively and precisely discriminate population clusters in high dimensional analysis.[10]

Finally, it should be mentioned that physiologic clones exist. Given that a lymphocyte's normal response to antigen is clonal expansion, this should not be surprising. Specifically, germinal center populations in lymph nodes with florid follicular hyperplasia may show a skewing of the kappa to lambda ratios or even the appearance of light chain restriction.[3,11,12] Key in differentiating physiologic from lymphomatous B-cell

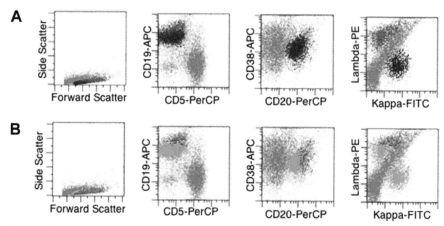

Fig. 1. (*A*) In this orbital biopsy, the B cells have been isolated and the kappa and lambda clusters have been rendered in blue and violet, respectively, with a kappa to lambda ratio of 0.9. However, note that the kappa and lambda clusters are not entirely superimposable, with differences in forward scatter, CD19, and CD20 noted between the two populations. Also note the asymmetry of the lambda cluster in the light chain plot. (*B*) When this case is reanalyzed using a multidimensional cluster analysis approach, it is evident that there is a lambda-restricted population of B cells (*red*) that can be distinguished by higher forward scatter and brighter CD19 and CD20. This population represented 4.2% of events, whereas the background polyclonal B cells (*green*) represented 18% of events. The histologic features were characteristic of extranodal marginal zone lymphoma.

clones in these circumstances is that the physiologic clones will lack immunophenotypic aberrancy, in contrast to their neoplastic counterparts (**Fig. 2**). Therefore, it can be argued that in the lymphoid realm, aberrancy is a more direct and specific expression of the neoplastic phenotype than clonality.

Light Chain Negative Lymphomas

It has been argued that lymphoma cannot be diagnosed without light chain expression. Two basic arguments have been proposed to support this proposition. The first is that demonstration of clonality is necessary to establish a diagnosis of lymphoma. This argument, of course, is clearly not the case, as anyone who has made a histologic diagnosis of lymphoma without the aid of clonality studies (which is the norm) can readily attest. The basis of the histologic diagnosis of lymphoma is morphologic aberrancy that exceeds acceptable limits. By analogy, the immunophenotypic diagnosis of lymphoma is based on aberrancy that exceeds acceptable limits.

A more compelling argument is that lack of light chain expression in B cells is not strictly aberrant.[13] Specifically, normal germinal center cells downregulate surface immunoglobulin. However, when specifically discriminated from nongerminal center cells (for example, based on a combination of CD20 and CD38 or CD10 and CD38), they show a pattern of limited polytypic antigen expression rather than a total absence of surface light chain (see **Fig. 2B**).[3] Consequently, a complete lack of light chain expression can be used as an indication of a lymphomatous proliferation.[14] Also, of course, germinal center cells will show otherwise normal patterns of antigen expression for that subset (see **Fig. 2B**). It is also worth noting at this point that lack of light chain expression may represent a technical artifact. Specifically, B cells in serous body fluids often seem to lack light chain expression.[10] This lack of expression can

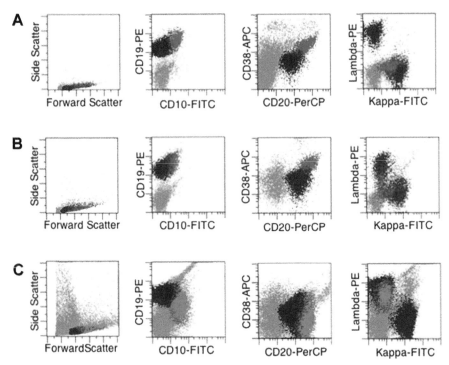

Fig. 2. (*A*) This cervical lymph node from a 19-year-old man demonstrates a 13% population of cells with a germinal center immunophenotype; they are CD10(+) but also bright for CD19, CD20, and CD38 when compared with primary follicle/mantle zone cells (*blue*, 39%). Note, however, that most of this population expresses kappa light chain (kappa to lambda ratio of 14:1). However, histology revealed conventional florid follicular hyperplasia, with no morphologic indication of lymphoma. Such a light chain skew is rarely seen in florid follicular hyperplasia. (*B*) In this typical case of florid follicular hyperplasia, the germinal center cells (*violet*) demonstrate the same immunophenotypic characteristics as those illustrated in (*A*), with the exception of a pattern of partial polytypic light chain expression. (*C*) Contrast both (*A*) and (*B*) with this example of follicular lymphoma in which there was a prominent background polytypic B-cell population. The neoplastic cells (*red*) constituted 4.8% of events; although they are CD10(+), they differ from normal germinal center cells by underexpression of CD19 and CD38 (in addition to being light chain restricted). Dim CD19 is a common finding in follicular lymphoma.

be mitigated by technical maneuvers, such as 37°C incubation and/or increasing the amount of light chain reagent (**Fig. 3**). Finally, it has been demonstrated that some lymphomas will seem to not express light chains with one set of light chain reagents but be clearly restricted with another.[15]

Other Analysis Considerations

As mentioned earlier, gross B-cell gating with determination of kappa/lambda ratios may be insufficient to identify small populations. Cluster analysis with color eventing (arbitrary assignment of colors to simultaneously visualized populations) can help identify subtle findings. When kappa and lambda clusters are assigned different colors, lack of complete overlap of these clusters in other fluorescent plots will usually be evident when an abnormal population is present (see **Fig. 1**). It is also important to

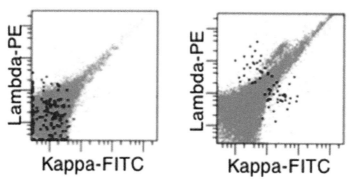

Fig. 3. This analysis of pleural fluid seems to show a lack of light chain expression on the small population of B cells (*blue*) present (*left*). However, after a 37°C incubation step and increasing the amount of light chain reagent, distinct kappa and lambda clusters can be resolved (*right*).

not rely strictly on scatter gating or CD45/side scatter gating but also to review ungated fluorescence plots to identify populations that scatter in unusual locations, have diminished CD45 expression, or do not form distinct clusters. For example, heavily vacuolated cells may have higher side scatter than expected for lymphocytes and mimic monocytes or granulocytes in scatter plots.[16] These considerations are particularly important for lymphoblastic processes, which frequently do not reside in the CD45/side scatter blast gate, either because of small cell size or diminished or absent CD45 expression.

Finally, a few words regarding the criteria for calling antigens positive or negative is warranted, as this can affect both classification and prognostication. Many practitioners use a threshold of 20% of events beyond a negative control, although this is arbitrary; some investigators have suggested 10% might be more appropriate on precisely gated neoplastic populations.[17] It is certain, however, that the optimal threshold will vary based on choices of antibodies, fluorochromes, instrument settings, and processing protocols; in most situations it is impractical or impossible to validate such thresholds. Therefore, this will likely remain arbitrary and, thus, represent a challenge for harmonization across laboratories. More important, perhaps, than the threshold used is the negative control that is used. Some investigators use internal negative populations (eg, T cells as a negative control for B-cell antigens). This practice is appropriate when the populations being compared have similar physical characteristics (eg, both are small lymphocyte populations) but not when they differ. Large cells, for example, have higher autofluorescence than small cells in some fluorescence channels, necessitating the use of autofluorescence controls (no antibodies), isotype controls, or fluorescence minus one controls, with the same populations gated in the control and the experimental tubes (ensuring an apples-to-apples comparison) (see **Fig. 5**).

SMALL B-CELL LYMPHOMAS AND CHRONIC LYMPHOPROLIFERATIVE DISORDERS
Classification

The application of flow cytometry to the classification of neoplasms of small B cells ranges from providing supportive information (eg, in the case of follicular lymphoma [FL]) to delineating immunophenotypes that are essentially definitional (eg, in the cases of chronic lymphocytic leukemia/small lymphocytic lymphoma [CLL/SLL] and hairy cell leukemia). The immunophenotypic profiles of the various small B-cell malignancies are provided in **Table 1**.

Chronic lymphocytic leukemia/small lymphocytic lymphoma versus mantle cell lymphoma

The diagnosis of CLL/SLL has, for practical purposes, become an immunophenotypic one, given the lack of defining genetic markers. Although characteristic lymph node histology may substitute for a complete immunophenotype, in blood and bone marrow the disease definition rests on flow cytometry. The defining immunophenotype is CD5(+), CD10(−), CD19(+), CD20(dim+), CD22(dim+), CD23(+), FMC7(−), surface immunoglobulin(dim+) (**Fig. 4**).[18,19] In 1994, Matutes and colleagues[18] proposed a scoring system that incorporated 5 markers: CD5, CD22, CD23, FMC7, and sIg. A score of 1 was assigned when the proper immunophenotypic pattern was seen and 0 when it was absent; CLL/SLL was diagnosed when the score was 4 or 5. The investigators reported an 87% sensitivity and greater than 99% specificity for the diagnosis of CLL/SLL. The same group later reported that the classification was improved with the addition of CD79b in the scheme or the replacement of CD22 with CD79b (CD79b is negative in most cases of CLL/SLL and positive in most other small B-cell disorders).[20] This modification improved the accuracy of the scoring system from 92% to 97%.

The proportion of CLL/SLL cases that show atypical immunophenotypic features varies across studies. This variation likely relates to both differences in definition

Table 1	
Typical immunophenotypic features of small B-cell disorders	
Disorder	**Typical Immunophenotype (Key Diagnostic Features Italicized)**
CLL/SLL	*CD5(+)*, CD10(−), CD11c(−/+), CD19(+), *CD20(dim+)*, *CD22(dim+)*, *CD23(+)*, *FMC7(−)*, *CD79b(−)*, CD200(+), *surface immunoglobulin(dim+)*[19,20,39,42–45,47]
Mantle cell lymphoma	*CD5(+)*, CD10(−), CD19(+), *CD20(+)*, CD22(+), *CD23(−)*, *FMC7(+)*, *CD79b(+)*, CD200(−), *surface immunoglobulin(+)*[30–34,39,42–45]
FL	CD5(−), *CD10(+)*, *CD19(dim+)*, CD20(+), CD23(+/−), FMC7(+), CD38(+)[9,17,69–71,169]
Lymphoplasmacytic lymphoma	CD5(−), CD10(−), CD11c(+), CD19(+), CD20(+), CD22(+), CD23(+/−), FMC7(+), CD79b(+)[25,28,170]
Extranodal marginal zone lymphoma	CD5(−), CD10(−), CD11c(−), CD19(+), CD20(+), CD23(−), FMC7(−)[169,171]
Nodal marginal zone lymphoma	CD5(−), CD10(−), CD11c(−), CD19(+), CD20(+), CD23(−)[169,172]
Hairy cell leukemia	CD5(−), CD10(−), *CD11c(bright+)*, CD19(+), CD20(+), *CD22(bright+)*, CD23(−), FMC7(+), *CD25(+)*, *CD103(+)*, *CD123(+)*, CD200(bright+)[42,52–56]
Splenic marginal zone lymphoma	CD5(−), CD10(+), CD11c(+/−), CD19(+), CD20(+), CD22(+), CD23(−/+), FMC7(+), *CD25(−)*, *CD103(−)*, *CD123(−)*[54,67,68,169,172,173]
Hairy cell leukemia variant	CD5(−), CD10(+), *CD11c(bright+)*, CD19(+), CD20(+), *CD22(bright+)*, CD23(−), FMC7(+), *CD25(−)*, *CD103(+)*, *CD123(−)*[53,54,63–66,68]
Splenic diffuse red pulp small B-cell lymphoma	CD5(−), CD10(−), CD11c(moderately bright+), CD19(+), CD20(+), CD22(moderately bright+), CD25(−), CD103(−/+), CD123(−)[67,68]

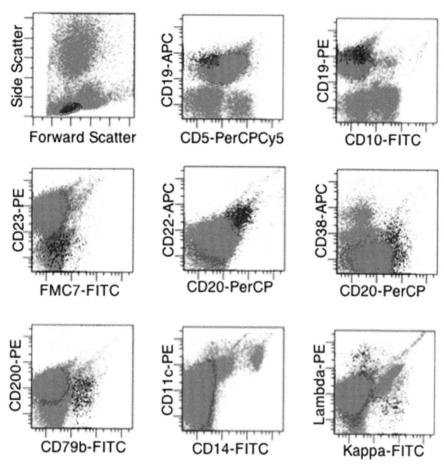

Fig. 4. Chronic lymphocytic leukemia/small lymphocytic lymphoma, characteristic immunophenotype. The neoplastic cells (*red*) are CD19(+), CD5(+), CD10(−), CD23(+), FMC7(−), CD79b(−), and CD200(+). Additionally, the neoplastic cells show dim expression of CD20, CD22, and surface immunoglobulin compared with normal B cells in the sample (*blue*). Finally, this example shows a lack of CD38 expression, a favorable prognostic feature.

(eg, what constitutes dim vs bright sIg) as well as the lack of a clear gold standard for the diagnosis of CLL/SLL. Clearly, a minority of CLL/SLL cases can deviate from the typical pattern for each of the antigens described earlier, as detailed in **Table 2**. Obviously, immunophenotypic variability is problematic for a disease that effectively has an immunophenotypic definition, and it complicates the distinction of CLL/SLL from mantle cell lymphoma (MCL), the other major CD5(+) small B-cell disorder as well as from uncommon CD5(+) variants of other small B-cell disorders that are usually CD5(−).[21–29] MCL, although CD5(+) like CLL/SLL, differs immunophenotypically in that it demonstrates strong CD20 and surface immunoglobulin (that is, similar intensity of expression as normal B cells), and is characteristically CD23(−) and FMC7(+).[30–34] However, some MCLs may be CD23(+) (though usually of dim intensity) and/or FMC7(−), further complicating this immunophenotypic distinction.[35–41] Consequently, investigators have sought additional markers to aid in the discrimination of CLL/SLL from other small B-cell disorders. CD200 has been shown to be

Table 2 Percentage of chronic lymphocytic leukemia/small lymphocytic lymphoma cases deviating from classic antigen patterns	
Classic Antigen Pattern	Percentage of Cases Deviating
CD20 dim-positive	11%–38%[20,174–177]
CD22 dim-positive	0%–8%[7,8,20,175]
CD23 positive	3%–5%[20,175]
FMC7 negative	7%–14%[20,174,177]
CD79b negative	5%–18%[20,177,178]
Surface immunoglobulin dim-positive	5%–42%[20,175,176]

moderately brightly expressed in virtually all cases of CLL/SLL, including cases with an otherwise atypical immunophenotype, whereas it is dim or negative in greater than 95% of MCLs.[39,42–45] Note that CD200 is not useful to distinguish CLL/SLL from marginal zone lymphomas, which show a wide range of CD200 expression.[46] Expression of CD11c has been shown to have a high negative predictive value for MCL, although the literature indicates a low sensitivity (27%) for CLL/SLL.[47] In the authors' experience, most CLL/SLL cases express partial or variable CD11c (see **Fig. 4**), whereas MCLs usually completely lack expression of this antigen (Kroft SH, 2017, unpublished data). Finally, it is worth noting that occasional CD5(+) small B-cell disorders are unclassifiable.[35]

Hairy cell leukemia versus splenic small B-cell lymphomas

Hairy cell leukemia (HCL), like CLL/SLL, has been traditionally defined based on immunophenotype. The recent discovery of a highly sensitive and specific genetic marker for this disease, BRAF V600E mutation,[48–50] has provided a new gold standard for the diagnosis of this entity. Nevertheless, flow cytometric immunophenotyping remains the first diagnostic modality used in this disorder; the specificity of the immunophenotype and other clinicopathologic features arguably obviates proceeding with molecular analysis to make this diagnosis. The importance of making an accurate diagnosis of HCL should also be stressed, given the availability of very specific and highly effective therapy for this disorder.[51]

The classic immunophenotype of HCL was established in 1993 by Robbins and colleagues[52]: strong expression of CD19, CD20, and surface immunoglobulin; very bright coexpression of CD11c and CD22; and expression of CD25 and CD103 (**Fig. 5**). More recently it has been recognized that CD123 expression and bright CD200 are also characteristic features of HCL.[42,53–55] Additionally, HCL is usually CD23(−) and FMC7(+).[56] This immunophenotype describes most HCL cases. However, deviations from this classic pattern have been described. Chen and colleagues[57] described a lack of CD25 in 3% of cases, a lack of CD103 in 6%, and expression of CD23 in 17%. Notably, no individual case showed more than one of these uncommon features.

Most cases of HCL are CD5(−) and CD10(−). However, CD10 is expressed in 10% to 20% of HCL cases; these do not seem to differ in other respects from CD10(−) cases.[58] Rare cases of CD5(+) HCL exist, but too few have been reported to assess whether they differ clinically from those with a classic immunophenotype.[27,52,59,60]

The main differential diagnoses with HCL, both clinically and pathologically, are the group of splenic small B-cell lymphomas, which includes splenic marginal zone lymphoma (SMZL), HCL variant (HCV), and splenic diffuse red pulp small B-cell lymphoma (SDRPL). The first is a moderately well-characterized clinicopathologic entity, whereas

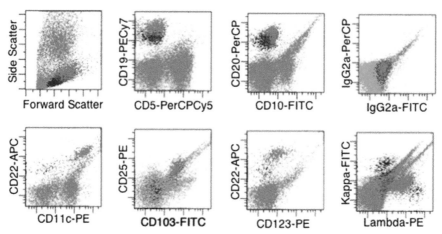

Fig. 5. Hairy cell leukemia, characteristic immunophenotype. The neoplastic cells (*red*) in hairy cell leukemia characteristically show light scatter characteristics more similar to mono-cytes than mature lymphocytes (compare with the normal B cells, *blue*). Most cases of hairy cell leukemia lack expression of CD5 and CD10. Note that the leukemia cells in this example seem to express CD10 when compared with the mature B cells. However, it is evident in the isotypic control that the neoplastic cells have higher autofluorescence in the FITC channel than small lymphocytes (*green*) and that in fact the hairy cells are CD10(−). Other character-istic features illustrated in this case are bright coexpression of CD11c and CD22 and expres-sion of CD25, CD103, and CD123.

the other two remain provisional entities in the World Health Organization's (WHO) classification.[61] All of these typically CD5(−)/CD10(−) disorders show some immuno-phenotypic features suggestive of HCL, and all need to be distinguished from HCL because of poor response to agents that are highly active in that disorder. Whether they need to be (and, in fact, reliably can be) distinguished from one another is unclear now, and it is difficult to pin down their immunophenotypes precisely because of over-lapping clinicopathologic features and lack of good gold standards for diagnosis.[62] Nevertheless, some generalizations can be made.

The closest immunophenotypic mimic of HCL is HCV. This entity characteristically shows bright coexpression of CD11c and CD22 and expression of CD103 (**Fig. 6**).[53,54,63–66] However, the lack of CD25 and CD123 will distinguish it from HCL. SMZLs typically coexpress CD11c and CD22 but do not show bright coexpres-sion of these markers. CD25 is expressed in a minority of cases, and both CD103 and CD123 will be negative.[54,67] SDRPL is the least well characterized of all of these en-tities and has been reported to have heterogeneous immunophenotypic features. Although CD11c and CD22 may be brightly coexpressed, they tend to be less bright than in HCL.[67] Although CD103 is expressed in approximately 40%, and CD123 dimly expressed in 16%, CD25 is negative in most reported cases.[68]

Other classification issues

Expression of CD10 is an immunophenotypic hallmark of FL (see **Fig. 2**). However, roughly 10% of low-grade FLs lack expression of this antigen by flow cytome-try.[17,69–71] Conversely, other low-grade B-cell processes that are characteristically CD10(−) may occasionally be CD10(+). As mentioned earlier, this is a feature of 10% of HCLs[58]; but rare cases of CLL/SLL, MCL, and lymphoplasmacytic lymphoma may express CD10.[28,29,41,72]

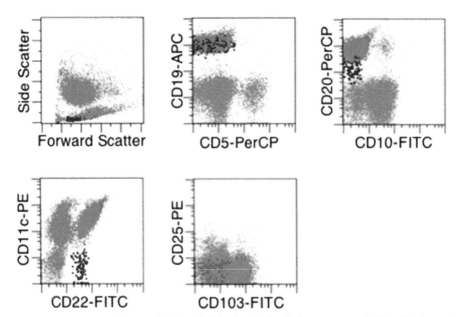

Fig. 6. HCL variant. This CD5(−)/CD10(−) leukemia (*red*) demonstrates bright CD11c and CD22 and is predominantly positive for CD103. However, it is CD25(−). Also, compare the light scatter properties with the HCL illustrated in **Fig. 5**. Normal B cells are illustrated in blue.

Just as CD10 defines FL, CD5 is a defining feature of CLL/SLL and MCL. However, roughly 10% of MCLs lack CD5.[41,73] CD5(−) CLL/SLL probably exists,[74] but establishing this diagnosis is extremely difficult.

Finally, it is worth mentioning that immunophenotypic variation in lymphomas may be seen across different tissue sites and over time in individual patients, although these are uncommonly of sufficient magnitude to affect classification.[40,75–77]

Prognostic Markers

Chronic lymphocytic leukemia/small lymphocytic lymphoma

By far the most work on the impact of immunophenotypic features on prognosis has been performed in CLL/SLL. In the wake of the discovery that lack of somatic hypermutation in Ig VH genes was associated with poor outcomes in CLL/SLL,[78,79] it became desirable to identify an easily measurable surrogate laboratory test for mutational status. CD38 was immediately identified as a candidate, with expression associated with an unmutated status.[79] Additional investigation clearly identified CD38 expression as an adverse prognostic indicator in CLL/SLL, although it has turned out not to be a useful surrogate for Ig VH mutation.[80–84] Furthermore, because expression of CD38 often does not show an all-or-none pattern of expression, thresholds for the percentage of cells expressing CD38 beyond a control must be established. Unfortunately, optimal thresholds vary based on the technical differences, such as processing protocols, reagent choices, and instrument settings; thus, different investigators have used different values.[80,83–91] This difference essentially means that thresholds cannot be blindly adopted from the literature for clinical use. Yet, few laboratories have the ability to establish their own thresholds based on outcome data. Finally, concern has been expressed that CD38 levels can change during the course of the disease,[80,85,92,93] although this has not been a consistent finding.[88] It also has been shown that the level of CD38 expression depends on the tumor microenvironment.[94]

After identification of the differential expression of the gene encoding the T-cell signaling protein ZAP-70 between mutated and unmutated CLL/SLL (expression being associated with lack of somatic mutation),[95] investigators began assessing this protein by flow cytometry and suggested that it predicted mutational status in most cases.[96,97] As in the case of CD38, ZAP-70 was found to be a less useful surrogate for mutational status than originally hoped (~75% concordance); but it is clearly a potent prognostic factor.[98–101] In fact, there is some evidence that it is a stronger predictor of outcome than mutational status.[100] However, as in the case of CD38, the continuous expression patterns of ZAP-70 in CLL/SLL require the establishment of thresholds; various approaches to establishing these have been proposed.[99,102–110] As with CD38 though, thresholds have proven to be extremely different to standardize across laboratories. The utility of ZAP-70 expression by flow cytometry as a clinical laboratory test (as opposed to a research test) is further compromised by the lability of this protein; expression seems to depend on the type of specimen handling and the time to processing.[108,109,111] Ultimately, ZAP-70 by flow cytometry seems to lack sufficient robustness to be suitable as a routine clinical test; consequently, many clinical laboratories have discontinued testing for this biomarker.

Most recently, expression of CD49d has been investigated and found to be a strong, independent indicator of more aggressive disease.[112–116] Importantly, this marker seems to be analytically stable, and stable over time in individual patients; in most cases expression is either bright or absent, presumably allowing for a more robust, reproducible clinical assay.[112,114,117]

Finally, it should be noted that these 3 immunophenotypic markers show correlations with one another but have been demonstrated to provide independent prognostic information. Therefore, approaches using combinations of the markers have been proposed.[88,92,118]

Other small B-cell processes

Little information is available on the impact of immunophenotype on the clinical course in other small B-cell neoplasms. Kelemen and colleagues[40] reported that CD23 expression was associated with better outcomes in MCL. Similarly, CD23 expression in FL has been linked to better outcomes.[119] Recently, CD38 has been reported to be a poor prognostic marker in HCL.[120]

Minimal Residual Disease

Flow cytometry has emerged as an effective means of monitoring minimal residual disease (MRD) following therapy in CLL/SLL, MCL, and HCL and should be applicable to other small B-cell disorders, such as FL.[121–126] The details of the approach to MRD analysis and clinical utility in these disorders is beyond the scope of this review.

AGGRESSIVE MATURE B-CELL NEOPLASMS

Flow cytometry plays a smaller role in aggressive B-cell non-Hodgkin lymphoma than in small B-cell neoplasms. However, flow cytometry is used as a first-line diagnostic modality in many centers; productive flow cytometry analyses may eliminate the need for subsequent immunohistochemistry in many cases. Flow cytometry is particularly useful in the case of fine-needle aspirations, in which material may not be available for immunohistochemical evaluation. Finally, as described later, immunophenotypic features detected by flow cytometry may be of value in prognostication or prediction of genetic lesions.

Diffuse Large B-Cell Lymphoma

Although it commonly stated that DLBCL is difficult to diagnose by flow cytometry because of losses in processing,[127] in the authors' experience, most DLBCLs can be identified by flow cytometry, independent of the site of involvement.[128] DLBCLs most commonly show expression of CD19, CD20, CD22, and bright CD45.[127,129] In one report, diminished CD20 expression by flow cytometry was described in roughly 15% of all DLBCLs and was notably discordant with strong positivity by immunohistochemistry in this subset. Further, this decreased CD20 expression was associated with a poorer prognosis, though cytogenetic and molecular factors were not studied in this analysis.[129] Most DLBCLs show monotypic light chain expression by flow cytometry; however, nearly a quarter of cases lack both kappa and lambda surface staining.[15,130] CD23 is expressed in approximately one-third of DLBCL and FMC7 in two-thirds (unpublished observations). CD200 is observed in 22% of cases.[131]

Immunophenotypic subsets of DLBCL have prognostic and therapeutic relevance. CD10 expression may be observed in 30% to 60% of DLBCLs by flow cytometry and/or immunohistochemistry, with expression of this marker establishing germinal center origin per the Han criteria[132,133] Of note, the Han criteria are based on immunohistochemical assessment; flow cytometry may be more sensitive for the detection of CD10 than immunohistochemistry in DLBCL.[134] CD5 expression is present in approximately 5% to 10% of DLBCLs and may indicate either de novo CD5(+) DLBCL or a Richter transformation of CLL/SLL. The de novo subset has been shown to have a poorer outcome compared with CD5(–) DLBCLs.[135] Immunophenotypically, the large cell lymphomas arising out of CLL/SLL have similar antigen expression patterns to the CLL/SLL.[136]

Burkitt Lymphoma

Burkitt lymphoma (BL) has the following immunophenotype by flow cytometry: CD5(–), CD10(+), CD19(+), CD20(+), CD38 bright(+), surface light chain(+), and terminal deoxynucleotidyl transferase (TdT)(–) (**Fig. 7**). Several groups have described patterns of antigen expression helpful in distinguishing BL from CD10(+) DLBCL, including diminished or absent expression of CD18, CD44, CD54, CD79b, and CD200, and increased expression of CD38 and CD43, in BL compared with CD10(+) DLBCL.[42,137–140] Of note, bright CD38 expression on CD10(+) B-cell neoplasms, at a similar intensity to plasma cells, is predictive for *MYC* rearrangements generally, with enhanced specificity when there is expression of FMC7 in the absence of CD23.[139]

High-Grade B-Cell Lymphoma with MYC and BCL2 and/or BCL6 Rearrangements (Double/Triple-Hit Lymphomas)

In the WHO's 2016 classification of tumors of hematopoietic and lymphoid tissues update, large B-cell lymphomas with *MYC* and *BCL2* and/or *BCL6* rearrangements and a mature immunophenotype will all be classified in one category, independent of morphology.[61] Approximately 5% to 10% of DLBCLs are double-hit lymphomas (DHLs) with *MYC* and *BCL2/BCL6* rearrangements.[141] These high-grade neoplasms have a poorer prognosis compared with DLBCLs without such rearrangements; therefore, their identification is critical to clinical management.[142–145] Multiple studies have

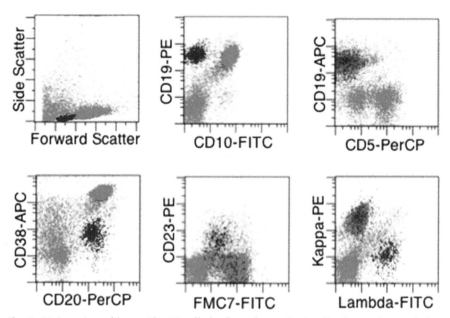

Fig. 7. BL in a tissue biopsy. The BL cells (*red*) are larger in size (*by forward scatter*) than mature B cells (*blue*) and are CD5(−), CD10(+), CD19(+), CD20 bright(+), CD23(−), FMC7(+), CD38 bright(+), and kappa light chain restricted. Bright CD38 expression has been associated with *MYC* rearrangements.

examined clinical, morphologic, genetic, and immunophenotypic features of these lymphomas in an effort to identify characteristics predictive of the presence of these rearrangements and, therefore, optimize cytogenetic testing for maximum cost-effectiveness.[146,147]

Flow cytometry can play a role in predicting the double or triple hits. Most DHLs are CD10(+) and, therefore, of germinal center origin. They have the following characteristic immunophenotype, as compared with normal resting or germinal center B cells, as confirmed across multiple studies: diminished CD19 (30%–67%), diminished CD20 (36%–70%), diminished CD19 and CD20 (28%–56%), and decreased CD45 (30%–45%) expression (**Fig. 8**).[148–150] Surface light chain is also dim or absent in 47% to 67% of DHLs.[148,150] Finally, bright CD38 expression is also characteristic.[139,148]

B-LYMPHOBLASTIC LEUKEMIA/LYMPHOMA

The diagnosis of B-lymphoblastic leukemia/lymphoma (B-ALL) is established by blast immunophenotyping via flow cytometry or immunohistochemistry, with flow cytometry being the preferred modality given its increased sensitivity. A thorough, diagnostic immunophenotype by flow cytometry is recommended for assigning B-lineage specificity, excluding mixed phenotype leukemias, predicting cytogenetic or molecular abnormalities, and monitoring disease with MRD assessment. Recommended antibodies at diagnosis include cytoplasmic TdT, myeloperoxidase, CD22, IgM, and CD79a; surface CD10, CD19, CD20, CD22, CD34, CD38, CD45, kappa, and lambda; myeloid antigens, such as CD11b, CD13, CD14, CD15, CD33, CD64, and CD65; and T-cell antigens.[151,152]

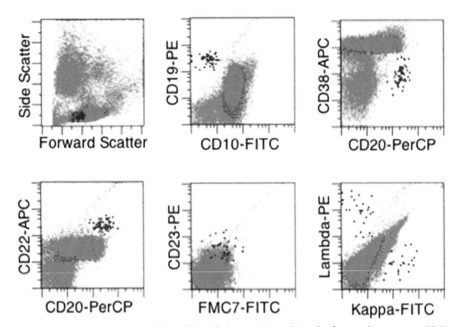

Fig. 8. DHL in bone marrow. DHL cells (*red*) show enlarged size by forward scatter, positivity for CD10, bright expression of CD38, and frequent underexpression of CD19, CD20, and light chain. Normal B cells are illustrated in blue.

B-ALLs have a characteristic immunophenotype, showing expression of CD19, HLA-DR and cytoplasmic CD22, CD79a, and TdT in nearly all cases.[153] Most B-ALLs also express CD10 (75%–90%), CD38 (85%), and CD34 (80%). When compared with their normal counterpart, hematogones, leukemic B-lymphoblasts show immunophenotypic aberrancy in nearly all cases (**Fig. 9**).[154] Such aberrancies can manifest as asynchronous antigen expression (such as coexpression of CD34 and CD20), lineage infidelity (such as expression of myeloid or T-cell antigens), or underexpression/overexpression of normally expressed antigens (see discussion of the immunophenotype of hematogones, the normal counterpart of B-ALL, later). Among the most frequent aberrancies are uniform or continuous expression of TdT or CD34 (73%–93%), overexpression of CD10 (61%–86%), and underexpression of CD38 and CD45 (52%–80%).[154,155] Aberrant myeloid antigen expression may be observed in up to 86% of B-ALLs when multiple antigens are tested.[154] Light chain expression is rarely observed.[151,154] Notably, it is well documented that B-ALL blast immunophenotypes can change to varying degrees over time and/or as a result of therapy (30%–78% of cases).[155–157]

The major immunophenotypic differential diagnosis of B-ALL in bone marrow is hematogone hyperplasia. Hematogones can be recognized by their highly reproducible maturation pattern toward mature B cells (see **Fig. 9**; **Fig. 10**).[10,158,159] The most immature forms are CD10(bright+), CD19(+), CD20(−), CD22(moderately+), CD38(moderately bright+), CD45(dim+), TdT(+), CD123(−), and CD34(+). As they mature, hematogones slightly downregulate CD10, slightly upregulate CD19 and CD38, upregulate CD45 and CD123 expression, lose CD34 and TdT, and progressively gain CD20. Acquisition of polytypic surface immunoglobulin is seen during hematogone maturation; interestingly, this begins before CD20 is acquired. Deviations

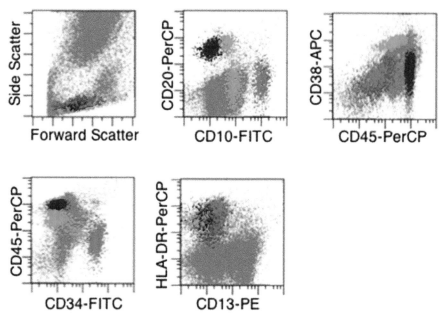

Fig. 9. Recurrent B-ALL with hematogones. The neoplastic B-lymphoblasts (*red*) show aberrant bright CD10 and CD34 expression with dim CD38 and CD45 expression, as compared with the hematogones (*green*), which show a normal, reproducible maturation pattern (also see **Fig. 10**). CD13 is additionally expressed aberrantly by the neoplastic B-lymphoblasts. Mature B cells are illustrated in blue.

from this maturation pattern represent immunophenotypic aberrancy and are evidence for a neoplastic proliferation of lymphoblasts. Other markers that have been shown to have characteristic expression patterns in hematogones and, thus, potential utility in distinguishing B-ALL from hematogones are CD58, CD81, CD123, and BCL-2.[160–163]

Hematogones may be arbitrarily divided into 3 maturational stages.[159] Stage 1 comprises the CD20(−), CD34(+), TdT(+) subset, stage 3 the most mature subset, with CD20 expression at or exceeding that seen in mature B cells, and stage 2 everything in between stages 1 and 3. Normally, stage 2 hematogones predominate, averaging roughly two-thirds of the hematogone population, with the remaining one-third equally divided between stages 1 and 3.[153] However, both right shifts and left shifts may be seen in hematogone maturation in reactive states. However, the qualitative maturation pattern will remain unchanged.

The concomitant presence of hematogones and neoplastic blasts is unusual at B-ALL diagnosis but may be occasionally seen at the time of recurrence (see **Fig. 9**). However, these populations should be easily distinguished based on the invariant maturation pattern of hematogones coupled with the various aberrancies seen in B-ALL. Follow-up analyses for residual B-ALL require an antibody panel designed to interrogate the most common B-ALL aberrancies relative to hematogones. A detailed discussion of minimal residual disease analysis in B-ALL is presented in Aaron C. Shaver and Adam C. Seegmiller's article "B Lymphoblastic Leukemia Minimal Residual Disease Assessment by Flow Cytometric Analysis," in this issue.

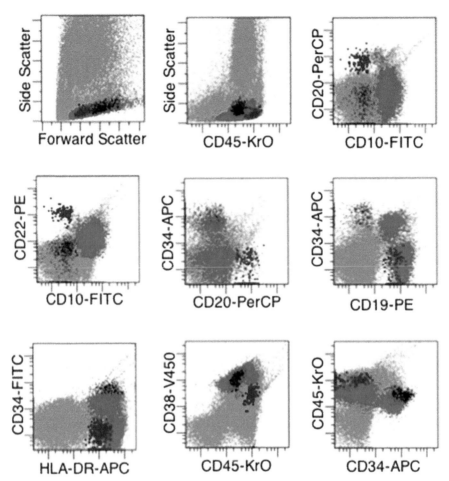

Fig. 10. Hematogone maturation patterns. Hematogones (*magenta*) show a characteristic maturation pattern. The most immature hematogones are CD10(bright+), CD19(+), CD20(−), CD34(+), and CD45 dim(+). As they mature, they slightly downregulate CD10, lose CD34, and show increases in intensity of CD19 (slightly), CD20, and CD45. Hematogones maintain moderately bright CD38 and HLA-DR and dim CD22 expression (relative to mature B cells) throughout maturation. Final maturation to mature B cells (*blue*) is associated with loss of CD10 and downregulation of CD38. Myeloblasts are illustrated in black.

Some B-ALL immunophenotypes are predictive of recurring cytogenetic and molecular abnormalities and, thus, prognosis. In the good cytogenetics category, blasts usually express CD10, CD22, CD34, and CD123 in hyperdiploidy states and CD10(bright), CD27, CD34, and CD13 and/or CD33 in t(12;21) B-ALLs.[164–168] Blasts with *MLL* rearrangements show expression of NG2 (highly specific), CD15, CD34, and TdT and have diminished CD10 and CD24 **(Fig. 11)**.[154,164] Most Philadelphia chromosome(+) B-ALLs express bright CD10, CD25, TdT and CD34 and show CD13 and/or CD33 expression.[154,164] Finally, B-ALLs with the t(1;19) characteristically show negativity for both CD10 and CD34 in the blasts.[154,164]

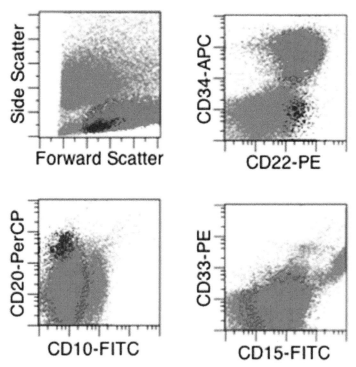

Fig. 11. B-ALL with *MLL* gene rearrangement. The neoplastic B-lymphoblasts (*red*) show multiple aberrancies, including bright, uniform CD34 and CD22 expression, lack of CD10, partial CD20 expression, and CD15 positivity. The lack of CD10 and expression of CD34 and CD15 is characteristic *MLL*-rearranged B-ALL. Mature B cells are illustrated in blue.

REFERENCES

1. Chen HI, Akpolat I, Mody DR, et al. Restricted kappa/lambda light chain ratio by flow cytometry in germinal center B cells in Hashimoto thyroiditis. Am J Clin Pathol 2006;125(1):42–8.
2. Chizuka A, Kanda Y, Nannya Y, et al. The diagnostic value of kappa/lambda ratios determined by flow cytometric analysis of biopsy specimens in B-cell lymphoma. Clin Lab Haematol 2002;24(1):33–6.
3. Reichard KK, McKenna RW, Kroft SH. Comparative analysis of light chain expression in germinal center cells and mantle cells of reactive lymphoid tissues. A four-color flow cytometric study. Am J Clin Pathol 2003;119(1):130–6.
4. Geary WA, Frierson HF, Innes DJ, et al. Quantitative criteria for clonality in the diagnosis of B-cell non- Hodgkin's lymphoma by flow cytometry. Mod Pathol 1993;6(2):155–61.
5. Taylor CR. Results of multiparameter studies of B-cell lymphomas. Am J Clin Pathol 1979;72(4 Suppl):687–98.
6. Ray S, Craig FE, Swerdlow SH. Abnormal patterns of antigenic expression in follicular lymphoma: a flow cytometric study. Am J Clin Pathol 2005;124(4): 576–83.
7. Huang J, Fan G, Zhong Y, et al. Diagnostic usefulness of aberrant CD22 expression in differentiating neoplastic cells of B-Cell chronic lymphoproliferative

disorders from admixed benign B cells in four-color multiparameter flow cytometry. Am J Clin Pathol 2005;123(6):826–32.

8. Sanchez ML, Almeida J, Vidriales B, et al. Incidence of phenotypic aberrations in a series of 467 patients with B chronic lymphoproliferative disorders: basis for the design of specific four-color stainings to be used for minimal residual disease investigation. Leukemia 2002;16(8):1460–9.

9. Yang W, Agrawal N, Patel J, et al. Diminished expression of CD19 in B-cell lymphomas. Cytometry B Clin Cytom 2005;63(1):28–35.

10. Reichard KK, Kroft SH. Flow cytometry in the assessment of hematologic disorders. In: Orazi A, Foucar K, Knowles DM, et al, editors. Neoplastic hematopathology. Baltimore (MD): Lippincott, Williams and Wilkins; 2013. p. 119–45.

11. Kussick SJ, Kalnoski M, Braziel RM, et al. Prominent clonal B cell populations identified by flow cytometry in histologically-reactive lymphoid proliferations. Am J Clin Pathol 2004;121(4):464–72.

12. Kroft SH. Monoclones, monotypes, and neoplasia pitfalls in lymphoma diagnosis. Am J Clin Pathol 2004;121(4):457–9.

13. Zhao XF, Cherian S, Sargent R, et al. Expanded populations of surface membrane immunoglobulin light chain-negative B cells in lymph nodes are not always indicative of B-cell lymphoma. Am J Clin Pathol 2005;124(1):143–50.

14. Li S, Eshleman JR, Borowitz MJ. Lack of surface immunoglobulin light chain expression by flow cytometric immunophenotyping can help diagnose peripheral B-cell lymphoma. Am J Clin Pathol 2002;118(2):229–34.

15. Horna P, Olteanu H, Kroft SH, et al. Flow cytometric analysis of surface light chain expression patterns in B-cell lymphomas using monoclonal and polyclonal antibodies. Am J Clin Pathol 2011;136(6):954–9.

16. Kesler MV, Paranjape GS, Asplund SL, et al. Anaplastic large cell lymphoma: a flow cytometric analysis of 29 cases. Am J Clin Pathol 2007;128(2):314–22.

17. Xu Y, McKenna RW, Kroft SH. Assessment of CD10 in the diagnosis of small B-cell lymphomas: a multiparameter flow cytometric study. Am J Clin Pathol 2002;117(2):291–300.

18. Matutes E, Owusu-Ankomah K, Morilla R, et al. The immunological profile of B-cell disorders and proposal of a scoring system for the diagnosis of CLL. Leukemia 1994;8(10):1640–5.

19. Almasri NM, Duque RE, Iturraspe J, et al. Reduced expression of CD20 antigen as a characteristic marker for chronic lymphocytic leukemia. Am J Hematol 1992;40(4):259–63.

20. Moreau EJ, Matutes E, A'Hern RP, et al. Improvement of the chronic lymphocytic leukemia scoring system with the monoclonal antibody SN8 (CD79b). Am J Clin Pathol 1997;108(4):378–82.

21. Baseggio L, Traverse-Glehen A, Petinataud F, et al. CD5 expression identifies a subset of splenic marginal zone lymphomas with higher lymphocytosis: a clinico-pathological, cytogenetic and molecular study of 24 cases. Haematologica 2010;95(4):604–12.

22. Ballesteros E, Osborne BM, Matsushima AY. CD5+ low-grade marginal zone B-cell lymphomas with localized presentation. Am J Surg Pathol 1998;22(2):201–7.

23. Ferry JA, Yang WI, Zukerberg LR, et al. CD5+ extranodal marginal zone B-cell (MALT) lymphoma. A low grade neoplasm with a propensity for bone marrow involvement and relapse. Am J Clin Pathol 1996;105(1):31–7.

24. Dronca RS, Jevremovic D, Hanson CA, et al. CD5-positive chronic B-cell lymphoproliferative disorders: diagnosis and prognosis of a heterogeneous disease entity. Cytometry B Clin Cytom 2010;78(Suppl 1):S35–41.
25. Morice WG, Chen D, Kurtin PJ, et al. Novel immunophenotypic features of marrow lymphoplasmacytic lymphoma and correlation with Waldenstrom's macroglobulinemia. Mod Pathol 2009;22(6):807–16.
26. Li Y, Hu S, Zuo Z, et al. CD5-positive follicular lymphoma: clinicopathologic correlations and outcome in 88 cases. Mod Pathol 2015;28(6):787–98.
27. Jain D, Dorwal P, Gajendra S, et al. CD5 positive hairy cell leukemia: a rare case report with brief review of literature. Cytometry B Clin Cytom 2016;90(5):467–72.
28. Konoplev S, Medeiros LJ, Bueso-Ramos CE, et al. Immunophenotypic profile of lymphoplasmacytic lymphoma/Waldenstrom macroglobulinemia. Am J Clin Pathol 2005;124(3):414–20.
29. Dong HY, Gorczyca W, Liu Z, et al. B-cell lymphomas with coexpression of CD5 and CD10. Am J Clin Pathol 2003;119(2):218–30.
30. Kilo MN, Dorfman DM. The utility of flow cytometric immunophenotypic analysis in the distinction of small lymphocytic lymphoma/chronic lymphocytic leukemia from mantle cell lymphoma. Am J Clin Pathol 1996;105(4):451–7.
31. Huh YO, Pugh WC, Kantarjian HM, et al. Detection of subgroups of chronic B-cell leukemias by FMC7 monoclonal antibody. Am J Clin Pathol 1994; 101(3):283–9.
32. Molot RJ, Meeker TC, Wittwer CT, et al. Antigen expression and polymerase chain reaction amplification of mantle cell lymphomas. Blood 1994;83(6): 1626–31.
33. Zukerberg LR, Medeiros LJ, Ferry JA, et al. Diffuse low-grade B-cell lymphomas. Four clinically distinct subtypes defined by a combination of morphologic and immunophenotypic features. Am J Clin Pathol 1993;100(4):373–85.
34. Argatoff LH, Connors JM, Klasa RJ, et al. Mantle cell lymphoma: a clinicopathologic study of 80 cases. Blood 1997;89(6):2067–78.
35. Asplund SL, McKenna RW, Doolittle JE, et al. CD5-positive B-cell neoplasms of indeterminate immunophenotype: a clinicopathologic analysis of 26 cases. Appl Immunohistochem Mol Morphol 2005;13(4):311–7.
36. Schlette E, Fu K, Medeiros LJ. CD23 expression in mantle cell lymphoma: clinicopathologic features of 18 cases. Am J Clin Pathol 2003;120(5):760–6.
37. Dorfman DM, Pinkus GS. Distinction between small lymphocytic and mantle cell lymphoma by immunoreactivity for CD23. Mod Pathol 1994;7(3):326–31.
38. Gong JZ, Lagoo AS, Peters D, et al. Value of CD23 determination by flow cytometry in differentiating mantle cell lymphoma from chronic lymphocytic leukemia/small lymphocytic lymphoma. Am J Clin Pathol 2001;116(6):893–7.
39. Palumbo GA, Parrinello N, Fargione G, et al. CD200 expression may help in differential diagnosis between mantle cell lymphoma and B-cell chronic lymphocytic leukemia. Leuk Res 2009;33(9):1212–6.
40. Kelemen K, Peterson LC, Helenowski I, et al. CD23+ mantle cell lymphoma: a clinical pathologic entity associated with superior outcome compared with CD23- disease. Am J Clin Pathol 2008;130(2):166–77.
41. Gao J, Peterson L, Nelson B, et al. Immunophenotypic variations in mantle cell lymphoma. Am J Clin Pathol 2009;132(5):699–706.
42. Challagundla P, Medeiros LJ, Kanagal-Shamanna R, et al. Differential expression of CD200 in B-cell neoplasms by flow cytometry can assist in diagnosis, subclassification, and bone marrow staging. Am J Clin Pathol 2014;142(6): 837–44.

43. Sandes AF, de Lourdes Chauffaille M, Oliveira CR, et al. CD200 has an important role in the differential diagnosis of mature B-cell neoplasms by multiparameter flow cytometry. Cytometry B Clin Cytom 2014;86(2):98–105.

44. Alapat D, Coviello-Malle J, Owens R, et al. Diagnostic usefulness and prognostic impact of CD200 expression in lymphoid malignancies and plasma cell myeloma. Am J Clin Pathol 2012;137(1):93–100.

45. Fan L, Miao Y, Wu YJ, et al. Expression patterns of CD200 and CD148 in leukemic B-cell chronic lymphoproliferative disorders and their potential value in differential diagnosis. Leuk Lymphoma 2015;56(12):3329–35.

46. Challagundla P, Jorgensen JL, Kanagal-Shamanna R, et al. Utility of quantitative flow cytometry immunophenotypic analysis of CD5 expression in small B-cell neoplasms. Arch Pathol Lab Med 2014;138(7):903–9.

47. Kraus TS, Sillings CN, Saxe DF, et al. The role of CD11c expression in the diagnosis of mantle cell lymphoma. Am J Clin Pathol 2010;134(2):271–7.

48. Tiacci E, Trifonov V, Schiavoni G, et al. BRAF mutations in hairy-cell leukemia. N Engl J Med 2011;364(24):2305–15.

49. Tiacci E, Schiavoni G, Forconi F, et al. Simple genetic diagnosis of hairy cell leukemia by sensitive detection of the BRAF-V600E mutation. Blood 2012;119(1):192–5.

50. Arcaini L, Zibellini S, Boveri E, et al. The BRAF V600E mutation in hairy cell leukemia and other mature B-cell neoplasms. Blood 2012;119(1):188–91.

51. Else M, Dearden CE, Matutes E, et al. Long-term follow-up of 233 patients with hairy cell leukaemia, treated initially with pentostatin or cladribine, at a median of 16 years from diagnosis. Br J Haematol 2009;145(6):733–40.

52. Robbins BA, Ellison DJ, Spinosa JC, et al. Diagnostic application of two-color flow cytometry in 161 cases of hairy cell leukemia. Blood 1993;82(4):1277–87.

53. Venkataraman G, Aguhar C, Kreitman RJ, et al. Characteristic CD103 and CD123 expression pattern defines hairy cell leukemia: usefulness of CD123 and CD103 in the diagnosis of mature B-cell lymphoproliferative disorders. Am J Clin Pathol 2011;136(4):625–30.

54. Del Giudice I, Matutes E, Morilla R, et al. The diagnostic value of CD123 in B-cell disorders with hairy or villous lymphocytes. Haematologica 2004;89(3):303–8.

55. Pillai V, Pozdnyakova O, Charest K, et al. CD200 flow cytometric assessment and semiquantitative immunohistochemical staining distinguishes hairy cell leukemia from hairy cell leukemia-variant and other B-cell lymphoproliferative disorders. Am J Clin Pathol 2013;140(4):536–43.

56. Matutes E, Morilla R, Owusu-Ankomah K, et al. The immunophenotype of hairy cell leukemia (HCL). Proposal for a scoring system to distinguish HCL from B-cell disorders with hairy or villous lymphocytes. Leuk Lymphoma 1994;14(Suppl 1):57–61.

57. Chen YH, Tallman MS, Goolsby C, et al. Immunophenotypic variations in hairy cell leukemia. Am J Clin Pathol 2006;125(2):251–9.

58. Jasionowski TM, Hartung L, Greenwood JH, et al. Analysis of CD10+ hairy cell leukemia. Am J Clin Pathol 2003;120(2):228–35.

59. Chen D, Morice WG, Viswanatha DS, et al. CD5-positive hairy cell leukemia: a rare but distinct variant. Mod Pathol 2009;22:258A.

60. Dong HY, Weisberger J, Liu Z, et al. Immunophenotypic analysis of CD103+ B-lymphoproliferative disorders: hairy cell leukemia and its mimics. Am J Clin Pathol 2009;131(4):586–95.

61. Swerdlow SH, Campo E, Pileri SA, et al. The 2016 revision of the World Health Organization classification of lymphoid neoplasms. Blood 2016;127(20): 2375–90.

62. Traverse-Glehen A, Baseggio L, Callet-Bauchu E, et al. Hairy cell leukaemia-variant and splenic red pulp lymphoma: a single entity? Br J Haematol 2010; 150(1):113–6.

63. Cessna MH, Hartung L, Tripp S, et al. Hairy cell leukemia variant: fact or fiction. Am J Clin Pathol 2005;123(1):132–8.

64. Matutes E, Wotherspoon A, Brito-Babapulle V, et al. The natural history and clinico-pathological features of the variant form of hairy cell leukemia. Leukemia 2001;15(1):184–6.

65. Sainati L, Matutes E, Mulligan S, et al. A variant form of hairy cell leukemia resistant to alpha-interferon: clinical and phenotypic characteristics of 17 patients. Blood 1990;76(1):157–62.

66. de Totero D, Tazzari PL, Lauria F, et al. Phenotypic analysis of hairy cell leukemia: "variant" cases express the interleukin-2 receptor beta chain, but not the alpha chain (CD25). Blood 1993;82(2):528–35.

67. Baseggio L, Traverse-Glehen A, Callet-Bauchu E, et al. Relevance of a scoring system including CD11c expression in the identification of splenic diffuse red pulp small B-cell lymphoma (SRPL). Hematol Oncol 2011;29(1):47–51.

68. Traverse-Glehen A, Baseggio L, Bauchu EC, et al. Splenic red pulp lymphoma with numerous basophilic villous lymphocytes: a distinct clinicopathologic and molecular entity? Blood 2008;111(4):2253–60.

69. Kaleem Z, White G, Vollmer RT. Critical analysis and diagnostic usefulness of limited immunophenotyping of B-cell non-Hodgkin lymphomas by flow cytometry. Am J Clin Pathol 2001;115(1):136–42.

70. Almasri NM, Iturraspe JA, Braylan RC. CD10 expression in follicular lymphoma and large cell lymphoma is different from that of reactive lymph node follicles. Arch Pathol Lab Med 1998;122(6):539–44.

71. Kurtin PJ, Hobday KS, Ziesmer S, et al. Demonstration of distinct antigenic profiles of small B-cell lymphomas by paraffin section immunohistochemistry. Am J Clin Pathol 1999;112(3):319–29.

72. Zanetto U, Dong H, Huang Y, et al. Mantle cell lymphoma with aberrant expression of CD10. Histopathology 2008;53(1):20–9.

73. Liu Z, Dong HY, Gorczyca W, et al. CD5- mantle cell lymphoma. Am J Clin Pathol 2002;118(2):216–24.

74. Huang JC, Finn WG, Goolsby CL, et al. CD5- small B-cell leukemias are rarely classifiable as chronic lymphocytic leukemia. Am J Clin Pathol 1999;111(1): 123–30.

75. Xu Y, McKenna RW, Asplund SL, et al. Comparison of immunophenotypes of small B-cell neoplasms in primary lymph node and concurrent blood or marrow samples. Am J Clin Pathol 2002;118(5):758–64.

76. Onciu M, Berrak SG, Medeiros LJ, et al. Discrepancies in the immunophenotype of lymphoma cells in samples obtained simultaneously from different anatomic sites. Am J Clin Pathol 2002;117(4):644–50.

77. Echeverri C, Fisher S, King D, et al. Immunophenotypic variability of B-cell non-Hodgkin lymphoma: a retrospective study of cases analyzed by flow cytometry. Am J Clin Pathol 2002;117(4):615–20.

78. Hamblin TJ, Davis Z, Gardiner A, et al. Unmutated Ig V(H) genes are associated with a more aggressive form of chronic lymphocytic leukemia. Blood 1999;94(6): 1848–54.

79. Damle RN, Wasil T, Fais F, et al. Ig V gene mutation status and CD38 expression as novel prognostic indicators in chronic lymphocytic leukemia. Blood 1999; 94(6):1840–7.

80. Hamblin TJ, Orchard JA, Ibbotson RE, et al. CD38 expression and immunoglobulin variable region mutations are independent prognostic variables in chronic lymphocytic leukemia, but CD38 expression may vary during the course of the disease. Blood 2002;99(3):1023–9.

81. Oscier DG, Gardiner AC, Mould SJ, et al. Multivariate analysis of prognostic factors in CLL: clinical stage, IGVH gene mutational status, and loss or mutation of the p53 gene are independent prognostic factors. Blood 2002;100(4): 1177–84.

82. Jelinek DF, Tschumper RC, Geyer SM, et al. Analysis of clonal B-cell CD38 and immunoglobulin variable region sequence status in relation to clinical outcome for B-chronic lymphocytic leukaemia. Br J Haematol 2001;115(4):854–61.

83. Ghia P, Guida G, Stella S, et al. The pattern of CD38 expression defines a distinct subset of chronic lymphocytic leukemia (CLL) patients at risk of disease progression. Blood 2003;101(4):1262–9.

84. Krober A, Seiler T, Benner A, et al. V(H) mutation status, CD38 expression level, genomic aberrations, and survival in chronic lymphocytic leukemia. Blood 2002; 100(4):1410–6.

85. Ibrahim S, Keating M, Do KA, et al. CD38 expression as an important prognostic factor in B-cell chronic lymphocytic leukemia. Blood 2001;98(1):181–6.

86. Rassenti LZ, Jain S, Keating MJ, et al. Relative value of ZAP-70, CD38, and immunoglobulin mutation status in predicting aggressive disease in chronic lymphocytic leukemia. Blood 2008;112(5):1923–30.

87. Durig J, Naschar M, Schmucker U, et al. CD38 expression is an important prognostic marker in chronic lymphocytic leukaemia. Leukemia 2002;16(1): 30–5.

88. Schroers R, Griesinger F, Trumper L, et al. Combined analysis of ZAP-70 and CD38 expression as a predictor of disease progression in B-cell chronic lymphocytic leukemia. Leukemia 2005;19(5):750–8.

89. Boonstra JG, van Lom K, Langerak AW, et al. CD38 as a prognostic factor in B cell chronic lymphocytic leukaemia (B-CLL): comparison of three approaches to analyze its expression. Cytometry B Clin Cytom 2006;70(3):136–41.

90. Mainou-Fowler T, Dignum H, Taylor PR, et al. Quantification improves the prognostic value of CD38 expression in B-cell chronic lymphocytic leukaemia. Br J Haematol 2002;118(3):755–61.

91. Thornton PD, Fernandez C, Giustolisi GM, et al. CD38 expression as a prognostic indicator in chronic lymphocytic leukaemia. Hematol J 2004;5(2):145–51.

92. Del Giudice I, Morilla A, Osuji N, et al. Zeta-chain associated protein 70 and CD38 combined predict the time to first treatment in patients with chronic lymphocytic leukemia. Cancer 2005;104(10):2124–32.

93. Chevallier P, Penther D, Avet-Loiseau H, et al. CD38 expression and secondary 17p deletion are important prognostic factors in chronic lymphocytic leukaemia. Br J Haematol 2002;116(1):142–50.

94. Patten PE, Buggins AG, Richards J, et al. CD38 expression in chronic lymphocytic leukemia is regulated by the tumor microenvironment. Blood 2008;111(10): 5173–81.

95. Rosenwald A, Alizadeh AA, Widhopf G, et al. Relation of gene expression phenotype to immunoglobulin mutation genotype in B cell chronic lymphocytic leukemia. J Exp Med 2001;194(11):1639–47.

96. Crespo M, Bosch F, Villamor N, et al. ZAP-70 expression as a surrogate for immunoglobulin-variable-region mutations in chronic lymphocytic leukemia. N Engl J Med 2003;348(18):1764–75.
97. Wiestner A, Rosenwald A, Barry TS, et al. ZAP-70 expression identifies a chronic lymphocytic leukemia subtype with unmutated immunoglobulin genes, inferior clinical outcome, and distinct gene expression profile. Blood 2003;101(12): 4944–51.
98. Orchard JA, Ibbotson RE, Davis Z, et al. ZAP-70 expression and prognosis in chronic lymphocytic leukaemia. Lancet 2004;363(9403):105–11.
99. Hassanein NM, Perkinson KR, Alcancia F, et al. A single tube, four-color flow cytometry assay for evaluation of ZAP-70 and CD38 expression in chronic lymphocytic leukemia. Am J Clin Pathol 2010;133(5):708–17.
100. Rassenti LZ, Huynh L, Toy TL, et al. ZAP-70 compared with immunoglobulin heavy-chain gene mutation status as a predictor of disease progression in chronic lymphocytic leukemia. N Engl J Med 2004;351(9):893–901.
101. Durig J, Nuckel H, Cremer M, et al. ZAP-70 expression is a prognostic factor in chronic lymphocytic leukemia. Leukemia 2003;17(12):2426–34.
102. Slack GW, Wizniak J, Dabbagh L, et al. Flow cytometric detection of ZAP-70 in chronic lymphocytic leukemia: correlation with immunocytochemistry and Western blot analysis. Arch Pathol Lab Med 2007;131(1):50–6.
103. Chen YH, Peterson LC, Dittmann D, et al. Comparative analysis of flow cytometric techniques in assessment of ZAP-70 expression in relation to IgVH mutational status in chronic lymphocytic leukemia. Am J Clin Pathol 2007;127(2): 182–91.
104. Gibbs G, Bromidge T, Howe D, et al. Comparison of flow cytometric methods for the measurement of ZAP-70 expression in a routine diagnostic laboratory. Clin Lab Haematol 2005;27(4):258–66.
105. Zucchetto A, Bomben R, Bo MD, et al. ZAP-70 expression in B-cell chronic lymphocytic leukemia: evaluation by external (isotypic) or internal (T/NK cells) controls and correlation with IgV(H) mutations. Cytometry B Clin Cytom 2006;70(4): 284–92.
106. Wilhelm C, Neubauer A, Brendel C. Discordant results of flow cytometric ZAP-70 expression status in B-CLL samples if different gating strategies are applied. Cytometry B Clin Cytom 2006;70(4):242–50.
107. Shults KE, Miller DT, Davis BH, et al. A standardized ZAP-70 assay–lessons learned in the trenches. Cytometry B Clin Cytom 2006;70(4):276–83.
108. Letestu R, Rawstron A, Ghia P, et al. Evaluation of ZAP-70 expression by flow cytometry in chronic lymphocytic leukemia: a multicentric international harmonization process. Cytometry B Clin Cytom 2006;70(4):309–14.
109. Bakke AC, Purtzer Z, Leis J, et al. A robust ratio metric method for analysis of Zap-70 expression in chronic lymphocytic leukemia (CLL). Cytometry B Clin Cytom 2006;70(4):227–34.
110. Best OG, Ibbotson RE, Parker AE, et al. ZAP-70 by flow cytometry: a comparison of different antibodies, anticoagulants, and methods of analysis. Cytometry B Clin Cytom 2006;70(4):235–41.
111. Sheikholeslami MR, Jilani I, Keating M, et al. Variations in the detection of ZAP-70 in chronic lymphocytic leukemia: comparison with IgV(H) mutation analysis. Cytometry B Clin Cytom 2006;70(4):270–5.
112. Gattei V, Bulian P, Del Principe MI, et al. Relevance of CD49d protein expression as overall survival and progressive disease prognosticator in chronic lymphocytic leukemia. Blood 2008;111(2):865–73.

113. Rossi D, Cerri M, Capello D, et al. Biological and clinical risk factors of chronic lymphocytic leukaemia transformation to Richter syndrome. Br J Haematol 2008; 142(2):202–15.

114. Baumann T, Delgado J, Santacruz R, et al. CD49d (ITGA4) expression is a predictor of time to first treatment in patients with chronic lymphocytic leukaemia and mutated IGHV status. Br J Haematol 2016;172(1):48–55.

115. Dal Bo M, Bulian P, Bomben R, et al. CD49d prevails over the novel recurrent mutations as independent prognosticator of overall survival in chronic lymphocytic leukemia. Leukemia 2016;30(10):2011–8.

116. Shanafelt TD, Geyer SM, Bone ND, et al. CD49d expression is an independent predictor of overall survival in patients with chronic lymphocytic leukaemia: a prognostic parameter with therapeutic potential. Br J Haematol 2008;140(5): 537–46.

117. Gooden CE, Jones P, Bates R, et al. CD49d shows superior performance characteristics for flow cytometric prognostic testing in chronic lymphocytic leukemia/small lymphocytic lymphoma. Cytometry B Clin Cytom 2016. [Epub ahead of print].

118. Zucchetto A, Bomben R, Dal Bo M, et al. CD49d in B-cell chronic lymphocytic leukemia: correlated expression with CD38 and prognostic relevance. Leukemia 2006;20(3):523–5 [author reply: 528–9].

119. Olteanu H, Fenske TS, Harrington AM, et al. CD23 expression in follicular lymphoma: clinicopathologic correlations. Am J Clin Pathol 2011;135(1):46–53.

120. Poret N, Fu Q, Guihard S, et al. CD38 in hairy cell leukemia is a marker of poor prognosis and a new target for therapy. Cancer Res 2015;75(18): 3902–11.

121. Rawstron AC, Bottcher S, Letestu R, et al. Improving efficiency and sensitivity: European Research Initiative in CLL (ERIC) update on the international harmonised approach for flow cytometric residual disease monitoring in CLL. Leukemia 2013;27(1):142–9.

122. Strati P, Keating MJ, O'Brien SM, et al. Eradication of bone marrow minimal residual disease may prompt early treatment discontinuation in CLL. Blood 2014; 123(24):3727–32.

123. Sausville JE, Salloum RG, Sorbara L, et al. Minimal residual disease detection in hairy cell leukemia. Comparison of flow cytometric immunophenotyping with clonal analysis using consensus primer polymerase chain reaction for the heavy chain gene. Am J Clin Pathol 2003;119(2):213–7.

124. Cheminant M, Derrieux C, Touzart A, et al. Minimal residual disease monitoring by 8-color flow cytometry in mantle cell lymphoma: an EU-MCL and LYSA study. Haematologica 2016;101(3):336–45.

125. Ladetto M, Lobetti-Bodoni C, Mantoan B, et al. Persistence of minimal residual disease in bone-marrow predicts outcome in follicular lymphomas treated with a rituximab-intensive program. Blood 2013;122(23):3759–66.

126. Sanchez ML, Almeida J, Gonzalez D, et al. Incidence and clinicobiologic characteristics of leukemic B-cell chronic lymphoproliferative disorders with more than one B-cell clone. Blood 2003;102(8):2994–3002.

127. Bertram HC, Check IJ, Milano MA. Immunophenotyping large B-cell lymphomas. Flow cytometric pitfalls and pathologic correlation. Am J Clin Pathol 2001;116(2):191–203.

128. Harrington AM, Olteanu H, Kroft SH. Most diffuse large B-cell lymphomas are identified by flow cytometry. Mod Pathol 2012;24:339A.

129. Johnson NA, Boyle M, Bashashati A, et al. Diffuse large B-cell lymphoma: reduced CD20 expression is associated with an inferior survival. Blood 2009; 113(16):3773–80.
130. Tomita N, Takeuchi K, Hyo R, et al. Diffuse large B cell lymphoma without immunoglobulin light chain restriction by flow cytometry. Acta Haematol 2009;121(4): 196–201.
131. Sorigue M, Junca J, Granada I. CD200 in high-grade lymphoma, chronic lymphocytic leukemia, and chronic lymphocytic leukemia-phenotype monoclonal B-cell lymphocytosis. Am J Clin Pathol 2015;144(4):677–9.
132. Swerdlow SH, Campo E, Harris NL, et al, editors. WHO classification of tumors of haematopoietic and lymphoid tissues. Lyon (France): IARC; 2008.
133. Hans CP, Weisenburger DD, Greiner TC, et al. Confirmation of the molecular classification of diffuse large B-cell lymphoma by immunohistochemistry using a tissue microarray. Blood 2004;103(1):275–82.
134. Xu Y, McKenna RW, Kroft SH. Comparison of multiparameter flow cytometry with cluster analysis and immunohistochemistry for the detection of CD10 in diffuse large B-cell lymphomas. Mod Pathol 2002;15(4):413–9.
135. Yamaguchi M, Seto M, Okamoto M, et al. De novo CD5+ diffuse large B-cell lymphoma: a clinicopathologic study of 109 patients. Blood 2002;99(3):815–21.
136. Kroft SH, Dawson DB, McKenna RW. Large cell lymphoma transformation of chronic lymphocytic leukemia/small lymphocytic lymphoma. A flow cytometric analysis of seven cases. Am J Clin Pathol 2001;115(3):385–95.
137. Schniederjan SD, Li S, Saxe DF, et al. A novel flow cytometric antibody panel for distinguishing Burkitt lymphoma from CD10+ diffuse large B-cell lymphoma. Am J Clin Pathol 2010;133(5):718–26.
138. McGowan P, Nelles N, Wimmer J, et al. Differentiating between Burkitt lymphoma and CD10+ diffuse large B-cell lymphoma: the role of commonly used flow cytometry cell markers and the application of a multiparameter scoring system. Am J Clin Pathol 2012;137(4):665–70.
139. Maleki A, Seegmiller AC, Uddin N, et al. Bright CD38 expression is an indicator of MYC rearrangement. Leuk Lymphoma 2009;50(6):1054–7.
140. Kesler MV, Xu Y, Karandikar NJ, et al. Flow cytometric comparison of Burkitt and CD10(+) large B-cell lymphomas [Abstract]. Mod Pathol 2005;18(Supp 1):237A.
141. Horn H, Ziepert M, Becher C, et al. MYC status in concert with BCL2 and BCL6 expression predicts outcome in diffuse large B-cell lymphoma. Blood 2013; 121(12):2253–63.
142. Johnson NA, Savage KJ, Ludkovski O, et al. Lymphomas with concurrent BCL2 and MYC translocations: the critical factors associated with survival. Blood 2009;114(11):2273–9.
143. Le Gouill S, Talmant P, Touzeau C, et al. The clinical presentation and prognosis of diffuse large B-cell lymphoma with t(14;18) and 8q24/c-MYC rearrangement. Haematologica 2007;92(10):1335–42.
144. Tomita N, Tokunaka M, Nakamura N, et al. Clinicopathological features of lymphoma/leukemia patients carrying both BCL2 and MYC translocations. Haematologica 2009;94(7):935–43.
145. Kanungo A, Medeiros LJ, Abruzzo LV, et al. Lymphoid neoplasms associated with concurrent t(14;18) and 8q24/c-MYC translocation generally have a poor prognosis. Mod Pathol 2006;19(1):25–33.
146. Snuderl M, Kolman OK, Chen YB, et al. B-cell lymphomas with concurrent IGH-BCL2 and MYC rearrangements are aggressive neoplasms with clinical and

pathologic features distinct from Burkitt lymphoma and diffuse large B-cell lymphoma. Am J Surg Pathol 2010;34(3):327–40.

147. Green TM, Young KH, Visco C, et al. Immunohistochemical double-hit score is a strong predictor of outcome in patients with diffuse large B-cell lymphoma treated with rituximab plus cyclophosphamide, doxorubicin, vincristine, and prednisone. J Clin Oncol 2012;30(28):3460–7.

148. Harrington AM, Olteanu H, Kroft SH, et al. The unique immunophenotype of double-hit lymphomas. Am J Clin Pathol 2011;135(4):649–50.

149. Wu D, Wood BL, Dorer R, et al. "Double-Hit" mature B-cell lymphomas show a common immunophenotype by flow cytometry that includes decreased CD20 expression. Am J Clin Pathol 2010;134(2):258–65.

150. Roth CG, Gillespie-Twardy A, Marks S, et al. Flow cytometric evaluation of double/triple hit lymphoma. Oncol Res 2016;23(3):137–46.

151. Dworzak MN, Buldini B, Gaipa G, et al. AIEOP-BFM consensus guidelines 2016 for flow cytometric immunophenotyping of pediatric acute lymphoblastic leukemia. Cytometry B Clin Cytom 2017. [Epub ahead of print].

152. Sedek L, Bulsa J, Sonsala A, et al. The immunophenotypes of blast cells in B-cell precursor acute lymphoblastic leukemia: how different are they from their normal counterparts? Cytometry B Clin Cytom 2014;86(5):329–39.

153. Kroft SH, Karandikar NJ. Flow cytometry in the diagnosis of acute leukemias and myelodysplastic/myeloproliferative disorders. In: Keren DF, McCoy JP, Carey JL, editors. Flow cytometry in clinical diagnosis. Chicago: ASCP Press; 2007. p. 151–98.

154. Seegmiller AC, Kroft SH, Karandikar NJ, et al. Characterization of immunophenotypic aberrancies in 200 cases of B acute lymphoblastic leukemia. Am J Clin Pathol 2009;132(6):940–9.

155. Chen W, Karandikar NJ, McKenna RW, et al. Stability of leukemia-associated immunophenotypes in precursor B-lymphoblastic leukemia/lymphoma: a single institution experience. Am J Clin Pathol 2007;127(1):1–8.

156. Borowitz MJ, Pullen DJ, Winick N, et al. Comparison of diagnostic and relapse flow cytometry phenotypes in childhood acute lymphoblastic leukemia: implications for residual disease detection: a report from the children's oncology group. Cytometry B Clin Cytom 2005;68(1):18–24.

157. Gaipa G, Basso G, Maglia O, et al. Drug-induced immunophenotypic modulation in childhood ALL: implications for minimal residual disease detection. Leukemia 2005;19(1):49–56.

158. McKenna RW, Washington LT, Aquino DB, et al. Immunophenotypic analysis of hematogones (B-lymphocyte precursors) in 662 consecutive bone marrow specimens by 4-color flow cytometry. Blood 2001;98(8):2498–507.

159. McKenna RW, Asplund SL, Kroft SH. Immunophenoytpic analysis of hematogones (B-lymphocyte precursors) and neoplastic lymphoblasts by 4-color flow cytometry. Leuk Lymphoma 2004;45(2):277–85.

160. Hassanein NM, Alcancia F, Perkinson KR, et al. Distinct expression patterns of CD123 and CD34 on normal bone marrow B-cell precursors ("hematogones") and B lymphoblastic leukemia blasts. Am J Clin Pathol 2009;132(4):573–80.

161. Hartung L, Bahler DW. Flow cytometric analysis of BCL-2 can distinguish small numbers of acute lymphoblastic leukaemia cells from B-cell precursors. Br J Haematol 2004;127(1):50–8.

162. Lee RV, Braylan RC, Rimsza LM. CD58 expression decreases as nonmalignant B cells mature in bone marrow and is frequently overexpressed in adult and

pediatric precursor B-cell acute lymphoblastic leukemia. Am J Clin Pathol 2005; 123(1):119–24.

163. Muzzafar T, Medeiros LJ, Wang SA, et al. Aberrant underexpression of CD81 in precursor B-cell acute lymphoblastic leukemia: utility in detection of minimal residual disease by flow cytometry. Am J Clin Pathol 2009;132(5):692–8.

164. Hrusak O, Porwit-MacDonald A. Antigen expression patterns reflecting genotype of acute leukemias. Leukemia 2002;16(7):1233–58.

165. Djokic M, Bjorklund E, Blennow E, et al. Overexpression of CD123 correlates with the hyperdiploid genotype in acute lymphoblastic leukemia. Haematologica 2009;94(7):1016–9.

166. Pui CH, Rubnitz JE, Hancock ML, et al. Reappraisal of the clinical and biologic significance of myeloid- associated antigen expression in childhood acute lymphoblastic leukemia. J Clin Oncol 1998;16(12):3768–73.

167. Mancini M, Scappaticci D, Cimino G, et al. A comprehensive genetic classification of adult acute lymphoblastic leukemia (ALL): analysis of the GIMEMA 0496 protocol. Blood 2005;105(9):3434–41.

168. Borowitz MJ, Rubnitz J, Nash M, et al. Surface antigen phenotype can predict TEL-AML1 rearrangement in childhood B-precursor ALL: a Pediatric Oncology Group study. Leukemia 1998;12(11):1764–70.

169. Kost CB, Holden JT, Mann KP. Marginal zone B-cell lymphoma: a retrospective immunophenotypic analysis. Cytometry B Clin Cytom 2008;74(5):282–6.

170. Carlile B, McKenna RW, Kroft SH. Lymphoplasmacytoid lymphoma: an immunophenotypic re-evaluation [abstract]. Mod Pathol 2001;14:157A.

171. Garcia DP, Rooney MT, Ahmad E, et al. Diagnostic usefulness of CD23 and FMC-7 antigen expression patterns in B-cell lymphoma classification. Am J Clin Pathol 2001;115(2):258–65.

172. Berger F, Felman P, Thieblemont C, et al. Non-MALT marginal zone B-cell lymphomas: a description of clinical presentation and outcome in 124 patients. Blood 2000;95(6):1950–6.

173. Matutes E, Morilla R, Owusu-Ankomah K, et al. The immunophenotype of splenic lymphoma with villous lymphocytes and its relevance to the differential diagnosis with other B-cell disorders. Blood 1994;83(6):1558–62.

174. Delgado J, Matutes E, Morilla AM, et al. Diagnostic significance of CD20 and FMC7 expression in B-cell disorders. Am J Clin Pathol 2003;120(5):754–9.

175. Rathke SK, Chang JC, Harrington AM, et al. The immunophenotype of prolymphocytoid transformation of chronic lymphocytic leukemia/small lymphocytic lymphoma (CLL/SLL) revisited. Mod Pathol 2013;26:356A–7A.

176. Tefferi A, Bartholmai BJ, Witzig TE, et al. Heterogeneity and clinical relevance of the intensity of CD20 and immunoglobulin light-chain expression in B-cell chronic lymphocytic leukemia. Am J Clin Pathol 1996;106(4):457–61.

177. Monaghan SA, Peterson LC, James C, et al. Pan B-cell markers are not redundant in analysis of chronic lymphocytic leukemia (CLL). Cytometry B Clin Cytom 2003;56(1):30–42.

178. Schlette E, Medeiros LJ, Keating M, et al. CD79b expression in chronic lymphocytic leukemia. Association with trisomy 12 and atypical immunophenotype. Arch Pathol Lab Med 2003;127(5):561–6.

Flow Cytometry of T cells and T-cell Neoplasms

Jeffrey W. Craig, MD, PhD, David M. Dorfman, MD, PhD*

KEYWORDS

- Flow cytometry • T-cell neoplasia • Immunophenotypic analysis
- Pan T-cell antigens

KEY POINTS

- Flow cytometry is advantageous in the evaluation of T-cell neoplasia for multiple reasons.
- Immunophenotypic features of normal T-cell biology and development are retained by T-cell neoplasms and aid in their diagnostic classification.
- Aberrant flow cytometric features are exhibited by the majority of lesional T-cell populations, but may also be seen in a variety of benign and reactive conditions.
- Characteristic immunophenotypic profiles and aberrant immunophenotypes are known for virtually all T-cell neoplasms.

INTRODUCTION

Immunophenotypic characterization is an essential component of the diagnostic workup of T-cell neoplasia.[1–3] To this end, flow cytometry is one of pathology's most powerful tools, offering the ability to simultaneously profile multiple antigens on individual cells. Although the routine flow cytometry panels used in clinical practice lack reliable markers of T-cell clonality, characteristic immunophenotypic profiles and aberrant immunophenotypes are known for virtually all T-cell neoplasms. The value of flow cytometry is not limited to the immunoprofiling performed at the time of initial diagnosis, however, as variations of flow cytometric methods offer other potential benefits (**Box 1**).[4] The range of clinical indications that warrant flow cytometry with the evaluation of T-cell lineage markers is exceedingly broad (**Box 2**).[5] Many of the markers considered most useful for the initial and secondary evaluations of suspected T-cell neoplasia are found in guidelines provided by the 2006 Bethesda International Consensus Conference (**Table 1**).[6]

Disclosure Statement: The authors have nothing to disclose.
Department of Pathology, Brigham and Women's Hospital, Harvard Medical School, 75 Francis Street, Boston, MA 02115, USA
* Corresponding author.
E-mail address: ddorfman@bwh.harvard.edu

Clin Lab Med 37 (2017) 725–751
http://dx.doi.org/10.1016/j.cll.2017.07.002
0272-2712/17/© 2017 Elsevier Inc. All rights reserved.

Box 1
Potential uses and benefits of flow cytometry in the evaluation of T-cell neoplasia

- Provides immunophenotypic data for routine disease diagnosis and classification
- May provide rapid confirmation that lesional tissue is present (eg, via fine needle aspiration evaluation)
- Provides important staging information (eg, central nervous system involvement)
- Assists in the detection of minimal residual disease (eg, monitoring treatment response in T-lymphoblastic leukemia/lymphoma)
- May provide evidence of relapse or progression of known T-cell malignancies (eg, leukemic evolution of cutaneous T-cell lymphoma)
- May identify prognostic markers and targets of molecular therapies (eg, CD52)

Data from Kaleem Z. Flow cytometric analysis of lymphomas: current status and usefulness. Arch Pathol Lab Med 2006;130(12):1850–8.

T-cell neoplasia often recapitulates the various stages of normal T-cell development and differentiation, permitting disease classification according to similarities with benign T-cell subsets and precursors. Thus, in conjunction with flow cytometry data, an understanding of normal T-cell biology can lead to many diagnostic inferences. For example, the varying stages of early T-cell maturation are readily evident from the immunophenotypic spectrum of T-lymphoblastic leukemia/lymphoma (T-ALL/LBL). The $\gamma\delta$ T cells and natural killer (NK) cells of the innate immune system also share immunophenotypic features with their neoplastic counterparts, as do the more heterogeneous and functionally complex $\alpha\beta$ T cells of the adaptive immune system. Herein, we review the spectrum of flow cytometric findings associated with T-cell neoplasia and its mimics, and discuss the most common immunophenotypic features associated with specific disease entities.

Box 2
Indications for T-cell flow cytometry

- Cytopenia(s) of any kind
- Lymphocytosis
- Eosinophilia
- Lymphadenopathy
- Extranodal mass
- Splenomegaly
- Skin rash
- Circulating or increased bone marrow blasts
- Atypical cells in body fluid specimens
- Staging and monitoring known T-cell malignancies

Data from Davis BH, Holden JT, Bene MC, et al. 2006 Bethesda International Consensus recommendations on the flow cytometric immunophenotypic analysis of hematolymphoid neoplasia: medical indications. Cytometry B Clin Cytom 2007;72(Suppl 1):S5–13.

Table 1
Common T-cell markers for initial and secondary flow cytometry evaluations

Initial Panel	Secondary Reagents
CD2, CD3, CD4, CD5, CD7, CD8, CD45, and CD56	CD1a, cCD3, CD10, CD16, CD25, CD26, CD30, CD34, CD45RA, CD45RO, CD57, αβ TCR, γδ TCR, cTIA-1, TCR Vβ chain isoforms, and TdT

Data from Wood BL, Arroz M, Barnett D, et al. 2006 Bethesda International Consensus recommendations on the immunophenotypic analysis of hematolymphoid neoplasia by flow cytometry: optimal reagents and reporting for the flow cytometric diagnosis of hematopoietic neoplasia. Cytometry B Clin Cytom 2007;72(Suppl 1):S14–22.

FLOW CYTOMETRIC FEATURES OF NEOPLASTIC T-CELL POPULATIONS

Most precursor and peripheral T-cell and NK-cell lymphomas can be readily identified by multiparameter flow cytometry.[7] To achieve maximal benefit, flow cytometry users will routinely search for a diverse set of flow cytometric features, each of which potentially suggests the presence of an aberrant T-cell population (**Table 2**).[8] Among the items listed, the most broadly useful is the detection of aberrant T-cell populations as discrete immunophenotypic clusters exhibiting altered expression of pan T-cell antigens (**Fig. 1**). This general approach has been validated through comparison of

Table 2
Possible flow cytometric manifestations of T-cell neoplasia

Finding	Comment
Relative T-cell predominance (ie, T cells represent a significant majority of total events or total lymphocytes)	Considered a generally nonspecific finding seen in many non-neoplastic conditions
T-cell subset restriction (eg, CD4 vs CD8, predominance of γδ TCR over αβ TCR)	Low sensitivity due to large numbers of admixed reactive T cells in many instances
Distinct light-scatter properties (forward scatter, side scatter) compared with non-neoplastic T cells	All benign T-cell subsets show similar light-scatter properties under normal circumstances
Abnormal CD45 expression	Typically in the form of dim or negative expression
Coexpression or absence of both CD4 and CD8	Most commonly seen in precursor T-cell neoplasms
Expression of non–T-cell antigens (eg, CD13, CD33, and CD117), markers of T-cell activation or functional differentiation (eg, CD10, CD25 and CD30), or blastic markers (eg, CD34, TdT and CD1a)	Often helpful for disease classification and diagnosis
Altered expression of the pan T-cell antigens CD2, CD3, CD5, and CD7	Frequently in the form of complete or partial loss of fluorescence intensity; changes may only be present on a subset of cells; similar findings may be seen in certain reactive conditions

Data from Gorczyca W, Weisberger J, Liu Z, et al. An approach to diagnosis of T-cell lymphoproliferative disorders by flow cytometry. Cytometry 2002;50(3):177–90.

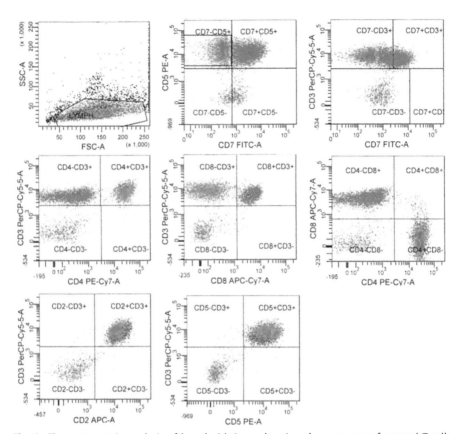

Fig. 1. Flow cytometric analysis of lymphoid tissue showing the presence of normal T cells (*red population*) that express pan T-cell markers CD2, CD3, CD5, and CD7, with subpopulations positive for CD4 and CD8, as well as an aberrant T-cell population (*green*) that is positive for pan T-cell markers CD3 and CD5 with decreased expression of pan T-cell marker CD7 and positivity for CD4 but not CD8.

neoplastic T-cell populations to established body site–specific normal and reactive T-cell subsets.[9] The diminished expression of 1 or more pan T-cell antigens is seen in approximately 90% of all T-cell neoplasms, and the complete loss of 1 or more pan T-cell antigens is seen in approximately 60%.[8] Multiple studies suggest that among mature T-cell neoplasms, CD7 and CD3 are the pan T-cell markers most frequently altered and CD2 the most frequently retained, whereas CD7 is typically expressed by immature T-cell neoplasms, which are typically negative for surface CD3 (sCD3) expression.[8–12] Although altered expression of pan T-cell antigens is a generally reliable feature of T-cell neoplasms, it is well established that small non-neoplastic T-cell subsets with aberrant immunophenotypes (eg, γδ T cells, CD4$^-$/CD8$^-$ αβ T-cells, CD4$^+$/CD8$^+$ T cells, and T cells lacking CD2, CD5, or CD7) may be seen under both normal and reactive conditions, including viral infections and non–T-cell malignancies.[8,9] For this reason, few flow cytometric criteria remain relatively specific for malignancy following statistical analysis (**Box 3**).[8] Once a neoplastic T-cell population has been identified, a preliminary differential diagnosis may be formulated based on the expression patterns of CD4 and CD8 (**Table 3**).[13]

Box 3
Flow cytometric findings with high specificity for T-cell neoplasia

- Complete loss or markedly diminished CD45 expression
- Complete loss of one or more pan T-cell antigen(s) (excluding NK cells and γδ T cells)
- Diminished expression of more than 2 pan T-cell antigens combined with altered light-scatter properties
- A majority of CD4$^+$/CD8$^+$ or CD4$^-$/CD8$^-$ T cells (excluding thymic lesions)

Data from Gorczyca W, Weisberger J, Liu Z, et al. An approach to diagnosis of T-cell lymphoproliferative disorders by flow cytometry. Cytometry 2002;50(3):177–90.

FLOW CYTOMETRY OF IMMATURE T CELLS
T-Lymphoblastic Leukemia/Lymphoma

T-ALL/LBL is an aggressive neoplasm of lymphoblasts committed to the T-lineage through expression of cytoplasmic CD3 ε chain (cCD3ε or simply cCD3) or sCD3 in the absence of lineage-defining myeloid or B-cell markers. The disease may primarily involve the bone marrow and/or blood (T-ALL) or present as a tissue-based mass involving the thymus, lymph nodes, or extranodal sites (T-LBL). The precursor nature of T-lymphoblasts is best indicated by the expression of terminal deoxynucleotidyl transferase (TdT), CD99, CD34, CD1a, or cCD3ε without sCD3.[14] The expression of TdT and CD1a on T cells outside of the thymus is notably abnormal and always indicative of an aberrant population.[15] CD10 expression has been reported in 15% to 63% of cases of T-ALL/LBL, and when paired with the expression of pan T-cell markers and the absence of follicular helper T-cell (TFH) markers, is suggestive of immaturity.[16] Occasionally T-ALL/LBL blasts are negative for TdT (<5% of cases), but only rarely are they negative for both TdT and CD34.[17]

T-ALL/LBL can be further classified into subtypes that correspond to the normal stages of thymocyte development (pro-T, pre-T, cortical-T, and medullary-T), although significant heterogeneity exists (**Table 4**).[18,19] In addition to TdT and cCD3,

---

Table 3
Differential diagnosis of T-cell neoplasms according to CD4 and CD8 expression

CD4$^-$/CD8$^-$	CD4$^+$/CD8$^-$
• T-lymphoblastic leukemia/lymphoma (T-ALL/LBL) • Natural killer (NK) or NK/T-cell neoplasms (eg, extranodal NK-/T-cell lymphoma, nasal type [ENK/TL-NT])	• Most cutaneous T-cell lymphomas (eg, Sézary syndrome [SS]) • T-cell prolymphocytic leukemia (T-PLL) (subset) • Adult T-cell leukemia/lymphoma (ATLL) • Anaplastic large-cell lymphoma (ALCL) • Nodal peripheral T-cell lymphomas with T follicular helper phenotype (NPTCL-TFH)
CD4$^-$/CD8$^+$	**CD4$^+$/CD8$^+$**
• T-cell large granular lymphocytic leukemia (T-LGL leukemia) • Certain lymphomas of γδ T cells (eg, hepatosplenic T-cell lymphoma [HSTL]) • T-cell prolymphocytic leukemia (T-PLL) (subset)	• T-lymphoblastic leukemia/lymphoma (T-ALL/LBL) • T-cell prolymphocytic leukemia (T-PLL) (subset) • Rare ATLL and T-LGL leukemias

Data from Craig FE, Foon KA. Flow cytometric immunophenotyping for hematologic neoplasms. Blood 2008;111(8):3941–67.

Table 4
Common immunophenotypic features of T-ALL/LBL subtypes

ALL	TdT	CD1a	CD34	HLA-DR	cCD3	sCD3	CD2	CD5	CD7	CD4	CD8
Pro-T	+	−	+/−	+/−	+	−	−	−	+	−	−
Pre-T	+	−	+/−	+/−	+	−	+	+	+	−	−
Cortical-T	+	+	−	−	+	−	+	+	+	+	+
Mature T	+	−	−	−	+	+	+	+	+	+/−	−/+

+, positive staining; −, negative staining.

the most sensitive marker of T-lineage precursors is CD7, which is expressed across all subtypes (>95% of T-ALL/LBL).[10] CD1a expression is often seen in the cortical-T subtype, whereas sCD3 is typically encountered in only the most mature medullary-T subtype. CD4 and CD8 expression are absent in the pro-T and pre-T subtypes, and doubly positive in the cortical-T subtype (**Fig. 2**). These expression patterns are

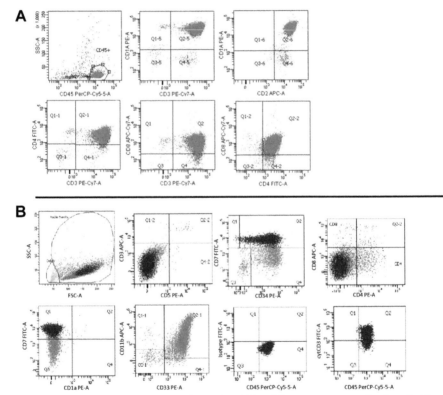

Fig. 2. (A) Flow cytometric analysis of peripheral blood from a patient with T-lymphoblastic leukemia/lymphoma with a cortical thymocyte phenotype, exhibiting positivity for CD45 and pan T-cell markers CD2, CD3, CD5 (not shown) and CD7 (not shown), coexpression of CD4 and CD8, expression of CD1a and TdT (not shown), and absence of staining for HLA-DR, B-cell, and myeloid markers (not shown). (B) Flow cytometric analysis of peripheral blood from a patient with early T-cell precursor (ETP) acute lymphoblastic leukemia, exhibiting positivity for CD45, T-cell markers CD7 (subset) and cytoplasmic CD3, and myeloid markers CD11b, CD33 and CD117 (not shown), with absence of staining for surface CD3, CD5, CD4, and CD8. (*Courtesy of* Dr Olga Weinberg, Boston Children's Hospital, Boston, MA.)

nonspecific, however, as CD4⁻/CD8⁻ and CD4⁺/CD8⁺ immunophenotypes may also be encountered in mature T-cell neoplasms.

CD45 expression is always positive, but may be dim (~30%), and T-cell receptor (TCR) expression is frequently absent (~50%) in T-ALL/LBL.[10] Aberrant expression of the B-cell marker CD79a, NK-cell markers (eg, CD16 and CD56), and myeloid markers (especially CD13 and/or CD33), are occasionally seen and do not preclude the diagnosis of T-ALL/LBL, although expression of myeloperoxidase (MPO), if present, suggests a diagnosis of mixed phenotype acute leukemia (see later in this article). Although T-ALL and T-LBL are considered different manifestations of the same disease, the immunophenotype of T-LBL tends to be slightly more mature than that of T-ALL, likely reflecting derivation from a more mature thymocyte counterpart.[20]

Early T-cell precursor acute lymphoblastic leukemia

Early T-cell precursor acute lymphoblastic leukemia (ETP-ALL) is a newly recognized subtype of T-ALL identified through gene expression profiling and included within the most recent World Health Organization (WHO) classification as a provisional diagnostic entity.[3,21] ETP-ALL encompasses a subset of the T-ALL cases described previously that are derived from early T-cell precursors that retain multilineage differentiation potential and thus respond poorly to lymphoid-directed chemotherapy.[22,23] The distinctly immature immunophenotype shared by most ETP-ALL cases includes the absence of CD1a and CD8 expression (<5% positive lymphoblasts), absent or weak CD5 expression (<75% positive lymphoblasts), and the expression of at least one of the following myeloid or stem-cell markers (≥25% positive lymphoblasts): CD117, CD34, HLA-DR, CD13, CD33, CD11b, or CD65 (see **Fig. 2**).[21] Substantial immunophenotypic variation is seen within ETP-ALL cases identified by gene expression profiling, including the expression of CD5 in the absence of myeloid or stem-cell markers, and the expression of surface CD3 and γδ TCR. For these reasons the boundaries of an acceptable ETP-ALL immunophenotype are yet to be defined.[19]

Mixed phenotype acute leukemia

Mixed phenotype acute leukemias (MPALs) are defined as those with blasts that express antigens of more than one lineage to such a degree that it is not possible to assign the leukemia to just one lineage with certainty.[24] These encompass both bilineal leukemias having 2 separate blast populations, each of a different lineage, and biphenotypic leukemias having a single blast population coexpressing antigens of more than one lineage (**Fig. 3**).[1] The 2016 WHO classification revision emphasizes that in cases in which 2 distinct blast populations can be resolved, it is not necessary that specific lineage-defining markers be present, but only that each individual population would otherwise be considered as either B, T, or myeloid leukemia.[3]

In all other cases, establishing the presence of a T-cell component requires strong expression of sCD3 or cCD3ε, with at least a fraction of blasts expressing cCD3 at the level of normal T cells (**Table 5**).[3,24] In both the bilineal and biphenotypic subtypes of MPAL, the T-cell lineage is most often seen in combination with the myeloid lineage rather than with the B-cell lineage.[17,25] In this setting, the diagnostic term "mixed phenotype acute leukemia, T/myeloid, not otherwise specified" is preferred. In a large series including all MPAL subtypes, 35% were T/myeloid, 4% were T/B, and 2% fulfilled criteria for acute trilineage leukemia.[26] Among the T/myeloid cohort, cCD3 was expressed in all cases, with the proportion of positive blasts ranging from 13% to

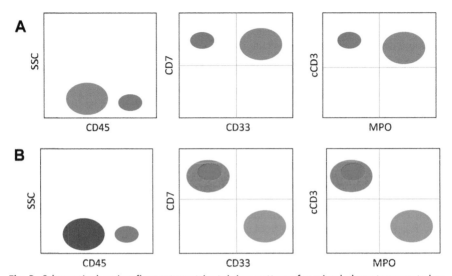

Fig. 3. Schematic showing flow cytometric staining patterns for mixed phenotype acute leukemia, T/myeloid. (*A*) Biphenotypic acute leukemia, with one population (*blue*) of CD45 dimly positive blasts that exhibit coexpression of T-cell markers CD7 and cytoplasmic CD3 and myeloid markers CD33 and MPO. (*B*) Bilineal acute leukemia with one population of CD45 dimly positive blasts (*red*) that exhibits expression of T-cell markers CD7 and cytoplasmic CD3 and a second population of CD45 dimly positive blasts (*blue*) that exhibits expression of myeloid markers CD33 and MPO. Note that in both examples, staining for cytoplasmic CD3 by the CD45 dimly positive blasts is comparable to staining observed for CD45 brightly positive mature T-cell markers (*green population*).

99%. CD2 and CD7 were variably expressed in approximately 70% and approximately 90% of cases, respectively.

Thymic Hyperplasia/Thymoma

Thymomas are neoplasms of thymic epithelial cells that are characteristically associated with large numbers of non-neoplastic T cells, presumably due to retention of normal thymic function.[27] By flow cytometry, thymic hyperplasia and lymphocyte-rich thymoma characteristically show a majority of immature T cells that express CD1a, TdT, and both CD4 and CD8 (ie, cortical thymocytes), and lack expression of CD10, CD34, and HLA-DR, without loss of expression of pan T-cell antigens CD2, CD5, and CD7.[28] Frequently this immature T-cell population consists of cells

Table 5		
Lineage markers for defining Mixed phenotype acute leukemia		
T-Lineage	**Myeloid Lineage**	**B-Lineage**
Strong cytoplasmic CD3ε or surface CD3	Myeloperoxidase or at least 2 monocytic markers (NSE, CD11C, CD14, CD64, lysozyme)	Strong CD19 plus 1 extra B-cell marker, or weak CD19 plus 2 extra B-cell markers (CD79a, cytoplasmic CD22, CD10)

From Swerdlow SH, Campo E, Harris NL, et al. WHO Classification of tumours of haematopoietic and lymphoid tissues. 4th Ed. 2008; with permission.

with variable coexpression of both CD4 and CD8, with one or the other predominating such that CD4 versus CD8 scattergrams display a characteristic double-tailed comet pattern (**Fig. 4**).[29] By comparison, cases of CD4+/CD8+ T-ALL/LBL with admixed benign T cells will not show this distinctive pattern, but will instead display discrete populations of doubly positive and singly positive cells. The abundant CD4+/CD8+ cortical thymocytes seen in thymic hyperplasia and thymoma are reliable markers of benignancy that are lost in cases of thymic carcinoma.[30] A predominant population of CD4−/CD8− T cells or T cells with subset restriction, which may be present in some cases of T-ALL/LBL, is not seen in cases of thymic hyperplasia or thymoma.

Most T cells from cases of thymic hyperplasia and thymoma (typically ~75%–90% CD4+/CD8+ thymocytes plus ~5%–15% mature T cells) should be small in size and express uniformly bright CD45 and moderate levels of CD2, CD5, and CD7. Aberrant dim expression of CD45 or disproportionate intensities of CD2, CD5, or CD7 in most cells is suspicious for T-ALL/LBL.[28] Surface CD3 should display an even spectrum of densities ranging from negative to bright, a finding considered one of the most reliable ways for differentiating populations of benign thymocytes from lymphoblasts (see **Fig. 4**).[29] A minority of T cells from cases of thymic hyperplasia and thymoma (2%–10%) are more immature, intermediate-sized cells with a CD34+/TdT+/CD3−/dim/CD2dim/CD5dim/CD7bright/CD10dim/CD4−/CD8− immunophenotype.[28] The lymphoblasts of T-ALL/LBL typically lack these 2 discrete cell populations, which are best seen on forward scatter (FSC) versus CD3 scattergrams.

FLOW CYTOMETRY OF MATURE T CELLS
Non-neoplastic T-cell Subsets in Peripheral Blood and Bone Marrow

T-cell large granular lymphocytes
In healthy adults, large granular lymphocytes (LGLs) account for roughly 10% to 15% of peripheral blood leukocytes, and can be classified as belonging to either NK-cell (sCD3−) or cytotoxic T-cell (sCD3+) lineage.[31] The T-cell subset (T-LGLs) exhibits an activated, cytotoxic, effector lymphocyte phenotype (sCD3+/CD4−/CD8+/CD57+/αβ TCR+) with production of cytotoxic granule proteins and conserved expression of pan T-cell antigens (although the level of CD5 expression may be slightly

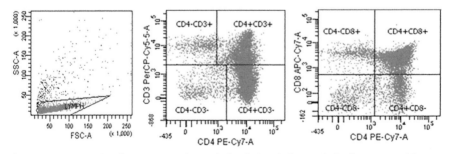

Fig. 4. Representative flow cytometric analysis of thymic hyperplasia/thymoma with most T-cells showing variable expression of pan T-cell marker CD3 and variable coexpression of CD4 and CD8 with subpopulations positive for only CD4 or CD8, or with absence of staining for CD4 and CD8. There is no loss of expression of pan T-cell markers CD5 and CD7 (not shown). Compare these findings with those in **Fig. 2**A, from a patient with T-lymphoblastic leukemia/lymphoma, in which the neoplastic cells are present as a discrete population of CD3-positive, CD4/CD8 double-positive cells.

lower than that of CD8⁻/CD57⁻ T cells), and very rarely with subset expression of additional NK-cell markers (eg, CD16, CD94, CD161 and occasionally CD56) (**Figs. 5** and **8**).[9,31–33] In addition, CD4⁺/CD56⁺ T-LGL cells may be present in patients who are immunosuppressed or have chronic inflammation or autoimmune disorders. T-LGLs are functionally heterogeneous and play significant roles in various disease states associated with chronic immune activation, including non-NK/T-cell malignancies, chronic intracellular infections, certain pulmonary diseases, autoimmune diseases, and following allogeneic transplantation.[34] Accordingly, T-LGLs are frequently increased in these conditions and may give rise to typically small clonal T-LGL populations.[35] Under certain circumstances (eg, T-LGL clones associated with inclusion body myositis) these presumably reactive T-LGL populations expand to meet formal diagnostic criteria for T-LGL leukemia.[36] In contrast to T-LGL leukemia, however, many reactive/polyclonal LGL proliferations will present as a composite of T-cell and NK-cell LGL subsets.[37]

Natural killer cells

NK cells are a distinct but heterogeneous lymphocyte subset of the innate immune system sharing certain similarities with cytotoxic T cells, including the cytomorphology of T-LGLs.[38] NK cells play important roles in host defense, cancer surveillance, and immune regulation, and their numbers in peripheral blood and secondary lymphoid tissue may be drastically altered by viral infections, autoimmune conditions, pregnancy,

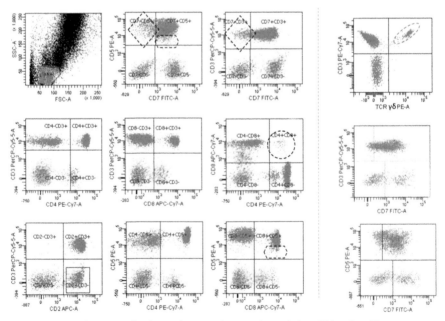

Fig. 5. Non-neoplastic T-cell subsets that may be seen in peripheral blood and bone marrow, including T-LGL cells (*dashed hexagon*) that are dimly positive for CD5 and positive for CD8; NK cells (*green population*) that are positive for CD2, CD7, and CD8 (variable staining), and negative for CD3, CD4, and CD5; CD7 dim/negative T cells (*dashed diamond*); and CD4/CD8 double-positive T cells (*dashed circle*). In addition, γδ T cells may be present (*right column*) with bright staining for CD3 (*green population*) and decreased staining for CD5. These cells were also positive for CD2 and CD16 (not shown).

malignancy, and following bone marrow transplantation.[39,40] By definition, they lack TCR gene rearrangements and a fully assembled TCR-CD3 complex.[41] The typical NK-cell immunophenotype is CD2+/sCD3−/CD5−/CD7+ with expression of NK-cell–associated antigens CD56 and CD16, which characteristically exhibit reciprocal and heterogeneous expression profiles under normal conditions, as well as CD94 and CD161 and variable expression of CD8 (30%–50% subset positivity) (see **Fig. 5**).[42–44] Expression of CD57 is normally restricted to more mature CD56[dim] NK cells.[45,46] The definitive identification of neoplastic NK cells by flow cytometry is limited by their occasionally normal immunophenotype coupled with the occasionally abnormal immunophenotype of benign NK-cell populations.[47]

T-cell receptor γδ T cells
T cells expressing the γδ TCR (γδ T cells) constitute a minority (1%–5%) of total T lymphocytes in healthy adults and differ from the more numerous αβ T cells in their capacity for major histocompatibility complex (MHC)-independent antigen recognition. Most are found in the spleen and epithelial-rich sites, including the skin and gastrointestinal and reproductive tracts, where they serve ill-defined but conserved roles in mucosal immunity.[48] γδ T cells express pan T-cell antigens at levels comparable to those of the αβ T-cell majority, but may display certain aberrancies under reactive conditions, including bright CD3, diminished CD7, and complete or partial loss of CD5, the latter of which frequently coincides with the aberrant expression of CD16 (see **Fig. 5**).[49] Outside of the thymus, virtually all γδ T cells are negative for CD4, whereas CD8 may be either negative or dimly positive in a subset of cells.[50] Expression of the NK/T-LGL markers CD16, CD56, CD57, and/or CD94 is a common finding.[49,50] Increased numbers of γδ T cells are frequently observed under conditions of immune activation, including infection, autoimmunity, and neoplastic conditions.[51] As double-negativity for CD4 and CD8 and absent CD5 expression are both associated with malignancy in mature αβ T cells, care must be taken not to overinterpret these features in reactive γδ T-cell populations.

T-cell lymphocytosis of undetermined significance
The detection of T-cell lymphocytosis may be the first indication of T-cell neoplasia, or may simply be a reflection of immune system activation. Results from a large study of T-cell lymphocytosis show that aberrant circulating T-cell populations are equally as likely to be reactive as they are neoplastic.[52] Further analysis shows that reactive and neoplastic T-cell populations with immunophenotypic aberrancies are also similar in terms of population size at the time of discovery, number of aberrantly expressed pan T-cell markers, and the repertoire of antigenic aberrancies encountered, which includes loss or diminished expression of all pan T-cell markers as well as intensity aberrations of CD4 and CD8 and the expression of TCR γδ. An elevated CD4-CD8 ratio (normal range 1–4) is more suggestive of autoimmunity or bacterial infection, whereas an inverted ratio is more suggestive of viral infections or cancer.[53] Peripheral populations of activated or reactive CD4+/CD8+ T cells are sometimes associated with viral infection, progressive transformation of germinal centers, and nodular lymphocyte-predominant Hodgkin lymphoma.[54,55]

Pan T-cell Antigen Loss in Non-Neoplastic Conditions
B-cell chronic lymphocytic leukemia/small lymphocytic lymphoma
Abnormalities of T-cell function occur regularly in patients with B-cell chronic lymphocytic leukemia (B-CLL).[56] The absolute number of circulating T cells is frequently increased, with relatively larger increases in CD8+ T cells compared with CD4+ T cells. Clonal or oligoclonal T-cell populations are present in most cases, where

they presumably represent tumor antigen-driven reactive T-cell proliferations or responses to persistent viral infections (eg, cytomegalovirus [CMV]).[57–59] By flow cytometry, these clonal T-cell populations are typically CD56$^+$ and/or CD57$^+$ and correspond to T-LGLs with CD4$^+$/CD8$^-$, CD4$^-$/CD8$^+$, and CD4$^-$/CD8$^-$ phenotypes.[60,61] Perturbations of specific T-cell compartments are not unique to B-CLL, however, as increases in the CD57$^+$, HLA-DR$^+$, CD16$^+$/CD56$^+$, CD62L$^-$, and CD28$^-$ subsets of both CD4$^+$ and CD8$^+$ T cells may be seen to varying degrees in all forms of hematologic neoplasia.[62]

Human immunodeficiency virus infection with decreased CD4 versus CD8

As a mechanism for viral entry into human cells, the human immunodeficiency virus (HIV) targets CD4 and the chemokine receptor CXCR4 on the surface of T lymphocytes, leading to the selective loss of CD4$^+$ T cells through a variety of mechanisms.[63] Peripheral blood CD4$^+$ T-cell levels decline to an average of 60% of their original levels within 12 to 18 months of seroconversion, whereas total circulating T-cell levels remain fairly constant during this time due to a robust and sustained CD8$^+$ T-cell lymphocytosis.[64] HIV infection is also linked to relative increases in $\gamma\delta$ T cells and decreases in NK cells.[65] The inverted CD4-CD8 T-cell ratio seen in patients with HIV infection also may be seen in other primary viral infections, and is thus nonspecific.[66] Care must be taken not to overinterpret apparent CD8$^+$ T-cell subset restriction in patients with known or suspected HIV infection.

Acute infectious mononucleosis and other viremias

Atypical lymphocytosis is a peripheral blood abnormality characterized by increased numbers of large reactive lymphocytes. Infectious mononucleosis (IM), a disease caused by the Epstein-Barr virus (EBV) and characterized by fever, sore throat, cervical adenopathy, and malaise, is the single most common clinical syndrome associated with atypical lymphocytosis.[67] EBV displays a marked tropism for B cells, which it targets through interactions with CD21 and/or CD35 in conjunction with HLA class II on the surface of resting B cells.[68] The immune response in IM includes increased circulating NK cells and a dramatic expansion of the peripheral CD8$^+$ T-cell compartment, primarily through increases in EBV-specific CD8$^+$ T-cell subsets.[69] Although the magnitude of these changes appears greatest in cases of atypical lymphocytosis caused by IM, similar findings are detected during other viral infections (eg, CMV, varicella zoster virus and viral hepatitis) and occasionally noninfectious causes.[70] Notably, the expanded CD8$^+$ T-cell populations seen in IM universally exhibit diminished CD7 expression (1-log below internal controls), slightly increased cells size by FSC, and occasional downregulation of CD5 (**Fig. 6**).[71]

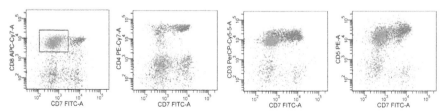

Fig. 6. Flow cytometric analysis of peripheral blood from a patient with acute IM, showing decreased staining for pan T-cell marker CD7 in a predominant population of activated CD3-positive, CD8-positive T cells (*green population*). Downregulation of CD7 may also be seen in patients with rheumatoid arthritis, inflammatory dermatoses, and with aging.

Immunophenotypic Patterns Associated With Specific Mature T-cell Neoplasms

T-cell prolymphocytic leukemia

T-cell prolymphocytic leukemia (T-PLL) is a rare aggressive T-cell neoplasm characterized by blood, bone marrow, lymph node, spleen, and liver involvement by small to intermediate-sized prolymphocytes.[72,73] T-PLL exhibits a mature post-thymic T-cell immunophenotype (CD2+/CD5+/CD7+) with occasionally dim surface CD3 expression and characteristic absence of CD25 and NK-cell markers.[13,74] T-PLL is most commonly CD4+/CD8− (65%), but may be CD4−/CD8+ (13%) or CD4+/CD8+ (21%) (**Fig. 7**).[75] The relatively high frequency of this latter group is unique among mature T-cell neoplasms. The prolymphocytes of T-PLL are consistently negative for CD34, TdT, and CD1a, in comparison with T-ALL/LBL; however, the CD3^{dim}/CD7^{bright} immunophenotype that may be seen in T-PLL, coupled with the relative propensity for CD4 and CD8 double-positivity, suggests that T-PLL may arise from T cells at an intermediate stage of differentiation between cortical thymocytes and mature T cells.[76] CD52 is usually expressed at high density and can be used as a target of therapy.[77] Although T-PLL most commonly presents as a single discrete population by flow cytometry, cases with 2 or more distinct subpopulations do occur.[78] Among mature T-cell neoplasms, T-PLL is the most likely to be immunophenotypically normal.[10] A variety of phenotypic abnormalities have been detected, however, including the aberrant expression of one or more pan T-cell antigens, the rare loss of CD45, and the rare aberrant expression of myeloid marker CD117.[78]

T cell large granular lymphocytic leukemia

T cell large granular lymphocytic leukemia (T-LGL leukemia) is a generally indolent disorder characterized by persistently increased numbers of circulating LGLs of cytotoxic T-cell phenotype.[79] Like most benign T-LGLs, most cases of T-LGL leukemia correspond to CD4−/CD8+ T cells that express αβ TCR and the activation marker CD57. Less common variants of T-LGL leukemia include those with CD4+/CD8−, CD4+/CD8+, and CD4−/CD8− immunophenotypes, the latter of which may be associated with γδ TCR expression.[35,80,81] The aberrant expression of at least one pan T-cell antigen, very frequently in the form of reduced or absent expression of CD5 or CD7

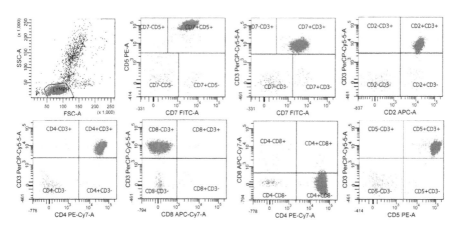

Fig. 7. Flow cytometric analysis of peripheral blood from a patient with T-PLL. In this case, the neoplastic cells show no loss of expression of pan T-cell markers CD2, CD3, CD5, or CD7. The neoplastic cells are positive for CD4 and negative for CD8, although other cases of T-PLL may be CD4/CD8 double-positive or CD4 negative and CD8 positive.

(approximately 90% and 80% of cases, respectively), is a near universal finding (**Fig. 8**).[43] Aberrant expression of 2 or more pan T-cell antigens is seen in 80% of cases.[82] The NK-cell markers CD16, CD56, and CD94 are frequently detected.[31,74] In the largest study to date, the immunophenotypic features most specific for T-LGL neoplasia, as opposed to reactive T-LGL proliferation, were the isolated presence of a distinct and expanded population of CD8^{dim}/CD57$^+$ T cells, complete or partial loss of CD5, and the expression of CD16.[33] In contrast, CD2 and CD7 loss were not specifically associated with clonal T-LGL leukemias.

Non-LGL γδ T-cell lymphomas

Lymphomas of γδ T-cell origin represent a rare subset of cytotoxic T-cell lymphomas typically associated with aggressive clinical behavior and extranodal presentation.[83] The best described examples (excluding γδ T-LGL leukemia) include hepatosplenic T-cell lymphoma (HSTL), primary cutaneous γδ T-cell lymphoma, and γδ T-cell lymphomas originating in mucosal sites such as the gastrointestinal tract (eg, monomorphic epitheliotropic intestinal T-cell lymphoma).[1,2] HSTL, which preferentially involves the liver, spleen and bone marrow, displays a common immunophenotype: CD2$^+$/CD3$^+$/CD4$^-$/CD5$^-$/CD8$^-$/γδ TCR$^+$.[84] CD5 is absent in most cases, in comparison with γδ T-LGL leukemia, which typically exhibits dim rather than absent CD5 expression, and CD7 is absent in 35% of cases.[85] CD8 is positive in 16% of cases, but CD4 is typically negative. The NK-cell–associated antigens CD16 and CD56 are frequently expressed (52% and 68%, respectively); however, CD57 is virtually always absent, in comparison with γδ T-LGL leukemia. Other activation-associated antigens may be expressed (eg, CD11b, CD11c, CD38, and CD43); however, CD25 and CD30 are usually negative.[86] The immunophenotypic features of nonhepatosplenic γδ T-cell lymphomas are generally very similar to those of HSTL (**Fig. 9**).[87]

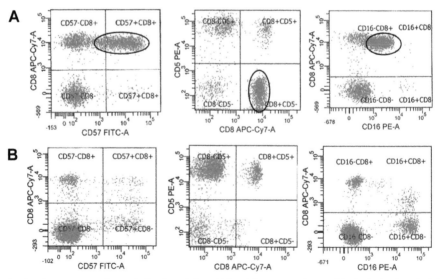

Fig. 8. Flow cytometric analysis of peripheral blood from a patient with T-LGL leukemia (A) compared with normal peripheral blood containing comparatively fewer T-LGLs that do not show significant clustering (B). The neoplastic cells show coexpression of CD8, CD16, and CD57 (circled population), with loss of expression of pan T-cell marker CD5.

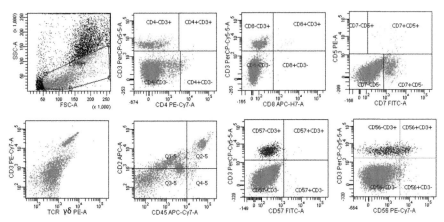

Fig. 9. Flow cytometric analysis of bone marrow from a patient with γδ T-cell lymphoma, in which the neoplastic cells are positive for CD2, CD3, CD7, CD56 (dim), CD94 (not shown), CD45, and TCR γδ, and negative for CD4, CD5, CD8, CD57, and TCR αβ (not shown).

Mature NK-cell neoplasms

Neoplastic disorders of NK cells include extranodal NK-/T-cell lymphoma, nasal type (ENK/TL-NT), aggressive NK-cell leukemia (ANKL), and chronic lymphoproliferative disorder of NK cells (CLPD-NK).[1,2] The "classic" immunophenotypic features of these NK-cell neoplasms are shared with most benign NK cells (CD2$^+$/CD56$^+$/cCD3ε$^+$/ sCD3$^-$/CD5$^-$/CD4$^-$/CD8$^-$), although aberrant phenotypes are not uncommon.[88,89] Abnormal expression of NK markers is frequent in neoplastic NK-cell populations, including absent or reduced expression of CD56, CD57, and CD161, and/or distinctively bright expression of CD16 and CD94.[43,90] Aberrantly dim expression of CD2 or CD7, aberrant gain of CD5, and uniform CD8 positivity may also indicate clonal NK-cell processes.[42]

ANKL is a rare form of LGL leukemia with an aggressive clinical course. The classic phenotype is sCD3$^-$/CD2$^+$/CD56$^+$/HLA-DR$^+$.[91] CD16 is positive in 75% of cases, whereas CD57 is only rarely expressed (13%) and CD25 is always absent, suggesting possible derivation from cytotoxic CD56^{dim} NK cells. CD7, CD8, and cCD3 are positive in 74%, 29%, and 43% of cases, respectively. Although normal NK cells typically overlap with benign lymphocytes on CD45/FSC/side scatter (SSC) gating, the neoplastic cell populations of ANKL frequently exhibit increased light-scatter characteristics and altered CD45 expression, with 41% of cases showing brighter and 10% showing dimmer CD45 than normal lymphocytes.[92]

CLPD-NK occurs in older adults and typically exhibits a prolonged, indolent course. The typical phenotype is sCD3$^-$/CD16$^{+(homogenous)}$/CD56$^{+(dim\ or\ bright)}$ **(Fig. 10)**.[93] CD2 and CD7 are present in a subset of cases, CD8 may occasionally be detected, and approximately half of cases express CD57. The neoplastic NK cells usually overlap with the normal lymphocytes on CD45/SSC gating.[92] Loss of CD16 and aberrant coexpression of CD5 may also occur.

Nodal peripheral T-cell lymphomas with T follicular helper phenotype

Nodal peripheral T-cell lymphomas with T follicular helper phenotype (NPTCL-TFH) represent a newly recognized class of peripheral CD4$^+$ T-cell lymphomas, including such entities as angioimmunoblastic T-cell lymphoma (AITCL) and follicular T-cell lymphoma. Members of this group share in the expression of at least 2 follicular helper

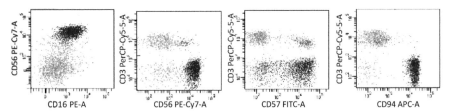

Fig. 10. Flow cytometric analysis of peripheral blood from a patient with chronic lympho-proliferative disorder of NK cells, in which the neoplastic cells (*blue population*) are positive for CD16, CD56, CD57, and CD 94, as well as pan T-cell markers CD2 and CD7 (not shown), and are negative for T-cell markers CD3, CD4, CD5, and CD8 (not shown). The neoplastic NK cells were present within the FSC/SSC lymphocyte gate (data not shown).

T-cell–associated antigens (CD279/PD1, CD10, BCL6, CXCL13, ICOS, SAP, and CCR5).[2] Of these antigens, CD10 is commonly found in routine flow cytometry panels and its expression on a significant population of T cells should raise suspicion for NPTCL-TFH. The most well-studied member of this group, AITCL, shows subset CD10 expression in 70% to 90% of cases, including those with peripheral blood involvement (**Fig. 11**).[94–100] CD10 positivity is not entirely specific for neoplasia, however, as small discrete populations of CD10[+] T cells, comprising 1% to 6% of total cells and up to 14% of all T cells, are found in 18% of reactive follicular hyperplasias and up to 50% of B-cell lymphomas.[101]

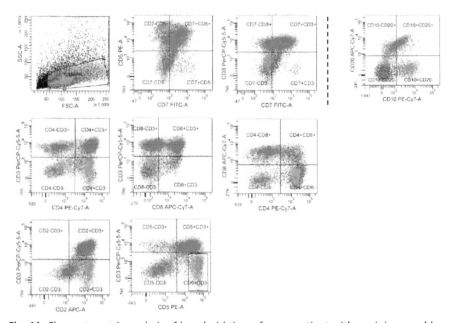

Fig. 11. Flow cytometric analysis of lymphoid tissue from a patient with angioimmunoblastic T-cell lymphoma, in which the neoplastic cells (*green population*) show positivity for pan T-cell markers CD2, CD5, and CD7 (decreased), as well as B-cell marker CD10, and are negative for CD3 and CD8. A background population of non-neoplastic lymphocytes (*red population*) is present, including T cells with expression of pan T-cell antigens, with subsets positive for CD4 and CD8, and non-neoplastic CD20-positive B cells.

Neoplastic AITCL cells show either similar or, more frequently, increased light-scatter properties compared with benign T cells.[95,96] CD2, CD4, and CD5 are expressed in virtually all cases, whereas CD8 and CD56 are absent. Surface CD3 expression is frequently lost or diminished (~50%–60% and 20%–30% of cases, respectively), CD7 expression patterns (complete, partial, or subset loss) are often abnormal (up to ~60%–70%), and αβ TCR expression is either lost or decreased in most cases (~70%).[94–96,98,100] Although circulating sCD3⁻/CD4⁺ T cells had been previously described in AITCL, more recent studies have demonstrated their seemingly universal presence in AITCL patients with leukemic blood involvement (ranging from <1% to >50% of circulating lymphocytes) and have shown this finding to have a 94% positive predictive value.[102,103] Similar populations of circulating sCD3⁻/CD4⁺ T cells have been described in the recently added WHO provisional entity follicular T-cell lymphoma.[104] When applied to the flow cytometric analysis of lymph node specimens, a cutoff of 3% sCD3⁻/CD4⁺ T cells (of total lymphocytes) is recommended for increased discrimination between NPTCL-TFH and plausible mimics (eg, reactive lymphoid tissues and Hodgkin lymphoma).[105]

Adult T-cell leukemia/lymphoma

Adult T-cell leukemia/lymphoma (ATLL) is a peripheral T-cell neoplasm of pleomorphic lymphocytes that arises in a small percentage of human T-cell leukemia virus type 1 (HTLV-1) carriers.[106] The characteristic immunophenotype is that of an activated mature T-lymphocyte with expression of CD2 and CD5, loss of CD7, and frequent downregulation of CD3 and αβ TCR.[107–109] The most characteristic immunophenotypic feature of this disease, however, is the uniformly strong expression of the alpha chain of the interleukin-2 receptor (CD25), in keeping with a regulatory T-cell phenotype that is further evidenced by the frequent expression of chemokine receptors CCR4 and FoxP3 (**Fig. 12**).[110] Although CD25 expression is not unique to ATLL, its presence on other T-cell neoplasms is typically more variable and of lower intensity. Most cases of ATLL are CD4⁺/CD8⁻, but cases with CD4⁻/CD8⁺ and CD4⁺/CD8⁺ phenotypes also may be encountered.[13]

Sézary syndrome

Sézary syndrome (SS) is an aggressive leukemic variant of cutaneous T-cell lymphoma characterized by erythroderma, lymphadenopathy, and numerous circulating T cells with atypical cytologic features.[111] A clonal population of T cells should be present in the peripheral blood and either ≥1000 Sézary cells/μL or a T-cell population with increased CD4-CD8 ratio (≥10) or an increase in CD4-positive T cells with an aberrant phenotype (≥40% CD4⁺/CD7⁻ cells or ≥30% CD4⁺CD26⁻ cells). Flow cytometric immunophenotypic analysis is able to detect an aberrant T-cell population in the vast majority of cases of SS (**Fig. 13**).[112–114] Sézary cells typically exhibit absence of staining for CD26 and expression of CD158k.[113,115–117]

Anaplastic large-cell lymphoma

Anaplastic large-cell lymphoma (ALCL) is an aggressive CD30⁺ T-cell non-Hodgkin lymphoma, which can be subdivided into cases associated with ALK translocations (NPM-ALK t[2;5] being most common) and those without.[118] The sensitivity and specificity of detecting ALK⁺ ALCL in flow cytometry specimens are high (~85% and 100%, respectively), owing to frequently increased FSC and SSC (similar to monocytes and granulocytes) in comparison with normal lymphocytes and CD45⁺/CD30⁺ phenotype coupled with the expression of one or more T-cell antigens (CD4 ≥ CD2 ≥ CD7 = CD3 > CD5 >> CD8; median approximately 3 T-cell antigens expressed) and multiple immunophenotypic aberrancies

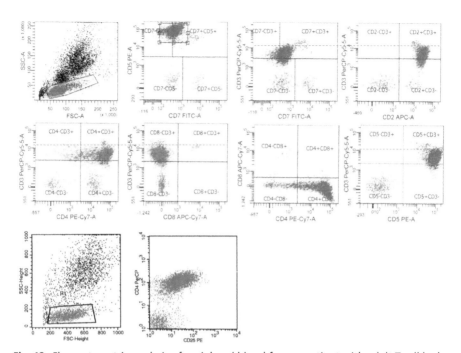

Fig. 12. Flow cytometric analysis of peripheral blood from a patient with adult T-cell leukemia/lymphoma, in which the neoplastic cells (*green population*) in upper two rows are positive for T-cell markers CD2, CD3, CD4, and CD5, with decreased staining for T-cell marker CD7, absence of staining for CD8, and coexpression of CD25 (*red population*) in bottom row. Note that the neoplastic cells show decreased staining for CD3 compared with normal T cells (*red population*) in the upper 2 rows.

(Fig. 14).[119–122] Other notable immunophenotypic features include the expression of CD56 in up to 60% of cases and bright CD25 in 75% to 90%, along with the consistent absence of B-cell markers.[119–122] The expression of myeloid antigens CD13 and CD33 is often seen in ALK⁺ ALCL, but is less common in ALK⁻

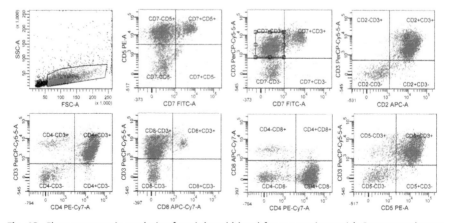

Fig. 13. Flow cytometric analysis of peripheral blood from a patient with Sezary syndrome, in which the neoplastic cells are positive for T-cell markers CD2, CD4, and CD5, with decreased CD3 expression, and are negative for CD7 and CD8. The CD4-CD8 ratio is 11:1.

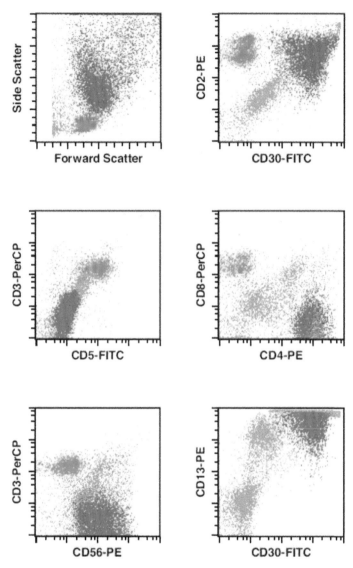

Fig. 14. Flow cytometric analysis of bone marrow from a patient with anaplastic large-cell lymphoma, in which the neoplastic cells (*red population*) show significantly increased forward scatter and side scatter compared with normal T cells (*green population*), and are positive for CD30, as well as T-cell markers CD2 and CD4, with coexpression of CD56 and myeloid marker CD13, and absence of expression of T-cell markers CD3, CD5, and CD8. (*From* Kesler MV, Paranjape GS, Asplund SL, et al. Anaplastic large-cell lymphoma: a flow cytometric analysis of 29 cases. Am J Clin Pathol 2007;128(2):314–22; with permission.)

ALCL, and, when present, should not be interpreted as evidence of a myeloid neoplasm.[123]

A compilation of the most characteristic flow cytometry patterns seen in T-cell lymphoproliferative disorders is provided in **Box 4**.

Box 4
Characteristic flow cytometric patterns in T-cell lymphoproliferative disorders

- Absent, decreased, or increased expression of pan T-cell markers, especially CD3 and CD7

- Specific neoplastic patterns
  - *T-cell prolymphocytic leukemia:* positive for pan T-cell markers CD2, CD3, CD5, and CD7, and negative for CD34, TdT, and CD1a (vs T-lymphoblastic leukemia/lymphoma); may be double-positive for CD4 and CD8 or singly positive for CD4 or CD8
  - *T-cell large granular lymphocytic leukemia:* positive for CD3, CD8, CD16, and CD57, with complete or partial loss of CD5
  - γδ *T-cell lymphoma:* positive for CD2, CD3, CD16, and CD56, and negative for CD4, CD5, and CD57 (vs γδ T-cell large granular lymphocytic leukemia)
  - *Natural killer (NK)-cell neoplasms:* positive for CD2 and CD16, and negative for surface CD3; aggressive NK-cell leukemia is typically CD56 positive and CD57 negative, whereas chronic lymphoproliferative disorder of NK cells has variable expression of CD56 and is often positive for CD57
  - *Angioimmunoblastic T-cell lymphoma/follicular helper T-cell lymphomas:* positive for CD4, and negative to dimly positive for CD3, with frequent coexpression of B-cell marker CD10
  - *Adult T-cell leukemia/lymphoma:* positive for CD2 and CD5, negative for CD7, with frequent downregulation of CD3; strong coexpression of CD25 (vs Sézary syndrome)
  - *Sézary syndrome:* positive for CD3, CD4, and CD5, and negative for CD7, CD8, and CD26; CD4:CD8 >10
  - *Anaplastic large-cell lymphoma:* large cells by forward and side scatter that are positive for CD30, often positive for myeloid antigens, and negative for 1 or more pan T-cell markers

---

REFERENCES

1. Swerdlow SH, Campo E, Harris NL, et al. WHO classification of tumours of haematopoietic and lymphoid tissues. 4th edition. Lyon (France): International Agency for Research on Cancer; 2008. p. 150.

2. Swerdlow SH, Campo E, Pileri SA, et al. The 2016 revision of the World Health Organization classification of lymphoid neoplasms. Blood 2016;127(20): 2375–90.

3. Arber DA, Orazi A, Hasserjian R, et al. The 2016 revision to the World Health Organization classification of myeloid neoplasms and acute leukemia. Blood 2016; 127(20):2391–405.

4. Kaleem Z. Flow cytometric analysis of lymphomas: current status and usefulness. Arch Pathol Lab Med 2006;130(12):1850–8.

5. Davis BH, Holden JT, Bene MC, et al. 2006 Bethesda International Consensus recommendations on the flow cytometric immunophenotypic analysis of hematolymphoid neoplasia: medical indications. Cytometry B Clin Cytom 2007; 72(Suppl 1):S5–13.

6. Wood BL, Arroz M, Barnett D, et al. 2006 Bethesda International Consensus recommendations on the immunophenotypic analysis of hematolymphoid neoplasia by flow cytometry: optimal reagents and reporting for the flow cytometric diagnosis of hematopoietic neoplasia. Cytometry B Clin Cytom 2007; 72(Suppl 1):S14–22.

7. Karube K, Aoki R, Nomura Y, et al. Usefulness of flow cytometry for differential diagnosis of precursor and peripheral T-cell and NK-cell lymphomas: analysis of 490 cases. Pathol Int 2008;58(2):89–97.

8. Gorczyca W, Weisberger J, Liu Z, et al. An approach to diagnosis of T-cell lymphoproliferative disorders by flow cytometry. Cytometry 2002;50(3):177–90.

9. Jamal S, Picker LJ, Aquino DB, et al. Immunophenotypic analysis of peripheral T-cell neoplasms. A multiparameter flow cytometric approach. Am J Clin Pathol 2001;116(4):512–26.

10. Gorczyca W. Differential diagnosis of T-cell lymphoproliferative disorders by flow cytometry multicolor immunophenotyping. Correlation with morphology. Methods Cell Biol 2004;75:595–621.

11. Jones D, Dorfman DM. Phenotypic characterization of subsets of T cell lymphoma: toward a functional classification of T cell lymphoma. Leuk Lymphoma 2001;40(5–6):449–59.

12. Chu PG, Chang KL, Arber DA, et al. Immunophenotyping of hematopoietic neoplasms. Semin Diagn Pathol 2000;17(3):236–56.

13. Craig FE, Foon KA. Flow cytometric immunophenotyping for hematologic neoplasms. Blood 2008;111(8):3941–67.

14. Cortelazzo S, Ponzoni M, Ferreri AJ, et al. Lymphoblastic lymphoma. Crit Rev Oncol Hematol 2011;79(3):330–43.

15. Jaffe ES, Arber DA, Campo E, et al. Hematopathology. 2nd edition. Philadelphia: Elsevier; 2017.

16. Conde-Sterling DA, Aguilera NS, Nandedkar MA, et al. Immunoperoxidase detection of CD10 in precursor T-lymphoblastic lymphoma/leukemia: a clinicopathologic study of 24 cases. Arch Pathol Lab Med 2000;124(5):704–8.

17. Han X, Bueso-Ramos CE. Precursor T-cell acute lymphoblastic leukemia/lymphoblastic lymphoma and acute biphenotypic leukemias. Am J Clin Pathol 2007;127(4):528–44.

18. Bene MC, Castoldi G, Knapp W, et al. Proposals for the immunological classification of acute leukemias. European Group for the Immunological Characterization of Leukemias (EGIL). Leukemia 1995;9(10):1783–6.

19. You MJ, Medeiros LJ, Hsi ED. T-lymphoblastic leukemia/lymphoma. Am J Clin Pathol 2015;144(3):411–22.

20. Patel JL, Smith LM, Anderson J, et al. The immunophenotype of T-lymphoblastic lymphoma in children and adolescents: a Children's Oncology Group report. Br J Haematol 2012;159(4):454–61.

21. Coustan-Smith E, Mullighan CG, Onciu M, et al. Early T-cell precursor leukaemia: a subtype of very high-risk acute lymphoblastic leukaemia. Lancet Oncol 2009;10(2):147–56.

22. Rothenberg EV, Moore JE, Yui MA. Launching the T-cell-lineage developmental programme. Nat Rev Immunol 2008;8(1):9–21.

23. Jain N, Lamb AV, O'Brien S, et al. Early T-cell precursor acute lymphoblastic leukemia/lymphoma (ETP-ALL/LBL) in adolescents and adults: a high-risk subtype. Blood 2016;127(15):1863–9.

24. Porwit A, Béné MC. Acute leukemias of ambiguous origin. Am J Clin Pathol 2015;144(3):361–76.

25. Weir EG, Ali Ansari-Lari M, Batista DA, et al. Acute bilineal leukemia: a rare disease with poor outcome. Leukemia 2007;21(11):2264–70.

26. Matutes E, Pickl WF, Van't Veer M, et al. Mixed-phenotype acute leukemia: clinical and laboratory features and outcome in 100 patients defined according to the WHO 2008 classification. Blood 2011;117(11):3163–71.

27. Fujii Y, Okumura M, Yamamoto S. Flow cytometric study of lymphocytes associated with thymoma and other thymic tumors. J Surg Res 1999;82(2):312–8.

28. Li S, Juco J, Mann KP, et al. Flow cytometry in the differential diagnosis of lymphocyte-rich thymoma from precursor T-cell acute lymphoblastic leukemia/lymphoblastic lymphoma. Am J Clin Pathol 2004;121(2):268–74.

29. Gorczyca W, Tugulea S, Liu Z, et al. Flow cytometry in the diagnosis of mediastinal tumors with emphasis on differentiating thymocytes from precursor T-lymphoblastic lymphoma/leukemia. Leuk Lymphoma 2004;45(3):529–38.

30. Nakajima J, Takamoto S, Oka T, et al. Flow cytometric analysis of lymphoid cells in thymic epithelial neoplasms. Eur J Cardiothorac Surg 2000;18(3):287–92.

31. Fischer L, Hummel M, Burmeister T, et al. Skewed expression of natural-killer (NK)-associated antigens on lymphoproliferations of large granular lymphocytes (LGL). Hematol Oncol 2006;24(2):78–85.

32. Gastl G, Schmalzl F, Huhn D, et al. Large granular lymphocytes: morphological and functional properties. I. Results in normals. Blut 1983;46(6):297–310.

33. Ohgami RS, Ohgami JK, Pereira IT, et al. Refining the diagnosis of T-cell large granular lymphocytic leukemia by combining distinct patterns of antigen expression with T-cell clonality studies. Leukemia 2011;25(9):1439–43.

34. Strioga M, Pasukoniene V, Characiejus D. CD8+ CD28- and CD8+ CD57+ T cells and their role in health and disease. Immunology 2011;134(1):17–32.

35. Singleton TP, Yin B, Teferra A, et al. Spectrum of clonal large granular lymphocytes (LGLs) of αβ T cells: T-cell clones of undetermined significance, T-cell LGL leukemias, and T-cell immunoclones. Am J Clin Pathol 2015;144(1):137–44.

36. Greenberg SA, Pinkus JL, Amato AA, et al. Association of inclusion body myositis with T cell large granular lymphocytic leukaemia. Brain 2016;139(Pt 5):1348–60.

37. Neff JL, Howard MT, Morice WG. Distinguishing T-cell large granular lymphocytic leukemia from reactive conditions: laboratory tools and challenges in their use. Surg Pathol Clin 2013;6(4):631–9.

38. Lanier LL, Spits H, Phillips JH. The developmental relationship between NK cells and T cells. Immunol Today 1992;13(10):392–5.

39. Orange JS, Ballas ZK. Natural killer cells in human health and disease. Clin Immunol 2006;118(1):1–10.

40. Caligiuri MA. Human natural killer cells. Blood 2008;112(3):461–9.

41. Lanier LL, Phillips JH, Hackett J, et al. Natural killer cells: definition of a cell type rather than a function. J Immunol 1986;137(9):2735–9.

42. Morice WG. The immunophenotypic attributes of NK cells and NK-cell lineage lymphoproliferative disorders. Am J Clin Pathol 2007;127(6):881–6.

43. Morice WG, Kurtin PJ, Leibson PJ, et al. Demonstration of aberrant T-cell and natural killer-cell antigen expression in all cases of granular lymphocytic leukaemia. Br J Haematol 2003;120(6):1026–36.

44. Farag SS, Caligiuri MA. Human natural killer cell development and biology. Blood Rev 2006;20(3):123–37.

45. Björkström NK, Riese P, Heuts F, et al. Expression patterns of NKG2A, KIR, and CD57 define a process of CD56dim NK-cell differentiation uncoupled from NK-cell education. Blood 2010;116(19):3853–64.

46. Lopez-Vergès S, Milush JM, Pandey S, et al. CD57 defines a functionally distinct population of mature NK cells in the human CD56dimCD16+ NK-cell subset. Blood 2010;116(19):3865–74.

47. Zambello R, Trentin L, Ciccone E, et al. Phenotypic diversity of natural killer (NK) populations in patients with NK-type lymphoproliferative disease of granular lymphocytes. Blood 1993;81(9):2381–5.

48. Carding SR, Egan PJ. Gammadelta T cells: functional plasticity and heterogeneity. Nat Rev Immunol 2002;2(5):336–45.

49. Roden AC, Morice WG, Hanson CA. Immunophenotypic attributes of benign peripheral blood gammadelta T cells and conditions associated with their increase. Arch Pathol Lab Med 2008;132(11):1774–80.
50. Inghirami G, Zhu BY, Chess L, et al. Flow cytometric and immunohistochemical characterization of the gamma/delta T-lymphocyte population in normal human lymphoid tissue and peripheral blood. Am J Pathol 1990;136(2):357–67.
51. McClanahan J, Fukushima PI, Stetler-Stevenson M. Increased peripheral blood gamma delta T-cells in patients with lymphoid neoplasia: a diagnostic dilemma in flow cytometry. Cytometry 1999;38(6):280–5.
52. Flammiger A, Bacher U, Christopeit M, et al. Multiparameter flow cytometry in the differential diagnosis of aberrant T-cell clones of unclear significance. Leuk Lymphoma 2015;56(3):639–44.
53. Béné MC, Le Bris Y, Robillard N, et al. Flow cytometry in hematological nonmalignant disorders. Int J Lab Hematol 2016;38(1):5–16.
54. Nascimbeni M, Shin EC, Chiriboga L, et al. Peripheral CD4(+)CD8(+) T cells are differentiated effector memory cells with antiviral functions. Blood 2004;104(2): 478–86.
55. Rahemtullah A, Reichard KK, Preffer FI, et al. A double-positive CD4+CD8+ T-cell population is commonly found in nodular lymphocyte predominant Hodgkin lymphoma. Am J Clin Pathol 2006;126(5):805–14.
56. Scrivener S, Goddard RV, Kaminski ER, et al. Abnormal T-cell function in B-cell chronic lymphocytic leukaemia. Leuk Lymphoma 2003;44(3):383–9.
57. Goolsby CL, Kuchnio M, Finn WG, et al. Expansions of clonal and oligoclonal T cells in B-cell chronic lymphocytic leukemia are primarily restricted to the CD3(+)CD8(+) T-cell population. Cytometry 2000;42(3):188–95.
58. Rezvany MR, Jeddi-Tehrani M, Wigzell H, et al. Leukemia-associated monoclonal and oligoclonal TCR-BV use in patients with B-cell chronic lymphocytic leukemia. Blood 2003;101(3):1063–70.
59. Mackus WJ, Frakking FN, Grummels A, et al. Expansion of CMV-specific CD8+CD45RA+CD27− T cells in B-cell chronic lymphocytic leukemia. Blood 2003;102(3):1057–63.
60. Serrano D, Monteiro J, Allen SL, et al. Clonal expansion within the CD4+CD57+ and CD8+CD57+ T cell subsets in chronic lymphocytic leukemia. J Immunol 1997;158(3):1482–9.
61. Martinez A, Pittaluga S, Villamor N, et al. Clonal T-cell populations and increased risk for cytotoxic T-cell lymphomas in B-CLL patients: clinicopathologic observations and molecular analysis. Am J Surg Pathol 2004;28(7):849–58.
62. Van den Hove LE, Vandenberghe P, Van Gool SW, et al. Peripheral blood lymphocyte subset shifts in patients with untreated hematological tumors: evidence for systemic activation of the T cell compartment. Leuk Res 1998;22(2): 175–84.
63. Levy JA. HIV pathogenesis: 25 years of progress and persistent challenges. AIDS 2009;23(2):147–60.
64. Giorgi JV, Detels R. T-cell subset alterations in HIV-infected homosexual men: NIAID Multicenter AIDS cohort study. Clin Immunol Immunopathol 1989;52(1): 10–8.
65. Margolick JB, Scott ER, Odaka N, et al. Flow cytometric analysis of gamma delta T cells and natural killer cells in HIV-1 infection. Clin Immunol Immunopathol 1991;58(1):126–38.
66. Zaunders J, Carr A, McNally L, et al. Effects of primary HIV-1 infection on subsets of CD4+ and CD8+ T lymphocytes. AIDS 1995;9(6):561–6.

67. Ebell MH, Call M, Shinholser J, et al. Does this patient have infectious mononucleosis? The rational clinical examination systematic review. JAMA 2016; 315(14):1502–9.

68. Shannon-Lowe C, Rowe M. Epstein Barr virus entry; kissing and conjugation. Curr Opin Virol 2014;4:78–84.

69. Taylor GS, Long HM, Brooks JM, et al. The immunology of Epstein-Barr virus-induced disease. Annu Rev Immunol 2015;33:787–821.

70. Hudnall SD, Patel J, Schwab H, et al. Comparative immunophenotypic features of EBV-positive and EBV-negative atypical lymphocytosis. Cytometry B Clin Cytom 2003;55(1):22–8.

71. Weisberger J, Cornfield D, Gorczyca W, et al. Down-regulation of pan-T-cell antigens, particularly CD7, in acute infectious mononucleosis. Am J Clin Pathol 2003;120(1):49–55.

72. Dearden CE. T-cell prolymphocytic leukemia. Med Oncol 2006;23(1):17–22.

73. Foucar K. Mature T-cell leukemias including T-prolymphocytic leukemia, adult T-cell leukemia/lymphoma, and Sézary syndrome. Am J Clin Pathol 2007; 127(4):496–510.

74. Cady FM, Morice WG. Flow cytometric assessment of T-cell chronic lymphoproliferative disorders. Clin Lab Med 2007;27(3):513–32, vi.

75. Matutes E, Brito-Babapulle V, Swansbury J, et al. Clinical and laboratory features of 78 cases of T-prolymphocytic leukemia. Blood 1991;78(12):3269–74.

76. Ginaldi L, Matutes E, Farahat N, et al. Differential expression of CD3 and CD7 in T-cell malignancies: a quantitative study by flow cytometry. Br J Haematol 1996; 93(4):921–7.

77. Ginaldi L, De Martinis M, Matutes E, et al. Levels of expression of CD52 in normal and leukemic B and T cells: correlation with in vivo therapeutic responses to Campath-1H. Leuk Res 1998;22(2):185–91.

78. Chen X, Cherian S. Immunophenotypic characterization of T-cell prolymphocytic leukemia. Am J Clin Pathol 2013;140(5):727–35.

79. O'Malley DP. T-cell large granular leukemia and related proliferations. Am J Clin Pathol 2007;127(6):850–9.

80. Lima M, Almeida J, Dos Anjos Teixeira M, et al. TCRalphabeta+/CD4+ large granular lymphocytosis: a new clonal T-cell lymphoproliferative disorder. Am J Pathol 2003;163(2):763–71.

81. Yabe M, Medeiros LJ, Wang SA, et al. Clinicopathologic, immunophenotypic, cytogenetic, and molecular features of γδ T-cell large granular lymphocytic leukemia: an analysis of 14 patients suggests biologic differences with αβ T-cell large granular lymphocytic leukemia. [corrected]. Am J Clin Pathol 2015; 144(4):607–19.

82. Lundell R, Hartung L, Hill S, et al. T-cell large granular lymphocyte leukemias have multiple phenotypic abnormalities involving pan-T-cell antigens and receptors for MHC molecules. Am J Clin Pathol 2005;124(6):937–46.

83. Garcia-Herrera A, Song JY, Chuang SS, et al. Nonhepatosplenic γδ T-cell lymphomas represent a spectrum of aggressive cytotoxic T-cell lymphomas with a mainly extranodal presentation. Am J Surg Pathol 2011;35(8):1214–25.

84. Weidmann E. Hepatosplenic T cell lymphoma. A review on 45 cases since the first report describing the disease as a distinct lymphoma entity in 1990. Leukemia 2000;14(6):991–7.

85. Ahmad E, Kingma DW, Jaffe ES, et al. Flow cytometric immunophenotypic profiles of mature gamma delta T-cell malignancies involving peripheral blood and bone marrow. Cytometry B Clin Cytom 2005;67(1):6–12.

86. Vega F, Medeiros LJ, Gaulard P. Hepatosplenic and other gammadelta T-cell lymphomas. Am J Clin Pathol 2007;127(6):869–80.
87. Arnulf B, Copie-Bergman C, Delfau-Larue MH, et al. Nonhepatosplenic gamma-delta T-cell lymphoma: a subset of cytotoxic lymphomas with mucosal or skin localization. Blood 1998;91(5):1723–31.
88. Hasserjian RP, Harris NL. NK-cell lymphomas and leukemias: a spectrum of tumors with variable manifestations and immunophenotype. Am J Clin Pathol 2007;127(6):860–8.
89. Jiang NG, Jin YM, Niu Q, et al. Flow cytometric immunophenotyping is of great value to diagnosis of natural killer cell neoplasms involving bone marrow and peripheral blood. Ann Hematol 2013;92(1):89–96.
90. Lima M, Spínola A, Fonseca S, et al. Aggressive mature natural killer cell neoplasms: report on a series of 12 European patients with emphasis on flow cytometry based immunophenotype and DNA content of neoplastic natural killer cells. Leuk Lymphoma 2015;56(1):103–12.
91. Suzuki R, Suzumiya J, Nakamura S, et al. Aggressive natural killer-cell leukemia revisited: large granular lymphocyte leukemia of cytotoxic NK cells. Leukemia 2004;18(4):763–70.
92. Li C, Tian Y, Wang J, et al. Abnormal immunophenotype provides a key diagnostic marker: a report of 29 cases of de novo aggressive natural killer cell leukemia. Transl Res 2014;163(6):565–77.
93. Cao F, Zhao H, Li Y, et al. Clinicopathological and phenotypic features of chronic NK cell lymphocytosis identified among patients with asymptomatic lymphocytosis. Int J Lab Hematol 2015;37(6):783–90.
94. Merchant SH, Amin MB, Viswanatha DS. Morphologic and immunophenotypic analysis of angioimmunoblastic T-cell lymphoma: emphasis on phenotypic aberrancies for early diagnosis. Am J Clin Pathol 2006;126(1):29–38.
95. Chen W, Kesler MV, Karandikar NJ, et al. Flow cytometric features of angioimmunoblastic T-cell lymphoma. Cytometry B Clin Cytom 2006;70(3):142–8.
96. Stacchini A, Demurtas A, Aliberti S, et al. The usefulness of flow cytometric CD10 detection in the differential diagnosis of peripheral T-cell lymphomas. Am J Clin Pathol 2007;128(5):854–64.
97. Yuan CM, Vergilio JA, Zhao XF, et al. CD10 and BCL6 expression in the diagnosis of angioimmunoblastic T-cell lymphoma: utility of detecting CD10+ T cells by flow cytometry. Hum Pathol 2005;36(7):784–91.
98. Baseggio L, Traverse-Glehen A, Berger F, et al. CD10 and ICOS expression by multiparametric flow cytometry in angioimmunoblastic T-cell lymphoma. Mod Pathol 2011;24(7):993–1003.
99. Baseggio L, Berger F, Morel D, et al. Identification of circulating CD10 positive T cells in angioimmunoblastic T-cell lymphoma. Leukemia 2006;20(2):296–303.
100. Loghavi S, Wang SA, Jeffrey Medeiros L, et al. Immunophenotypic and diagnostic characterization of angioimmunoblastic T-cell lymphoma by advanced flow cytometric technology. Leuk Lymphoma 2016;57(12):2804–12.
101. Cook JR, Craig FE, Swerdlow SH. Benign CD10-positive T cells in reactive lymphoid proliferations and B-cell lymphomas. Mod Pathol 2003;16(9):879–85.
102. Serke S, van Lessen A, Hummel M, et al. Circulating CD4+ T lymphocytes with intracellular but no surface CD3 antigen in five of seven patients consecutively diagnosed with angioimmunoblastic T-cell lymphoma. Cytometry 2000;42(3):180–7.

103. Singh A, Schabath R, Ratei R, et al. Peripheral blood sCD3⁻ CD4⁺ T cells: a useful diagnostic tool in angioimmunoblastic T cell lymphoma. Hematol Oncol 2014;32(1):16–21.

104. Moroch J, Copie-Bergman C, de Leval L, et al. Follicular peripheral T-cell lymphoma expands the spectrum of classical Hodgkin lymphoma mimics. Am J Surg Pathol 2012;36(11):1636–46.

105. Alikhan M, Song JY, Sohani AR, et al. Peripheral T-cell lymphomas of follicular helper T-cell type frequently display an aberrant CD3(-/dim)CD4(+) population by flow cytometry: an important clue to the diagnosis of a Hodgkin lymphoma mimic. Mod Pathol 2016;29(10):1173–82.

106. Qayyum S, Choi JK. Adult T-cell leukemia/lymphoma. Arch Pathol Lab Med 2014;138(2):282–6.

107. Matutes E. Adult T-cell leukaemia/lymphoma. J Clin Pathol 2007;60(12):1373–7.

108. Dahmoush L, Hijazi Y, Barnes E, et al. Adult T-cell leukemia/lymphoma: a cytopathologic, immunocytochemical, and flow cytometric study. Cancer 2002; 96(2):110–6.

109. Yokote T, Akioka T, Oka S, et al. Flow cytometric immunophenotyping of adult T-cell leukemia/lymphoma using CD3 gating. Am J Clin Pathol 2005;124(2): 199–204.

110. Ohshima K. Molecular pathology of adult T-cell leukemia/lymphoma. Oncology 2015;89(Suppl 1):7–15.

111. Kubica AW, Pittelkow MR. Sézary syndrome. Surg Pathol Clin 2014;7(2): 191–202.

112. Klemke CD, Brade J, Weckesser S, et al. The diagnosis of Sézary syndrome on peripheral blood by flow cytometry requires the use of multiple markers. Br J Dermatol 2008;159(4):871–80.

113. Bahler DW, Hartung L, Hill S, et al. CD158k/KIR3DL2 is a useful marker for identifying neoplastic T-cells in Sézary syndrome by flow cytometry. Cytometry B Clin Cytom 2008;74(3):156–62.

114. Morice WG, Katzmann JA, Pittelkow MR, et al. A comparison of morphologic features, flow cytometry, TCR-Vbeta analysis, and TCR-PCR in qualitative and quantitative assessment of peripheral blood involvement by Sézary syndrome. Am J Clin Pathol 2006;125(3):364–74.

115. Kelemen K, Guitart J, Kuzel TM, et al. The usefulness of CD26 in flow cytometric analysis of peripheral blood in Sézary syndrome. Am J Clin Pathol 2008;129(1): 146–56.

116. Lima M, Almeida J, dos Anjos Teixeira M, et al. Utility of flow cytometry immunophenotyping and DNA ploidy studies for diagnosis and characterization of blood involvement in CD4+ Sézary's syndrome. Haematologica 2003;88(8): 874–87.

117. Hristov AC, Vonderheid EC, Borowitz MJ. Simplified flow cytometric assessment in mycosis fungoides and Sézary syndrome. Am J Clin Pathol 2011;136(6): 944–53.

118. Hapgood G, Savage KJ. The biology and management of systemic anaplastic large cell lymphoma. Blood 2015;126(1):17–25.

119. Shen H, Tang Y, Xu X, et al. Simultaneous cytomorphological and multiparameter flow cytometric analysis of ALK-positive anaplastic large cell lymphoma in children. Oncol Lett 2013;5(2):515–20.

120. Muzzafar T, Wei EX, Lin P, et al. Flow cytometric immunophenotyping of anaplastic large cell lymphoma. Arch Pathol Lab Med 2009;133(1):49–56.

121. Kesler MV, Paranjape GS, Asplund SL, et al. Anaplastic large cell lymphoma: a flow cytometric analysis of 29 cases. Am J Clin Pathol 2007;128(2):314–22.
122. Juco J, Holden JT, Mann KP, et al. Immunophenotypic analysis of anaplastic large cell lymphoma by flow cytometry. Am J Clin Pathol 2003;119(2):205–12.
123. Bovio IM, Allan RW. The expression of myeloid antigens CD13 and/or CD33 is a marker of ALK+ anaplastic large cell lymphomas. Am J Clin Pathol 2008;130(4): 628–34.

Acute Myeloid Leukemia Immunophenotyping by Flow Cytometric Analysis

 CrossMark

Xueyan Chen, MD, PhD*, Sindhu Cherian, MD

KEYWORDS

- Flow cytometry • Acute myeloid leukemia • Mixed phenotype acute leukemia
- Minimal residual disease

KEY POINTS

- Immunophenotyping by flow cytometry plays a critical role in the diagnosis and classification of AML allowing for blast identification, lineage assignment, and immunophenotypic characterization.
- Flow cytometry can provide useful clues to underlying genetics, reliably distinguish AML from other precursor neoplasms that may be in the differential diagnosis, and provide insight to prognosis.
- AML MRD assessment has been demonstrated to be a particularly powerful tool in AML prognostication.

INTRODUCTION

Over the past 20 years, immunophenotyping by flow cytometry has become an essential laboratory tool in the diagnosis and classification of several hematologic malignancies. The role of this technology in evaluating acute leukemia and lymphoma is particularly well established and widely implemented.[1,2] In acute myeloid leukemia (AML), flow cytometry is crucial for detection of leukemic blasts, blast lineage assignment, and identification of aberrant immunophenotypic features that allow distinction of abnormal blast populations from normal progenitors.

With the elucidation of the antigen expression pattern of a given hematopoietic cell lineage during normal maturation,[3–5] assignment of individual cells to a specific lineage and stage of maturation is achieved with high confidence using a unique combination of markers. Leukemic blasts frequently show immunophenotypic deviation

Disclosure: The authors have no commercial or financial conflicts of interest or any funding sources relevant to this article.
Department of Laboratory Medicine, University of Washington, 1959 NE Pacific Street, Seattle, WA 98195, USA
* Corresponding author.
E-mail address: xchen1@uw.edu

from the antigenic expression pattern seen on normal hematopoietic progenitors of similar lineage and maturation stage. This basic principle allows for the recognition of leukemic blasts, determination of the immunophenotype, and subsequent classification in AML.

GENERAL APPROACH TO GATING
Population Identification

Specimens typically assessed by flow cytometry for involvement by AML include peripheral blood and bone marrow. In these specimens, the neoplastic blasts are often present in a background of normal hematopoietic progenitors. CD45 versus side scatter (SSC) gating is an initial strategy for blast identification in many clinical laboratories and provides a useful starting point to distinguish major hematopoietic cell populations (**Fig. 1**).[6,7] Based on the different intensity of CD45 expression and SSC on the hematopoietic lineages, this method allows for reliable identification of mature lymphocytes, monocytes, maturing granulocytes, myeloid blasts, and lymphoid blasts (hematogones). Although CD45 versus SSC gating is useful to guide initial assessment and allows tracking of a population of interest between tubes, the populations discriminated by this strategy are often not pure and additional lineage-specific markers must be used for definitive population identification.

Panel for Immunophenotyping

The expanded myeloid blasts in AML are often first recognized in a CD45 versus SSC defined "blast gate" with decreased CD45 expression and intermediate SSC.[4] However, several other populations fall within "blast gate" in addition to blasts, including basophils, plasmacytoid dendritic cells, hypogranular myeloid cells, and early monocytic cells. Therefore, additional markers are required to differentiate blasts from other populations in the blast gate.

The antibodies included in a panel used for the diagnosis of AML should be capable of confirming the immaturity of the suspected blast population, assigning the lineage, and delineating the aberrant antigenic expression pattern that distinguishes neoplastic blasts from normal progenitors. For myeloid blasts, a combination of CD34 and CD117 can usually be used to define immaturity. Accurate lineage assignment is a critical component in the diagnosis of acute leukemia. For this reason, the Bethesda International Consensus Conference recommends that the initial assessment of a new acute leukemia includes evaluation of myelomonocytic and lymphoid markers.[8] Myeloid lineage is suggested by expression of antigens including CD13, CD15, CD33, and MPO, whereas monocytic lineage is suggested by expression of antigens including CD4, CD14, bright CD33, and CD64. Assessment of lymphoid markers should be included in the initial evaluation of AML to confirm correct lineage assignment and to evaluate for aberrant expression of a nonlineage marker on an abnormal myeloid blast population. In this regard, a panel for acute leukemia evaluation should include B-cell markers (ie, CD19, CD22, and/or cytoplasmic CD79a) and T-cell markers (ie, CD2, surface and cytoplasmic CD3, CD5, and CD7). Once lineage is confidently assigned, a comprehensive assessment of antigens expressed by the blast population should be made to determine how the aberrant blast immunophenotype differs from that of normal progenitors. Aberrant antigenic expression on the leukemic blasts may include the following[4]: overexpression, underexpression, or loss of an antigen typically expressed by a myeloid blast; asynchronous antigen expression; cross-lineage antigen expression; and abnormally homogeneous antigen expression.

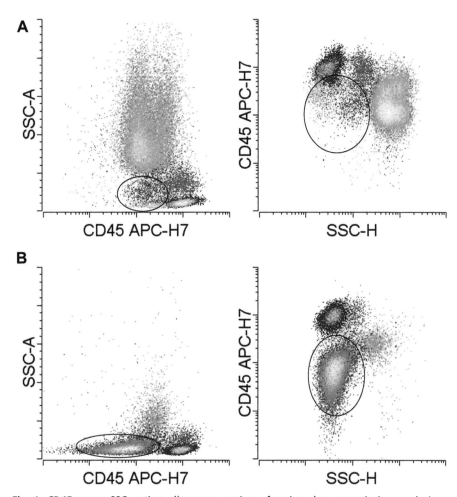

Fig. 1. CD45 versus SSC gating allows separation of various hematopoietic populations. Different laboratories display CD45 versus SSC in different ways with two common approaches being to either show SSC on the y-axis on a linear scale while displaying CD45 on the x-axis on a log scale (*left*), or to show CD45 on the y-axis on a log scale while showing SSC on the x-axis on a log scale (*right*). Both methods provide similar information and work well to separate relevant populations. (*A*) Normal bone marrow. CD45 is expressed with increasing intensity on hematopoietic cells as they mature, whereas SSC is increased on cells with more complex cytoplasm. The combination of these parameters allows separation of lymphocytes (*blue*), hematogones (*aqua*), monocytes (*pink*), granulocytes (*green*), and myeloid blasts (*red*). Using CD45 versus SSC, one can draw a CD45 versus SSC defined blast gate (*oval*). (*B*) Acute myeloid leukemia, not otherwise specified. Flow cytometry of the peripheral blood in this specimen demonstrates an expanded myeloid blast population (*colored red*; 67.3% of the white cells) in the CD45 versus SSC-defined blast gate. Neoplastic myeloid blasts typically have intermediate SSC with lower CD45 expression than mature hematopoietic populations and usually fall into the CD45 versus SSC defined blast gate (*oval*). Neutrophilic cells (*green*) are infrequent in this specimen and show aberrantly decreased SSC.

The panel of antibodies to assess a new acute leukemia in our laboratory is outlined in **Table 1**. This panel allows for the demonstration of normal maturation patterns of hematopoietic progenitors and thereby allows one to identify and characterize the abnormal immunophenotype of the leukemic blasts.

Blast Enumeration

Flow cytometry may assist in blast enumeration in the peripheral blood; however, enumeration of blasts in the bone marrow is confounded by several factors. Hemodilution artificially decreases the blast percentage and may be especially problematic in the setting of a fibrotic marrow. Additionally, processing of marrow specimens for flow cytometry often removes a subset of erythroid precursors. Excluding erythroid precursors from the denominator artificially increases the blast percentage. Therefore, the morphologic blast count is the most reliable method for blast enumeration.

Other Types of Blast Equivalents

In addition to myeloid blasts, other types of cells may represent blast equivalents for the purposes of diagnosing AML. These include abnormal promyelocytes that may be seen in acute promyelocytic leukemia (APL) and immature monocytic cells (monoblasts/promonocytes) that are seen in acute leukemia with monocytic differentiation. Abnormal promyelocytes have higher SSC than average myeloid blasts and are often excluded from a standard CD45 versus SSC defined blast gate. These are discussed in detail later (see section on AML with recurrent genetic abnormalities). Immature monocytic cells are typically characterized by expression of high levels of CD4, CD33, CD64, and HLA-DR, with intermediate CD15, and variable, often low, CD13. In contrast with more mature monocytic cells, monoblasts and promonocytes usually have low to absent CD14 (**Fig. 2**).[4,5] It is important to be familiar with the characteristics of the clone of CD14 used in the laboratory because different clones may recognize different proportions of immature monocytic cells.[9] Aberrant CD56 expression may be seen on immature monocytic populations, although this finding is not specific.[10–12]

Table 1
Immunophenotyping panel for the diagnosis of acute myeloid leukemia

Fluoro-chromes	PB or V450	FITC	PE	PETR	PeCy5, PECy5.5, or PERCP Cy5.5	PECy7	A594	APC	APCA700	APCCy7 or APCH7
Myeloid tube 1	HLA-DR	CD15	CD33	CD19	CD117	CD13	CD38	CD34	CD71	CD45
Myeloid tube 2	HLA-DR	CD64	CD123	CD4	CD14	CD13	CD38	CD34	CD16	CD45
B-cell tube	CD20	Kappa	Lambda		CD5	CD19	CD38	CD10		CD45
T-cell tube	CD8	CD2	CD5	CD34	CD56	CD3	CD4	CD7	CD30	CD45

Abbreviations: A594, Alexa Fluor 594; APC, allophycocyanin; APCA700, Allophycocyanin Alexa Fluor 700; APCCy7, Allophycocyanin cyanine-7; APCH7, Allophycocyanin H7; FITC, fluorescein isothiocyanate; PB, Pacific blue; PE, phycoerythrin; PECy5, Phycoerythrin cyanine-5; PECy5.5, Phycoerythrin cyanine-5.5; PECy7, Phycoerythrin cyanine-7; PerCPCy5.5, Peridinin chlorophyll protein cyanine 5.5; PETR, phycoerythrin Texas red; V450, BD Horizon dye V450.

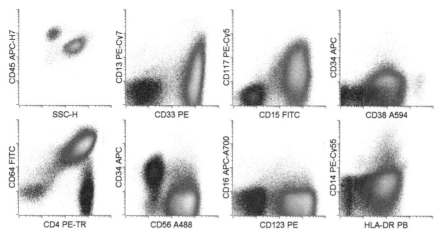

Fig. 2. Acute myeloid leukemia with monocytic differentiation. The monoblasts/promonocytes (*colored pink*; 76.7% of the white cells) in the bone marrow are characterized by increased SSC and expression of CD4, CD13 (heterogeneous), CD15, CD33 (bright), CD38, CD56, CD64, CD117 (heterogeneous), CD123, and HLA-DR without CD14, CD16, or CD34. Background reactive lymphoid cells are shown in *blue*.

Two unusual subtypes of AML include AML with erythroid or megakaryocytic differentiation. Early erythroid precursors (pronormoblasts) are recognized by expression of CD36, CD71, CD117, and CD235a.[13] Megakaryocytic blasts typically show expression of CD41 and/or CD61 on the surface.[14,15] Some studies suggest that use of intracellular CD61 maybe a more sensitive and specific marker.[16] It should be noted that evaluation of CD41 and CD61 can provide some technical challenges because adherence of platelets to blast populations may result in an artifact suggesting megakaryocytic differentiation when it is not present. Adequate washing to remove adherent platelets may be helpful in this regard.[17]

Acute Myeloid Leukemia With Recurrent Genetic Abnormalities

The 2008 World Health Organization (WHO) classification and 2016 Revision divide AML into four major categories: (1) AML with recurrent genetic abnormalities, (2) AML with myelodysplasia-related changes, (3) therapy-related myeloid neoplasms, and (4) AML, not otherwise specified.[18,19] A subset of AML subtypes show strong correlation between immunophenotype and underlying genetic abnormalities.

AML with t(8;21); *RUNX1-RUNX1T1* is a distinct clinicopathologic entity and displays a characteristic immunophenotypic profile by flow cytometry. The blasts typically show high levels of CD34, HLA-DR, and MPO expression with somewhat weaker expression of CD13 and CD33 (**Fig. 3**).[20–24] Coexpression of B-cell markers is frequently present, and may include CD19, PAX5, and/or cytoplasmic CD79a. CD56 is also expressed in 60% to 80% of cases in AML with t(8;21)[20,25,26]; in some studies, CD56 expression is correlated with an adverse prognosis.[26,27] CD56 is usually positive in t(8;21) AML with KIT-activating mutations, which occur in 20% to 25% of cases and are associated with an inferior outcome.[28,29] It is important to recognize this immunophenotypic pattern to avoid misclassification of this AML subtype as mixed phenotype acute leukemia (MPAL). Of note, AML with t(8;21) may sometimes present with fewer than 20% blasts by morphology. For this reason, the demonstration of coexpression of CD19 and CD56 on a myeloid blast population should raise

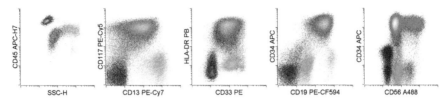

Fig. 3. Acute myeloid leukemia with t(8;21). The leukemic blasts (*colored red*; 36.3% of the white cells) in the bone marrow show expression of CD13 (heterogeneous), CD19, CD33, CD34 (increased), CD45 (decreased), CD56 (subset), CD117 (increased), and HLA-DR. Background reactive lymphoid cells are shown in *blue* and neutrophilic cells are shown in *green*.

the consideration of AML with t(8;21) even in cases with less than 20% blasts by morphology.

In APL with t(15;17), the typical blast equivalent is an abnormal promyelocyte. Characteristically, these blast equivalents have high SSC and express myeloid markers including heterogeneous CD13; low-to-absent CD15; uniformly bright CD33; heterogeneous CD117; and MPO without markers normally expressed at earlier stages of maturation, such as CD34 and HLA-DR (**Fig. 4**).[1,30,31] In the microgranular variant of APL, SSC may be lower and there is frequent variable expression of CD2 and CD34.[32,33] CD56 is expressed in 15% to 20% of APL cases and has been correlated with a poor prognosis.[34–36] Occasionally, basophilic differentiation with expression of basophil-specific marker CD203c is seen in APL during arsenic trioxide therapy.[37]

It is critical to distinguish APL from other AML subtypes lacking expression of CD34 and HLA-DR[38,39] because APL therapy differs from that of other subtypes of AML and typically incorporates all-*trans* retinoic acid.[40–42] Furthermore, APL is frequently associated with a life-threatening disseminated intravascular coagulation, and therefore needs prompt diagnosis and rapid and specific management. The major differential diagnostic considerations include AML with monocytic differentiation (which is most commonly HLA-DR positive allowing distinction of this entity in most cases) and AML with FLT3 and/or NPM1 mutations, which often lack expression of both CD34 and HLA-DR.[43] Although immunophenotype is characteristic, a definitive diagnosis of APL requires confirmatory genetic testing to demonstrate the presence of a PML-RARA fusion.

AML with *KMT2A* (*MLL*) rearrangements commonly shows some elements of monocytic differentiation by morphology and flow cytometry with monoblasts/promonocytes typically predominating as blast equivalents.[44–46] The monocytic blast

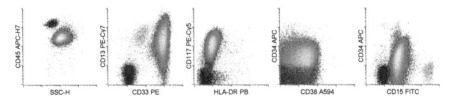

Fig. 4. Acute promyelocytic leukemia. The blast equivalents/abnormal promyelocytes (*colored red*; 90.9% of the white cells) in the bone marrow have increased SSC as compared with typical myeloid blasts. The blast equivalents express CD13 (heterogeneous), CD15 (dim), CD33 (bright), and CD117 without CD34, CD38, or HLA-DR. The dim CD15 expression helps distinguish this abnormal population from normal maturing myeloid cells (at the promyelocyte stage and beyond), which should have a high level of CD15 expression. Background reactive lymphoid cells are shown in *blue* and infrequent background neutrophilic cells are shown in *green*.

equivalents usually express myeloid-associated antigens and monocytic markers including CD4, CD33, CD64, and HLA-DR, whereas expression of CD13, CD14, and CD34 is often low to absent (see **Fig. 2**). Variable levels of CD56 and CD117 have also been described in AML with *KMT2A* (*MLL*) translocations.[45,47]

In addition to recurrent translocations and inversions, gene mutations also occur in AML. These include FLT3 internal tandem duplication, NPM1, and CEBPA mutations, which have been reported in patients with a normal karyotype and have prognostic significance.[48] NPM1 mutations occur in about one-third of adult AML cases and are frequently present in acute myelomonocytic and acute monocytic leukemia.[49,50] AML with NPM1 mutation commonly expresses myeloid-associated antigens and monocytic markers including CD13, CD14, CD33, and MPO, but lacks CD34 expression.[49,51] A subset of AML with cuplike nuclear morphology has been described that expresses CD123 without significant CD34 or HLA-DR, and is highly associated with FLT3 internal tandem duplication and NPM1 mutations (**Fig. 5**).[52]

CLASSIFICATION OF CHALLENGING CASES
Acute Leukemias of Ambiguous Lineage

In the 2008 WHO classification, acute leukemias of ambiguous lineage are defined as leukemias that show no clear evidence of differentiation along a single lineage.[1] They include acute undifferentiated leukemia (AUL) with no lineage-specific antigens on blasts and MPAL with blasts expressing antigens of more than one lineage. Flow cytometry is the preferred method to establish the diagnosis of acute leukemias of ambiguous lineage.

By definition, blasts in AUL do not express significant T, B, or myeloid lineage-specific markers, and lack markers for megakaryocytic, erythroid, and plasmacytoid dendritic cell lineages. MPAL is slightly more frequently than AUL and accounts for 2% to 5% of newly diagnosed AML.[53–57]

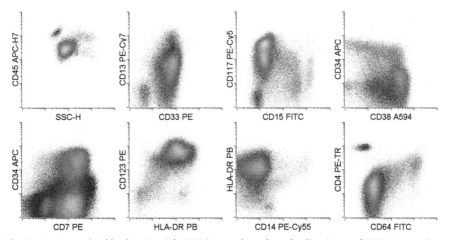

Fig. 5. Acute myeloid leukemia with FLT3 internal tandem duplication and NPM1 mutation. The leukemic blasts (*colored red*; 85.1% of the white cells) in the bone marrow show expression of CD7, CD13, CD33 (decreased), CD34 (variably decreased to absent), CD38 (variably decreased), CD117 (heterogeneous), HLA-DR (mildly decreased), and CD123 (increased) without CD4, CD14, or CD64. Some immunophenotypic features overlap with APL, although the SSC is lower than is typical for APL and in this case, the level of HLA-DR is higher than is typical for APL. Background reactive lymphoid cells are shown in *blue*, monocytic cells are shown in *pink*, and neutrophilic cells are shown in *green*.

Historically, MPAL includes acute bilineal leukemia, in which two distinct blast populations of different lineages are present, and acute biphenotypic leukemia, in which a single blast population coexpressing markers of more than one lineage is present. The diagnosis of MPAL is established in one of the three ways.[1,56] First, when two or more distinct blast populations are present, one of which would meet immunophenotypic criteria for AML and the other meet criteria for lymphoblastic leukemia (bilineal leukemia) (**Fig. 6**A). Second, a single blast population is present that meets criteria for B lymphoblastic leukemia or T lymphoblastic leukemia with coexpression of MPO (biphenotypic leukemia) (see **Fig. 6**B). Third, a single blast population is present that

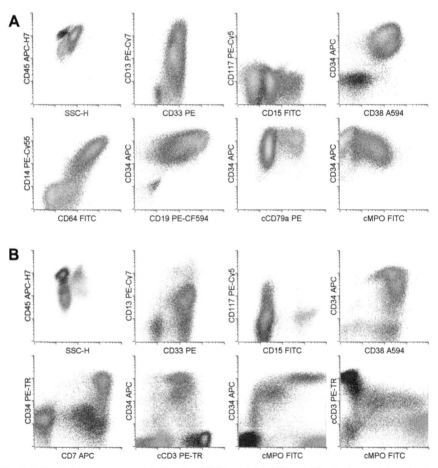

Fig. 6. Mixed phenotype acute leukemia. (*A*) B/myeloid, bilineal. The leukemic blasts in the peripheral blood are uniformly positive for CD34 and include two subsets. The dominant subset (*colored red*; 67% of the white cells) expresses CD13, CD14, CD15 (low, variable), CD19, CD33, CD34, and MPO without cCD79a or CD117. The minor subset (*colored aqua*; 10% of the white cells) expresses CD19, CD33, CD34, and cCD79a without CD13, CD14, CD15, CD64, CD117, or MPO. Background reactive lymphoid cells are shown in *blue*. (*B*) T/myeloid, biphenotypic. The leukemic blasts (*colored red*; 32.1% of the white cells) in the peripheral blood show expression of cCD3, CD7, CD13 (dim), CD33, CD34, CD38, CD117 (dim), and MPO (variable) without CD15. Background reactive lymphoid cells are shown in *blue*, monocytic cells are shown in *pink*, and neutrophilic cells are shown in *green*.

meets criteria for B lymphoblastic leukemia or T lymphoblastic leukemia and also shows evidence of monocytic differentiation (biphenotypic leukemia).

The WHO provides strict criteria for defining lineage in scenarios when a single blast population expressing markers of more than one lineage is identified. In this setting, the 2008 WHO classification and the 2016 Revision define myeloid lineage by expression of MPO or demonstration of monocytic differentiation (at least two of the following: nonspecific esterase, CD11c, CD14, CD64, lysozyme). T lineage is established by expression of strong cytoplasmic CD3 or surface CD3. B lineage assignment requires either strong expression of CD19 with strong expression of one additional B-cell marker (CD79a, cytoplasmic CD22, CD10), or weak expression of CD19 with strong expression of two additional B-cell markers. It is noted that to be considered strong, expression of CD19 or CD3 should be approaching that of a normal mature B or T cell, respectively. However, beyond that, no specific cutoff of aberrant blasts of a particular lineage is required by the WHO classification. It should be emphasized that these criteria only apply when one is considering a diagnosis of MPAL with a single blast population expressing markers of more than one lineage. These strict criteria need not be met when two distinct blast populations are identified that would each independently meet criteria for AML and acute lymphoblastic leukemia or in routine lineage assignment when making a diagnosis of a standard AML or acute lymphoblastic leukemia.

MPAL may be associated with recurrent cytogenetic abnormalities. Specifically, MPAL is further subdivided into MPAL with t(9;22); *BCR-ABL1* and MPAL with t(v;11q23); *KMT2A (MLL)* rearranged.[1,55,56] Most MPAL with t(9;22) have a B lymphoblast and a myeloid blast population. This category should not be diagnosed in patients with a known history of chronic myelogenous leukemia. MPAL with t(v;11q23) often contains a B lymphoblast and a monoblast population. The lymphoblast population generally expresses CD19 and is typically positive for CD15 without CD10.

Given that MPAL carries a worse prognosis than other acute leukemia subtypes, the accurate diagnosis of MPAL is critical and requires careful evaluation of available clinical, immunophenotypic, and genetic data. AML can frequently show aberrant nonlineage marker expression and some subtypes of AML characteristically show expression of nonlineage markers (eg, AML with t[8;21]). A diagnosis of MPAL should not be made in cases not meeting the strict definition as laid out by the WHO and should not be made if a different AML subcategory applies (eg, AML with recurrent genetic abnormalities, therapy-related myeloid neoplasms, AML with myelodysplasia-related changes).

Blastic Plasmacytoid Dendritic Cell Neoplasm

Blastic plasmacytoid dendritic cell neoplasm (BPDCN) is a rare form of hematopoietic neoplasm derived from the precursors of plasmacytoid dendritic cells. In the 2008 WHO classification, BPDCN is classified as a subtype of AML and related precursor neoplasms,[1] whereas the 2016 Revision defines BPDCN as a separate entity from AML.[18] BPDCN frequently involves skin and bone marrow with a leukemic dissemination and has an aggressive clinical course.[1,58–60]

By flow cytometry, BPDCN typically resides in the CD45 versus SSC defined blast gate (**Fig. 7**). Neoplastic cells express CD4, CD43, and CD56 with bright CD123 and HLA-DR. Expression of CD2, CD7, CD33, CD36, CD38, and TdT may be present in a subset of cases, but CD34 and other lineage-specific and associated markers are negative including CD3, CD5, CD19, CD20, CD13, CD14, CD16, CD64, and MPO. By immunohistochemistry, BPDCN expresses TCL-1 and BDCA-2 without lysozyme. The differentiation of BPDCN from AML with monocytic differentiation is challenging

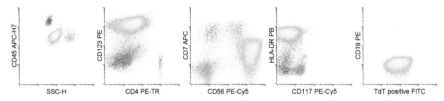

Fig. 7. Blastic plasmacytoid dendritic cell neoplasm. Flow cytometry reveals an expanded population of cells (*colored aqua*; 82% of the white cells) in the bone marrow with low CD45 and intermediate SSC. This population expresses CD4 (dim), CD7 (dim), CD56 (bright), CD123 (bright), HLA-DR, and TdT without CD34, CD117, or other B-cell or T-cell markers. Background reactive lymphoid cells are shown in *blue*, and neutrophilic cells are shown in *green*.

because both entities may express CD4, CD56, CD123, and HLA-DR. AML with monocytic differentiation typically has lower levels of CD123 and higher levels of CD64 by flow cytometry, and demonstrates expression of CD68 and lysozyme but lacks TCL-1 expression by immunohistochemistry.

DETECTION OF MINIMAL RESIDUAL DISEASE IN ACUTE MYELOID LEUKEMIA

Minimal residual disease (MRD) in acute leukemia is defined as the presence of leukemic blasts at a level lower than the limit of conventional morphologic detection. There is growing evidence that the presence of MRD after induction therapy is independently associated with an increased risk of relapse in AML.[61–69] Given the prognostic value of MRD, sensitive, accurate, and standardized methods are required for MRD detection and monitoring; however, the clinically relevant sensitivity of testing and optimal timing for MRD assessment vary in different patient populations and in different therapeutic protocols. In the United States, multiparametric flow cytometry is the most commonly used method to evaluate MRD in AML because of its assay availability, relative affordability, and rapid turnaround time. In greater than 95% of cases of AML, leukemic blasts have an aberrant immunophenotype that can be detected by a standard antibody panel with a sensitivity of 0.1% to 0.01%.[70]

The main challenge in performing MRD detection by flow cytometry is the lack of reproducibility across laboratories caused by considerable variability in instrumentation, reagents, data analysis, and reporting. Flow cytometry also has the disadvantage of requiring a high level of expertise for data interpretation. Therefore, in order for flow cytometry for AML MRD assessment to be widely implemented, interlaboratory standardization and demonstration of reproducibility is required.

Discriminating leukemic blasts from normal hematopoietic progenitors relies on the principle that the antigen expression patterns on the leukemic blasts differ from that seen on normal cells of a similar lineage and maturation stage.[71] At present, this fundamental principle is applied in two related methodologic approaches for detecting MRD by flow cytometry.

The first approach is based on identification of a combination of aberrant antigenic expression patterns on the leukemic blasts designated "leukemia-associated immunophenotypes" (LAIPs) that are absent in normal progenitors.[72–74] At diagnosis, an antibody panel is used to define LAIPs, or regions in multiparametric space that contain only leukemic blasts but not normal progenitors of the relevant lineage. After treatment, the informative antibody panel identified at diagnosis is used on subsequent samples and leukemic blasts present in the predefined LAIP regions are considered as MRD. An extensive list of LAIPs has been described[64,66,72,75] and includes such features as dyssynchronous antigen expression, cross-lineage antigen expression, antigen overexpression/underexpression, and aberrant light scatter. To increase sensitivity and specificity of MRD detection, all the LAIPs of the leukemic blasts detected at diagnosis should be followed in subsequent samples. Recognition of specific LAIPs may be improved by adding more fluorochromes and consequently including more simultaneous markers to define a leukemic blast with higher confidence.

Despite the successful application in some studies, this strategy has some limitations. First, LAIPs are not always stable during therapy and may shift because of leukemic blast heterogeneity.[76,77] In AML, immunophenotypic changes in expression of at least one antigen between diagnosis and relapse were observed in 88% to 91% of patients.[78,79] Such immunophenotypic shifts after treatment can lead to false-negative results. Second, similar to the leukemic blasts, the immunophenotype of the background normal or regenerating precursors may also change after therapy. Consequently, the normal precursors may appear in the regions defined for abnormal blasts, resulting in a false-positive result. Lastly, this strategy is highly dependent on the diagnostic immunophenotype. Without the knowledge of LAIPs at presentation, an individualized antibody panel cannot be constructed to accurately detect MRD.

An alternative strategy knows as the "difference from normal" approach relies on the assumption that the immunophenotype of the leukemic blasts differs from the patterns of antigen expression on normal hematopoietic progenitors of similar lineage and maturation stage.[3,80] At diagnosis, this method is similar to the identification of LAIPs, but there is no requirement to define regions for LAIPs. After treatment, using immunophenotypic aberrancies seen in the diagnostic sample as a starting point, all populations are evaluated for immunophenotypic deviations from the normal maturation pattern (**Fig. 8**). This approach avoids the limitations of LAIPs caused by immunophenotypic shift. In most cases, it is possible to detect leukemic blasts even when significant immunophenotypic changes are present in the relapsed/residual disease as compared with diagnosis. Additional advantages of the "difference form normal" approach over LAIP evaluation include that MRD is assessed without a diagnostic immunophenotype, and that a standard antibody panel is implemented.[80] However, this approach does require expert knowledge of antigen expression patterns during differentiation of normal hematopoietic progenitors in states of rest and recovery post therapy making standardization and implementation more challenging.

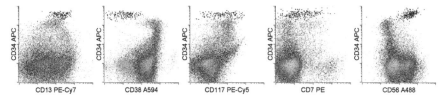

Fig. 8. The detection of MRD for acute myeloid leukemia following induction therapy by flow cytometry. The antibody combination allows the identification of residual leukemic blasts by deviation from normal hematopoietic precursors based on lineage and maturational stage. All plots show cells within the CD45 versus SSC defined blast gate. The leukemic blasts (*colored blue* and highlighted) that represent MRD are characterized by abnormal expression of CD7 (variable), CD13 (slightly increased), CD34 (increased), CD38 (decreased to absent), and CD56 as compared with the normal CD34-positive myeloid progenitors (*red*). The abnormal population is enumerated at 0.1% of the white cells. Background monocytes are shown in *pink*, and neutrophilic cells are shown in *green*.

In practice, components of both methods are commonly used simultaneously to a various degree to improve diagnostic accuracy. AML MRD assay sensitivity depends on the degree of immunophenotypic deviation of the leukemic blasts from normal progenitors, the number of normal progenitors of similar type, and the number of events acquired in each assay. The number of events recommended for acquisition and number of events to define a leukemic blast population vary significantly among groups and laboratories. In general, a sensitivity of 0.1% is achieved in AML for most patients with higher sensitivity possible for some aberrant immunophenotypes. The assay sensitivity can also vary at different time points of evaluation post therapy because some aberrant immunophenotypes may be challenging to differentiate from active marrow regeneration.

SUMMARY

Immunophenotyping by flow cytometry plays a critical role in the diagnosis and classification of AML allowing for blast identification, lineage assignment, and immunophenotypic characterization. Furthermore, flow cytometry can provide useful clues to underlying genetics, reliably distinguish AML from other precursor neoplasms that may be in the differential diagnosis, and provide insight to prognosis. AML MRD assessment has been demonstrated to be a particularly powerful tool in AML prognostication; however, this area also highlights the critical importance of standardization, which is needed to allow this modality to reach its full potential.

REFERENCES

1. Swerdlow SH, Campo E, Harris NL, et al. WHO classification of tumours of haematopoietic and lymphoid tissues. 4th edition. Lyon (France): IARC; 2008.
2. Cherian S, Wood BL. Flow cytometry in evaluation of hematopoietic neoplasms: a case based approach. Northfield (IL): CAP Press; 2012.
3. Wood B. Multicolor immunophenotyping: human immune system hematopoiesis. Methods Cell Biol 2004;75:559–76.
4. Wood BL. Myeloid malignancies: myelodysplastic syndromes, myeloproliferative disorders, and acute myeloid leukemia. Clin Lab Med 2007;27(3):551–75, vii.
5. Kussick SJ, Wood BL. Four-color flow cytometry identifies virtually all cytogenetically abnormal bone marrow samples in the workup of non-CML myeloproliferative disorders. Am J Clin Pathol 2003;120(6):854–65.
6. Borowitz MJ, Guenther KL, Shults KE, et al. Immunophenotyping of acute leukemia by flow cytometric analysis. Use of CD45 and right-angle light scatter to gate on leukemic blasts in three-color analysis. Am J Clin Pathol 1993;100(5):534–40.
7. Stelzer GT, Shults KE, Loken MR. CD45 gating for routine flow cytometric analysis of human bone marrow specimens. Ann N Y Acad Sci 1993;677:265–80.
8. Wood BL, Arroz M, Barnett D, et al. 2006 Bethesda International Consensus recommendations on the immunophenotypic analysis of hematolymphoid neoplasia by flow cytometry: optimal reagents and reporting for the flow cytometric diagnosis of hematopoietic neoplasia. Cytometry B Clin Cytom 2007;72(Suppl 1): S14–22.
9. Yang DT, Greenwood JH, Hartung L, et al. Flow cytometric analysis of different CD14 epitopes can help identify immature monocytic populations. Am J Clin Pathol 2005;124(6):930–6.
10. Kaleem Z, Crawford E, Pathan MH, et al. Flow cytometric analysis of acute leukemias. Diagnostic utility and critical analysis of data. Arch Pathol Lab Med 2003; 127(1):42–8.

11. Khalidi HS, Medeiros LJ, Chang KL, et al. The immunophenotype of adult acute myeloid leukemia: high frequency of lymphoid antigen expression and comparison of immunophenotype, French-American-British classification, and karyotypic abnormalities. Am J Clin Pathol 1998;109(2):211–20.

12. Zheng J, Wang X, Hu Y, et al. A correlation study of immunophenotypic, cytogenetic, and clinical features of 180 AML patients in China. Cytometry B Clin Cytom 2008;74(1):25–9.

13. Loken MR, Shah VO, Dattilio KL, et al. Flow cytometric analysis of human bone marrow: I. Normal erythroid development. Blood 1987;69(1):255–63.

14. Koike T, Aoki S, Maruyama S, et al. Cell surface phenotyping of megakaryoblasts. Blood 1987;69(3):957–60.

15. San Miguel JF, Gonzalez M, Canizo MC, et al. Leukemias with megakaryoblastic involvement: clinical, hematologic, and immunologic characteristics. Blood 1988; 72(2):402–7.

16. Kafer G, Willer A, Ludwig W, et al. Intracellular expression of CD61 precedes surface expression. Ann Hematol 1999;78(10):472–4.

17. Betz SA, Foucar K, Head DR, et al. False-positive flow cytometric platelet glycoprotein IIb/IIIa expression in myeloid leukemias secondary to platelet adherence to blasts. Blood 1992;79(9):2399–403.

18. Arber DA, Orazi A, Hasserjian R, et al. The 2016 revision to the World Health Organization classification of myeloid neoplasms and acute leukemia. Blood 2016; 127(20):2391–405.

19. Swerdlow SH, Campo E, Pileri SA, et al. The 2016 revision of the World Health Organization classification of lymphoid neoplasms. Blood 2016;127(20):2375–90.

20. De J, Zanjani R, Hibbard M, et al. Immunophenotypic profile predictive of KIT activating mutations in AML1-ETO leukemia. Am J Clin Pathol 2007;128(4):550–7.

21. Khoury H, Dalal BI, Nantel SH, et al. Correlation between karyotype and quantitative immunophenotype in acute myelogenous leukemia with t(8;21). Mod Pathol 2004;17(10):1211–6.

22. Khoury H, Dalal BI, Nevill TJ, et al. Acute myelogenous leukemia with t(8;21)–identification of a specific immunophenotype. Leuk Lymphoma 2003;44(10): 1713–8.

23. Porwit-MacDonald A, Janossy G, Ivory K, et al. Leukemia-associated changes identified by quantitative flow cytometry. IV. CD34 overexpression in acute myelogenous leukemia M2 with t(8;21). Blood 1996;87(3):1162–9.

24. Kita K, Nakase K, Miwa H, et al. Phenotypical characteristics of acute myelocytic leukemia associated with the t(8;21)(q22;q22) chromosomal abnormality: frequent expression of immature B-cell antigen CD19 together with stem cell antigen CD34. Blood 1992;80(2):470–7.

25. Chen SW, Li CF, Chuang SS, et al. Aberrant co-expression of CD19 and CD56 as surrogate markers of acute myeloid leukemias with t(8;21) in Taiwan. Int J Lab Hematol 2008;30(2):133–8.

26. Yang DH, Lee JJ, Mun YC, et al. Predictable prognostic factor of CD56 expression in patients with acute myeloid leukemia with t(8:21) after high dose cytarabine or allogeneic hematopoietic stem cell transplantation. Am J Hematol 2007; 82(1):1–5.

27. Baer MR, Stewart CC, Lawrence D, et al. Expression of the neural cell adhesion molecule CD56 is associated with short remission duration and survival in acute myeloid leukemia with t(8;21)(q22;q22). Blood 1997;90(4):1643–8.

28. Paschka P, Marcucci G, Ruppert AS, et al. Adverse prognostic significance of KIT mutations in adult acute myeloid leukemia with inv(16) and t(8;21): a Cancer and Leukemia Group B Study. J Clin Oncol 2006;24(24):3904–11.

29. Shimada A, Taki T, Tabuchi K, et al. KIT mutations, and not FLT3 internal tandem duplication, are strongly associated with a poor prognosis in pediatric acute myeloid leukemia with t(8;21): a study of the Japanese Childhood AML Cooperative Study Group. Blood 2006;107(5):1806–9.

30. Di Noto R, Mirabelli P, Del Vecchio L. Flow cytometry analysis of acute promyelocytic leukemia: the power of 'surface hematology'. Leukemia 2007;21(1):4–8.

31. Orfao A, Chillon MC, Bortoluci AM, et al. The flow cytometric pattern of CD34, CD15 and CD13 expression in acute myeloblastic leukemia is highly characteristic of the presence of PML-RARalpha gene rearrangements. Haematologica 1999;84(5):405–12.

32. Albano F, Mestice A, Pannunzio A, et al. The biological characteristics of CD34+ CD2+ adult acute promyelocytic leukemia and the CD34 CD2 hypergranular (M3) and microgranular (M3v) phenotypes. Haematologica 2006;91(3):311–6.

33. Biondi A, Luciano A, Bassan R, et al. CD2 expression in acute promyelocytic leukemia is associated with microgranular morphology (FAB M3v) but not with any PML gene breakpoint. Leukemia 1995;9(9):1461–6.

34. Ferrara F, Morabito F, Martino B, et al. CD56 expression is an indicator of poor clinical outcome in patients with acute promyelocytic leukemia treated with simultaneous all-trans-retinoic acid and chemotherapy. J Clin Oncol 2000;18(6): 1295–300.

35. Ito S, Ishida Y, Oyake T, et al. Clinical and biological significance of CD56 antigen expression in acute promyelocytic leukemia. Leuk Lymphoma 2004;45(9): 1783–9.

36. Murray CK, Estey E, Paietta E, et al. CD56 expression in acute promyelocytic leukemia: a possible indicator of poor treatment outcome? J Clin Oncol 1999;17(1): 293–7.

37. Masamoto Y, Nannya Y, Arai S, et al. Evidence for basophilic differentiation of acute promyelocytic leukaemia cells during arsenic trioxide therapy. Br J Haematol 2009;144(5):798–9.

38. Oelschlaegel U, Mohr B, Schaich M, et al. HLA-DRneg patients without acute promyelocytic leukemia show distinct immunophenotypic, genetic, molecular, and cytomorphologic characteristics compared to acute promyelocytic leukemia. Cytometry B Clin Cytom 2009;76(5):321–7.

39. Wetzler M, McElwain BK, Stewart CC, et al. HLA-DR antigen-negative acute myeloid leukemia. Leukemia 2003;17(4):707–15.

40. Fenaux P, Le Deley MC, Castaigne S, et al. Effect of all transretinoic acid in newly diagnosed acute promyelocytic leukemia. Results of a multicenter randomized trial. European APL 91 Group. Blood 1993;82(11):3241–9.

41. Kanamaru A, Takemoto Y, Tanimoto M, et al. All-trans retinoic acid for the treatment of newly diagnosed acute promyelocytic leukemia. Japan Adult Leukemia Study Group. Blood 1995;85(5):1202–6.

42. Tallman MS, Andersen JW, Schiffer CA, et al. All-trans retinoic acid in acute promyelocytic leukemia: long-term outcome and prognostic factor analysis from the North American Intergroup protocol. Blood 2002;100(13):4298–302.

43. Ferrari A, Bussaglia E, Ubeda J, et al. Immunophenotype distinction between acute promyelocytic leukaemia and CD15- CD34- HLA-DR- acute myeloid leukaemia with nucleophosmin mutations. Hematol Oncol 2012;30(3):109–14.

44. Baer MR, Stewart CC, Lawrence D, et al. Acute myeloid leukemia with 11q23 translocations: myelomonocytic immunophenotype by multiparameter flow cytometry. Leukemia 1998;12(3):317–25.

45. Munoz L, Nomdedeu JF, Villamor N, et al. Acute myeloid leukemia with MLL rearrangements: clinicobiological features, prognostic impact and value of flow cytometry in the detection of residual leukemic cells. Leukemia 2003;17(1):76–82.

46. Creutzig U, Harbott J, Sperling C, et al. Clinical significance of surface antigen expression in children with acute myeloid leukemia: results of study AML-BFM-87. Blood 1995;86(8):3097–108.

47. Chang H, Brandwein J, Yi QL, et al. Extramedullary infiltrates of AML are associated with CD56 expression, 11q23 abnormalities and inferior clinical outcome. Leuk Res 2004;28(10):1007–11.

48. Mrozek K, Marcucci G, Paschka P, et al. Clinical relevance of mutations and gene-expression changes in adult acute myeloid leukemia with normal cytogenetics: are we ready for a prognostically prioritized molecular classification? Blood 2007;109(2):431–48.

49. Falini B, Mecucci C, Tiacci E, et al. Cytoplasmic nucleophosmin in acute myelogenous leukemia with a normal karyotype. N Engl J Med 2005;352(3):254–66.

50. Falini B, Nicoletti I, Martelli MF, et al. Acute myeloid leukemia carrying cytoplasmic/mutated nucleophosmin (NPMc+ AML): biologic and clinical features. Blood 2007;109(3):874–85.

51. Haferlach C, Mecucci C, Schnittger S, et al. AML with mutated NPM1 carrying a normal or aberrant karyotype show overlapping biologic, pathologic, immunophenotypic, and prognostic features. Blood 2009;114(14):3024–32.

52. Kussick SJ, Stirewalt DL, Yi HS, et al. A distinctive nuclear morphology in acute myeloid leukemia is strongly associated with loss of HLA-DR expression and FLT3 internal tandem duplication. Leukemia 2004;18(10):1591–8.

53. Thalhammer-Scherrer R, Mitterbauer G, Simonitsch I, et al. The immunophenotype of 325 adult acute leukemias: relationship to morphologic and molecular classification and proposal for a minimal screening program highly predictive for lineage discrimination. Am J Clin Pathol 2002;117(3):380–9.

54. Bene MC. Biphenotypic, bilineal, ambiguous or mixed lineage: strange leukemias! Haematologica 2009;94(7):891–3.

55. Owaidah TM, Al Beihany A, Iqbal MA, et al. Cytogenetics, molecular and ultrastructural characteristics of biphenotypic acute leukemia identified by the EGIL scoring system. Leukemia 2006;20(4):620–6.

56. Weinberg OK, Arber DA. Mixed-phenotype acute leukemia: historical overview and a new definition. Leukemia 2010;24(11):1844–51.

57. Xu XQ, Wang JM, Lu SQ, et al. Clinical and biological characteristics of adult biphenotypic acute leukemia in comparison with that of acute myeloid leukemia and acute lymphoblastic leukemia: a case series of a Chinese population. Haematologica 2009;94(7):919–27.

58. Garnache-Ottou F, Feuillard J, Ferrand C, et al. Extended diagnostic criteria for plasmacytoid dendritic cell leukaemia. Br J Haematol 2009;145(5):624–36.

59. Garnache-Ottou F, Feuillard J, Saas P. Plasmacytoid dendritic cell leukaemia/lymphoma: towards a well defined entity? Br J Haematol 2007;136(4):539–48.

60. Herling M, Jones D. CD4+/CD56+ hematodermic tumor: the features of an evolving entity and its relationship to dendritic cells. Am J Clin Pathol 2007;127(5):687–700.

61. Buccisano F, Maurillo L, Gattei V, et al. The kinetics of reduction of minimal residual disease impacts on duration of response and survival of patients with acute myeloid leukemia. Leukemia 2006;20(10):1783–9.

62. Freeman SD, Virgo P, Couzens S, et al. Prognostic relevance of treatment response measured by flow cytometric residual disease detection in older patients with acute myeloid leukemia. J Clin Oncol 2013;31(32):4123–31.

63. Jourdan E, Boissel N, Chevret S, et al. Prospective evaluation of gene mutations and minimal residual disease in patients with core binding factor acute myeloid leukemia. Blood 2013;121(12):2213–23.

64. Kern W, Voskova D, Schoch C, et al. Determination of relapse risk based on assessment of minimal residual disease during complete remission by multiparameter flow cytometry in unselected patients with acute myeloid leukemia. Blood 2004;104(10):3078–85.

65. Kronke J, Schlenk RF, Jensen KO, et al. Monitoring of minimal residual disease in NPM1-mutated acute myeloid leukemia: a study from the German-Austrian acute myeloid leukemia study group. J Clin Oncol 2011;29(19):2709–16.

66. San Miguel JF, Vidriales MB, Lopez-Berges C, et al. Early immunophenotypical evaluation of minimal residual disease in acute myeloid leukemia identifies different patient risk groups and may contribute to postinduction treatment stratification. Blood 2001;98(6):1746–51.

67. Terwijn M, van Putten WL, Kelder A, et al. High prognostic impact of flow cytometric minimal residual disease detection in acute myeloid leukemia: data from the HOVON/SAKK AML 42A study. J Clin Oncol 2013;31(31):3889–97.

68. Venditti A, Buccisano F, Del Poeta G, et al. Level of minimal residual disease after consolidation therapy predicts outcome in acute myeloid leukemia. Blood 2000; 96(12):3948–52.

69. Yin JA, O'Brien MA, Hills RK, et al. Minimal residual disease monitoring by quantitative RT-PCR in core binding factor AML allows risk stratification and predicts relapse: results of the United Kingdom MRC AML-15 trial. Blood 2012;120(14): 2826–35.

70. Al-Mawali A, Gillis D, Lewis I. The role of multiparameter flow cytometry for detection of minimal residual disease in acute myeloid leukemia. Am J Clin Pathol 2009; 131(1):16–26.

71. Wood BL. Principles of minimal residual disease detection for hematopoietic neoplasms by flow cytometry. Cytometry B Clin Cytom 2016;90(1):47–53.

72. Feller N, van der Velden VH, Brooimans RA, et al. Defining consensus leukemia-associated immunophenotypes for detection of minimal residual disease in acute myeloid leukemia in a multicenter setting. Blood Cancer J 2013;3:e129.

73. Macedo A, Orfao A, Vidriales MB, et al. Characterization of aberrant phenotypes in acute myeloblastic leukemia. Ann Hematol 1995;70(4):189–94.

74. Reading CL, Estey EH, Huh YO, et al. Expression of unusual immunophenotype combinations in acute myelogenous leukemia. Blood 1993;81(11):3083–90.

75. Al-Mawali A, Gillis D, Hissaria P, et al. Incidence, sensitivity, and specificity of leukemia-associated phenotypes in acute myeloid leukemia using specific five-color multiparameter flow cytometry. Am J Clin Pathol 2008;129(6):934–45.

76. Borowitz MJ, Pullen DJ, Winick N, et al. Comparison of diagnostic and relapse flow cytometry phenotypes in childhood acute lymphoblastic leukemia: implications for residual disease detection: a report from the children's oncology group. Cytometry B Clin Cytom 2005;68(1):18–24.

77. Zeijlemaker W, Gratama JW, Schuurhuis GJ. Tumor heterogeneity makes AML a "moving target" for detection of residual disease. Cytometry B Clin Cytom 2014; 86(1):3–14.
78. Baer MR, Stewart CC, Dodge RK, et al. High frequency of immunophenotype changes in acute myeloid leukemia at relapse: implications for residual disease detection (Cancer and Leukemia Group B Study 8361). Blood 2001;97(11): 3574–80.
79. Langebrake C, Brinkmann I, Teigler-Schlegel A, et al. Immunophenotypic differences between diagnosis and relapse in childhood AML: implications for MRD monitoring. Cytometry B Clin Cytom 2005;63(1):1–9.
80. Wood BL. Flow cytometric monitoring of residual disease in acute leukemia. Methods Mol Biol 2013;999:123–36.

B Lymphoblastic Leukemia Minimal Residual Disease Assessment by Flow Cytometric Analysis

CrossMark

Aaron C. Shaver, MD, PhD*, Adam C. Seegmiller, MD, PhD

KEYWORDS

- Minimal residual disease • Flow cytometry • Acute lymphoblastic leukemia

KEY POINTS

- Minimal residual disease detection is of increasing clinical relevance, particularly in B-acute lymphoblastic leukemia.
- Multiparameter flow cytometry is a technique very well suited to detection of minimal residual disease.
- Interpretation of minimal residual disease flow cytometry is complicated, and immunophenotypic markers must often be evaluated in combination with each other.
- Differentiation from normal hematopoietic elements, such as hematogones, is the most important element of interpretation.
- Introduction of targeted therapy, particularly anti-CD19 therapy, is likely to complicate existing methods of minimal residual disease analysis, and will require new approaches.

INTRODUCTION

Disease recurrence is an important negative prognostic indicator in cancer. Thus, determining which patients are at greatest risk for relapse is an essential part of the diagnostic work-up because it has an impact on the therapeutic approach to many cancers. The basis of risk stratification differs among cancer types, but clinical stage, pathologic grade, and the presence of particular genetic abnormalities are common prognostic factors. Importantly, disease relapse generally occurs because a small number of residual tumor cells survives initial therapy and develops into a second tumor. In hematopoietic malignancies, classic descriptors for disease negativity, such as complete remission, are often relatively insensitive, relying on levels of disease

Disclosure Statement: The authors have nothing to disclose.
Department of Pathology, Microbiology, and Immunology, Vanderbilt University Medical Center, Nashville, TN, USA
* Corresponding author. C-3321A MCN, 1161 21st Avenue South, Nashville, TN 37232-2561.
E-mail address: aaron.shaver@vanderbilt.edu

burden of 1% to 5% of total cells. Modern methods of disease detection make it clear that, after treatment, populations of abnormal cells persist at a level much lower than can be readily detected, and that the presence or absence of this low-level disease involvement can play a major part in prognosis and relapse risk. Thus, in many cases, the best predictor of relapse is the persistence of these abnormal cells after therapy, often at levels below the sensitivity of conventional visual detection techniques. This is termed minimal residual disease (MRD).

The concept and utility of MRD detection is best developed in hematolymphoid malignancies. This is due to at least 2 factors: (1) easy access to sufficient tumor tissue using peripheral blood and/or bone marrow sampling and (2) highly sensitive immunologic techniques, primarily multiparameter flow cytometry (MFC), that can distinguish between leukemic cells and their non-neoplastic normal counterparts. Aside from MFC, other methods for MRD detection include polymerase chain reaction or methods based on next-generation sequencing for detection of disease-specific genetic abnormalities, including point mutations, chromosomal translocations, or clonal immunoglobulin or T-cell receptor gene VDJ rearrangements. Although these methods are equally or even, in many cases, more powerful for detecting very low levels of residual disease, their use depends on the presence of abnormalities that can be targeted by clinically validated genetic tests. In contrast, MFC has the advantage that it can be used on essentially any malignant population, regardless of the underlying genetics. In addition, the maturity of MFC as a clinical test has led to a large body of literature validating its use in the detection of MRD, which makes it easier to justify its application in routine clinical care.

Although MRD detection has been described and, to varying degrees, clinically validated in a wide variety of hematolymphoid malignancies, including acute myeloid leukemia, mature B-cell lymphoma, and plasma cell myeloma,[1–7] the disease with the longest history of MRD detection and the greatest degree of clinical applicability is B-acute lymphoblastic leukemia (B-ALL), a neoplasm of immature B-lineage precursor cells. Consequently, MRD detection by MFC has become a powerful tool in prognosis, monitoring, and treating B-ALL.[8] This review highlights the technical approach and clinical significance of MRD detection by MFC in B-ALL, and discusses recent developments and challenges in this important diagnostic tool.

TECHNICAL CONSIDERATIONS IN MINIMAL RESIDUAL DISEASE ASSESSMENT BY MULTIPARAMETER FLOW CYTOMETRY

There are several important technical principles associated with measurement of MRD by MFC.[9,10] First, it is critical to be able to distinguish neoplastic B lymphoblasts from their normal non-neoplastic counterparts. These normal B-lineage precursors are termed hematogones and they exhibit a distinctive pattern of cell surface marker expression, including predictable expression changes as the cells mature.[11–14] Leukemic B lymphoblasts almost always exhibit aberrant patterns of cell marker expression that allow them to be distinguished from hematogones.[11,13,15,16] These can include loss of markers normally expressed on hematogones, relative increase or decrease in expression of these markers, asynchronous expression of markers compared with normal temporal patterns, or abnormal expression of nonlineage markers, such as myeloid or T-cell markers.[15,16]

This unique pattern of aberrant marker expression is termed a leukemia-associated immunophenotype (LAIP). One approach to MRD detection is to use an initial diagnostic sample to determine the particular LAIP or fingerprint present in a patient's disease, and then to search for cells in a follow-up sample that match the LAIP seen in the diagnostic sample. The presence of immunophenotypic aberrancies allows the neoplastic cells to be distinguished from normal hematogones, which can be increased in marrows recovering from chemotherapy.[17,18] The effectiveness of this approach is roughly proportional to the number of aberrant markers seen.[16] Thus, it is important to carefully design MFC panels in such a way as to maximize detection of these aberrancies (see later discussion).

A limitation to this approach of detecting MRD is that it requires that the LAIP remain stable during the course of a patient's disease. However, several studies have demonstrated that B-ALL phenotypes can change in response to therapy, often in predictable ways, such that the immunophenotype of an MRD population can differ significantly from that seen at diagnosis.[19–23] These differences may hinder identification of MRD if it is focused solely on the diagnostic LAIP. Thus, a complementary difference from normal approach may also be required. This involves identifying each cell population and determining whether it significantly differs from the expected immunophenotypic pattern of normal cells, which could indicate MRD.[10,24]

A second technical consideration is sensitivity. There are variable estimates of the number of events or individual cells required to accurately identify an abnormal population in rare-event analyses, such as MRD detection, ranging from less than 10 to greater than 50.[1,9,25,26] However, reproducible quantification requires a higher threshold, with estimates ranging from 40 to 100 events in a well-controlled, reliable assay.[9,10,25,26] Because the lower threshold for clinical action is 0.01%,[27] at least 10^6 cells, much more than a typical diagnostic MFC assay, must be analyzed to ensure necessary sensitivity. The denominator for this percentage also varies in different studies, including mononuclear cells, total nucleated cells, or all CD45-positive leukocytes.[9,28]

Determining a lower cutoff for sensitivity is important not only for addressing the clinical needs of the test but also in meeting regulatory requirements. Regulatory agencies, such as the College of American Pathologists (CAP), the body responsible for regulating many American pathology laboratories, have specific requirements related to the lower limit of detection in rare event flow cytometric assays. In the CAP regulations, the lower limit of enumeration must be documented both in the laboratory procedure and the diagnostic report; this may be accomplished by including a line similar to, "This assay has been validated to a lower limit of detection of 0.01% of mononuclear cells," at the end of each clinical report. Validation of the lower limit of detection must be documented by the laboratory in a form available for inspection by the CAP. A combination of dilutional studies and proficiency testing is recommended to perform this validation. Dilutional studies offer the advantage of a known concentration of leukemic cells, but care is needed to make these studies reflect real practice. Diluting B-ALL blasts into peripheral blood, for example, may not reflect the actual challenge of interpreting bone marrow samples, and hematogone-rich bone marrow material is preferred for optimal testing. Proficiency testing material, such as from groups like United Kingdom National External Quality Assessment Service (UK NEQAS), also offers an opportunity for validation, and can be used in conjunction with laboratory-performed dilutional studies.

APPROACH TO INTERPRETATION OF MULTIPARAMETER FLOW CYTOMETRY FOR MINIMAL RESIDUAL DISEASE DETECTION

To determine whether a pattern of marker expression is abnormal, both for the LAIP and difference from normal approaches, the range of expression of the marker both in hematogones and in leukemic blasts must be fully understood. Normal hematogones do not express myeloid markers, such as CD13 or CD33, but these markers are frequently expressed aberrantly in B-ALL. Thus, for a marker with this expression pattern, it is sufficient to consider the marker on its own when describing a pattern of abnormal expression. In contrast, because CD20 expression in hematogones ranges from negative to as bright as a mature B cell, it is difficult to describe abnormal expression of CD20 as a marker considered on its own; the level of CD20 expression in B-ALL invariably falls somewhere in the range seen in normal hematogones. However, this does not mean that evaluation for CD20 is of no use in B-ALL MRD; instead, examination of CD20 is paired with another marker, such as CD10 or CD9, that shows variable expression during hematogone development (**Fig. 1**). In this approach, a low level of CD20 expression, such as would be seen in an early hematogone, would be aberrant when coupled with low-level CD10 expression, which is a marker of a later hematogone; thus it is the combination of markers that is aberrant, rather than the intensity of expression of either single marker on its own.

As a guide to the understanding of what role individual markers play in the detection of MRD, a list of some of the most common markers included in widely used MRD MFC panels follows, along with a brief discussion of their interpretation:

CD19

CD19 is invariably expressed in B-ALL (in the absence of specific anti-CD19 treatment; see later discussion) and thus is ubiquitous in MRD MFC panels. Remember that some non-B blastic malignancies, such as certain subtypes of AML, may also express CD19, so care must be taken to fully establish the lineage of a new blastic process.

CD45

A common marker for lymphocytes and lymphoid precursors, as well as other leukocytes, CD45 is commonly included in MFC panels. B-ALL is well known to present with

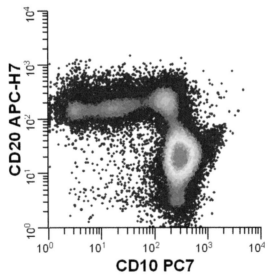

Fig. 1. Histogram of the normal maturation pattern of hematogones for CD10 and CD20. Hematogones begin at their earliest stage at the lower right: CD10 bright and CD20-negative. CD20 is steadily gained with little change in CD10 expression; then, once CD20 is expressed at a level similar to mature B cells, change in CD20 expression stops and loss of CD10 expression begins.

markedly lower CD45 than normal hematogones, which can be a very useful aid to initial diagnosis. However, this very low level of CD45 expression often disappears very rapidly on initiation of therapy and leukemic cells observed in day 28 bone marrows may have markedly increased CD45 expression compared with the patient's initial sample, at near-hematogone levels.[19,21] This makes CD45 less reliable than might be imagined as an abnormal marker for MRD detection, and illustrates the dangers in blindly following the LAIP approach.

CD20

This is another B-lineage specific marker with a wide range of expression in hematogones, from negative to brightly positive. Thus, as previously described, its primary use in MRD MFC comes when viewed in a 2-dimensional histogram with another variably expressed marker.

CD34

CD34 is a common marker of immaturity across lineages. In a manner analogous to the method described for CD20, abnormal persistence of CD34 at the same time that other markers are displaying a more mature phenotype (eg, loss of CD9 or CD10, or gain of CD20) can serve as a marker of malignancy. An important consideration in designing a gating strategy is that a significant subset of B-ALL lacks CD34 expression and, thus, using CD34 positivity as part of the gating scheme for downstream analysis is not recommended.

CD10

This is among most useful markers for B-ALL MRD detection because CD10 combines some of the most helpful attributes of both types of aberrant markers. CD10 goes through a range of expression during normal B cell maturation, similar to CD20 and CD34, and thus is useful as part of a multidimensional analysis: loss of CD10 alongside lack of expression of CD20 is not seen in normal hematogones and, in fact, is the hallmark of a particular subtype (KMT2A-rearranged) of B-ALL. In addition, CD10 may be expressed more brightly in B-ALL than in any normal stage of hematogone development and thus may be a diagnostic marker in its own right (**Fig. 2**), without needing to be combined with other markers for assessment of dyssynchronous maturation.

CD38

Normal hematogones uniformly express CD38 in a very bright and homogenous fashion until a very late stage of development. In B-ALL, CD38 typically remains positive but with a significantly reduced intensity and more heterogeneous distribution. Inclusion of CD38 in an MRD panel also allows plasma cells to be gated out of the analysis because neither hematogones nor B lymphoblasts express CD38 as brightly as plasma cells, thus removing them as a potential confounder.

CD58

Similar to CD10, CD58 may be useful in a multiparameter approach, in which persistent expression of CD58 (a marker of early hematogone development) alongside indicators of later maturation can be an indicator of aberrancy. A single parameter approach can also be effective because a significant subset of B-ALL expresses CD58 at a higher level than is ever seen during normal hematogone maturation.

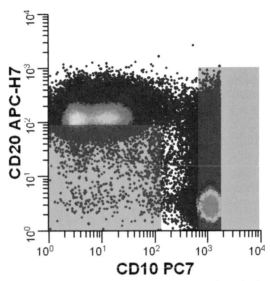

Fig. 2. Histogram of some of the subtleties involved in identifying leukemic blasts and distinguishing them from hematogones. At first glance, this pattern seems similar to the boomerang for CD10 and CD20 seen in **Fig. 1**, and could easily be misinterpreted as negative for residual disease. However, in this case, the CD10 bright, CD20-negative cells in the lower right corner have a CD10 intensity that is approximately half a log brighter than normal hematogones using the same instrument settings (compare to **Fig. 1**). The cells at the top left of the figure represent normal mature B cells. The red rectangles represent areas outside of the normal B-cell maturation curve, and thus areas in which any cell populations present are suspicious for leukemic blasts. Full evaluation for involvement requires backgating on populations in these areas and investigating their phenotype across all of the markers contained in the panel.

CD9, CD81

Expression of these markers, typically bright in hematogones and lost on maturation, may be aberrantly decreased in B-ALL,[29] thus making these markers part of the multiparameter group of useful markers.

CD13, CD33, CD15, CD2, and so forth

These myeloid and T-cell–specific markers are not seen on normal hematogones but are observed at varying frequencies in leukemic B lymphoblasts, making them useful markers of aberrancy when present.

Forward and Side Scatter

The scatter parameters may sometimes be overlooked in favor of more specific cluster of differentiation markers, but they serve an important role in B-ALL MRD detection. The most common abnormality is increased side scatter (SSC); normal hematogones have a significantly lower SSC than mature B cells until a very late stage of development. B-ALL blasts often have a subtle but reproducible increase in SSC that very specifically marks them as abnormal. One advantage of this SSC abnormality compared with some of the more obvious aberrancies, such as CD45 loss, is that the SSC abnormality rarely reverts over the course of treatment in which other abnormal patterns, such as loss of CD45, are subject to significant plasticity.

Many markers beyond those previously described have shown to be useful in B-ALL MRD detection, but the ones detailed here are among the most frequently used. Given the proliferation of different markers, designing an MFC panel that is optimized both for the detection of MRD and for ease of use and interpretation can be difficult. To address this issue, rigorous quantitative methods have recently been used to attempt to define optimal panel designs for MRD MFC, with different analyses converging on similar approaches.[16,26]

There are some considerations related to reporting the results of MRD MFC studies. In particular, the method by which the initial leukemic phenotype is described should be designed to provide useful information for follow-up studies, whether at the same institution or particularly if the patient is subsequently seen at another site and the diagnostic flow histograms are not available. Reporting a simple list of positive and negative markers is insufficient. "CD38-positive" fails to convey important details that help to determine whether the level of CD38 expression is different from normal. A fuller description of the phenotype should include modifiers that make the level of expression clearer. "CD38 heterogeneous" moderate or "CD81 dim" both convey that the level of expression is different than that typically seen in normal hematogones. An even more direct and useful method is to describe the phenotype and then to explicitly list which markers are aberrant and in which combinations (see later discussion for example reporting format). At the authors' institution, we use a single 8-color tube for MRD MFC, containing the markers CD9, CD10, CD19, CD20, CD34, CD38, CD45, and CD58, as reported elsewhere.[16] The advantage of a single-tube MRD panel is that it readily permits full immunophenotyping of small, sub-gated populations without needing to infer similar populations from tube to tube using a common phenotypic backbone of shared markers. However, other panels successfully use a common backbone to include a large number of markers[26] or to accommodate fewer colors.[11]

In the authors' laboratory, initial gating is performed on CD19-positive events (see later discussion for special notes on MRD testing in patients receiving anti-CD19 therapy). CD38^{++} plasma cells are removed from subsequent gates, being careful not to drop the plasma cell gate down into hematogone-level CD38 intensities, which could result in omitting blasts from analysis. This CD19-positive, nonplasma cell population, which should include normal hematogones and mature B cells, as well as possible leukemic blasts, is then analyzed with 2-dimensional histograms for every pairwise combination of CD9, CD10, CD20, CD34, CD38, and CD58, as well as combinations of forward scatter and SSC with CD10 and CD45, to assist in distinguishing high-SSC blasts (see previous note on SSC). All of these histograms are reviewed to determine which fits the phenotype of the initial sample (or is most abnormal, in cases in which no initial sample is available) while providing the best separation from normal maturing B cells. This approach provides important flexibility. If the blasts in a case are aberrantly bright for CD10, for example, that can be used as an approach for initial gating. However, in cases in which CD10 is only as bright as normal hematogones, or even negative, other gating approaches can be used (eg, bright CD58, decreased CD38, increased SSC). Alternative strategies that use fixed gates, on CD19 by CD10 or CD19 by CD34 histograms, for example, run the risk of missing small populations with less common phenotypes.

An important consideration in examining populations with the number of events necessary for assessing MRD is being careful to avoid false positives. Many of the markers used for MRD are not entirely specific for B lymphoblasts. For example, CD10 and CD58 are expressed strongly on granulocytes, and CD9 is expressed on basophils and some dendritic cells. Sub-gating on suspicious populations with careful examination by backgating into other histograms is necessary to rule out these and other confounders.

EXAMPLES OF MINIMAL RESIDUAL DISEASE ANALYSIS AND REPORTING

Carefully documenting the initial phenotype at diagnosis is a key feature for analysis of MRD, but allowances must be made for the kind of phenotypic shifts that are most frequently seen. In a diagnostic sample (**Fig. 3**A), the blast population has the following phenotype: positive for CD19, CD34, CD38, and CD58; and negative for CD10, CD20, and CD45. In this case, there are multiple useful markers or combinations of markers for MRD detection, particularly given the somewhat unusual negativity for CD10. In the histograms shown in the figure, the marked loss of CD45 and the double negativity for CD10 and CD20 (assuming a good initial gate excluding non-B cells and plasma cells, and no exposure to anti-CD20 agents) are not seen in hematogones and can be relied on. In addition, the combination of a relatively mature phenotype, such as CD10 negativity combined with the retained immature phenotype of positivity for CD34, CD38 (homogeneous), and CD58, provides more opportunities for gating away from hematogones. In a clinical report, this phenotype would best be described using the typical list of positive and negative markers, including qualifiers, such as heterogeneous, dim, and so forth, as appropriate. Furthermore, as previously discussed, an additional sentence highlighting informative markers for MRD can be useful to provide for the benefit of future interpreters. In this case, such as sentence might read, "Markers or combinations of markers suitable for future detection of MRD include CD10 by CD20, CD10 by CD34, CD10 by CD38, CD10 by CD58, and CD19 by CD45."

Analysis of MRD at day 28 of therapy for the same patient (see **Fig. 3**B) shows some of the phenotypic shifts that may occur during response to therapy. In this case, the leukemic blasts have retained portions of their phenotype. They continue to be positive for CD19, CD34, and CD58, and are negative for CD10 and CD20. However, the prior very dim CD45 has now increased to a level similar to hematogones, whereas CD38 has become much dimmer, similar to mature B cells. The increase in CD45 is a very common event in response to therapy[19,20,23] and, in this case, eliminates an initially aberrant marker combination. However, the loss of CD38 has created another set of abnormal marker pairs: retention of immature CD34 and CD58 in combination with the mature loss of CD38. Clinical reporting of this finding should include the new immunophenotype, along with a brief summary of the phenotypic shifts seen subsequent to diagnosis.

Fig. 4 demonstrates an example of the kind of false positive that may arise in MRD analysis and how to prevent it. In analyzing a CD38 by CD58 histogram gated on CD19-positive nonplasma cells, maturing hematogones (see **Fig. 4**A, teal) occupy a typical position, CD38 bright and CD58 heterogeneous positive. An apparently abnormal population of cells (see **Fig. 4**A) demonstrates a phenotype very frequently seen in B-ALL: retention of bright CD58 (in this case, even slightly brighter than normal; see previous discussion of CD58) coupled with loss of CD38. Relying on this histogram alone, this population is highly suspicious for MRD. However, the importance of backgating is demonstrated by inspection of the CD19 by CD45 histogram (see **Fig. 4**B), which clearly demonstrates that the concerning cells are actually non-B cells that have crept into the analysis due to imprecise positioning of the initial gate.

CLINICAL SIGNIFICANCE OF MINIMAL RESIDUAL DISEASE DETECTION IN B-ACUTE LYMPHOBLASTIC LEUKEMIA

MFC was first applied to MRD detection in B-ALL more than 20 years ago when Orfao and colleagues[30] showed that lymphoblasts with an aberrant phenotype could be detected by MFC in a subset of remission bone marrow samples before frank morphologic and clinical relapse. This led to a series of studies of pediatric B-ALL in the United

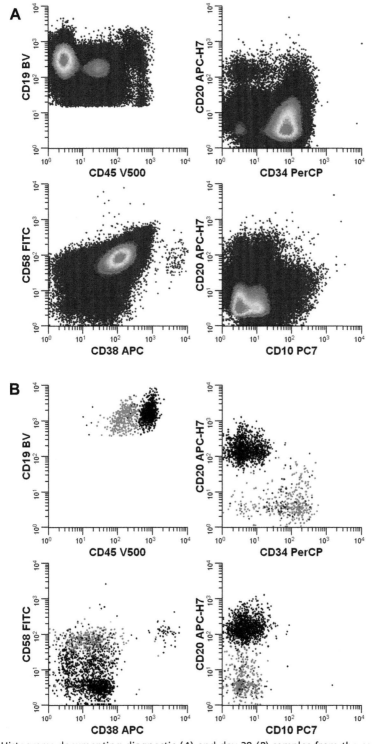

Fig. 3. Histograms documenting diagnostic (*A*) and day 28 (*B*) samples from the same patient. (*A*) The malignant blasts comprise most events and are highlighted by the warmer areas in the heat density contour map. (*B*) The leukemic blasts are red, whereas background normal B cells and hematogones are black. Note the shift in some elements of the phenotype (CD38 and CD45 intensity) between the 2 panels.

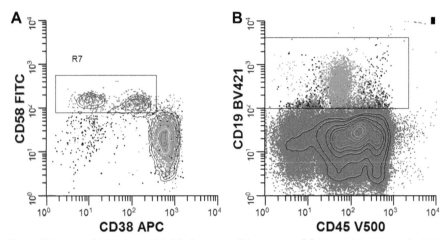

Fig. 4. This pair of histograms highlights a possible source of false positive errors in MRD analysis. Analysis of a CD38 by CD58 histogram (*A*) seems to show a population (*red*) with an immunophenotype markedly distinct from normal hematogones (*teal*) and strongly concerning for malignant blasts. Backgating to the original CD19 by CD45 histogram (*B*) makes it readily apparent that these apparently abnormal B cells are actually non-B cells creeping into the bottom of an overgenerous CD19 gate.

States and in Europe that established the prognostic value of MRD measurement.[31–34] Each of these studies measured bone marrow MRD at the end of induction chemotherapy and then at set intervals throughout therapy. They demonstrated that MRD by MFC could be applied to most patients (>90%) based on their diagnostic immunophenotype. In general, the presence of MRD was greatest at end of induction and steadily decreased throughout the course of therapy for patients who did not relapse. The presence of MRD correlated with other markers of high risk. For example, MRD was much more common in patients with *BCR/ABL1* or *KMT2A* (*MLL*) rearrangements, and less common in patients with *TEL/AML1* rearrangements or hyperdiploidy.[27,31,32] However, the presence of MRD at any point was a strong and independent predictor of relapse risk in all studies.

Further studies refined and extended these results. Coustan-Smith and colleagues[35] assayed bone marrow for MRD at an earlier time point (19 days after induction initiation) and showed that early clearance of leukemic blasts was a strong predictor of relapse-free survival. They also demonstrated that MRD could be detected in peripheral blood.[32] Although MRD was less frequent in blood than in bone marrow, its presence signaled even worse prognosis than when detected in marrow alone.

Building on these studies, the Children's Oncology Group (COG), a cooperative clinical trial group, incorporated MRD into their large clinical trials. This led to a seminal study that investigated the value of MRD detection in peripheral blood at day 8 after induction, and in bone marrow at day 29, in 2143 children with B-ALL.[36] The results confirmed the prognostic value of MRD, showing an inverse relationship between the amount of MRD and the probability of event-free survival for both early blood and later bone marrow samples. This held true even in subjects with favorable cytogenetic profiles, such that end-induction MRD was the strongest prognostic factor in multivariate analysis. These results were confirmed in subsequent large-scale trials.[37,38] Other studies have shown that this prognostic value holds for subjects who are retreated after relapse.[39,40]

Given the powerful risk-stratification afforded by MRD detection, a logical next step was application of MRD results to therapeutic strategies. Several trials have intensified therapy based on the presence or absence of MRD at the end of induction.[38,41,42] Each of these studies showed some evidence of benefit gained by giving more therapy to subjects with persistent MRD. Others have shown that the presence of MRD before hematopoietic stem cell transplant is a strong predictor of post-transplant relapse.[43–45]

Almost all of these studies have been performed on pediatric subjects, as would be expected given the higher prevalence of B-ALL in the pediatric population. Much less is known about the value of MRD detection in adults with B-ALL. However, at least 1 study demonstrated that presence of MRD is the only independent determinant of disease-free and overall survival in adolescents and adults (ages 15–60 years) with B-ALL.[46] This supports the use of MRD studies in nearly all patients and types of B-ALL.

As MRD detection by MFC has become more and more central to the clinical diagnosis and treatment of B-ALL, more attention has been paid to the logistics of coordinating methods and procedures between different institutions. As the COG undergoes a process to decentralize MFC MRD testing for B-ALL, efforts have begun to study the degree of training necessary to ensure that qualified clinical flow cytometry laboratories obtain similar results with standardized data.[47] The EuroFlow consortium has also released the results of their work on standardizing both the panels used for MFC and their interpretation.[26]

ACUTE LYMPHOBLASTIC LEUKEMIA MINIMAL RESIDUAL DISEASE IN TARGETED THERAPY

MFC detection of B-ALL MRD is complicated by 2 recent advances in therapy that target CD19. Chimeric antigen receptor T cells (CAR-T cells) are engineered to express a chimeric target-specific antibody (in this case, against CD19), such that binding of these cells to CD19-expressing B lymphoblasts (along with other, non-neoplastic CD19-expressing B cells) would result in activation of the T-cell response and destruction of the neoplastic cells.[48,49] Blinatumomab is an engineered protein that links the antigen-binding domains of anti-CD19 and anti-CD3 antibodies.[50–52] Known as a bispecific T-cell engager (BiTE), it binds both CD19-expressing B lymphoblasts with CD3-expressing T cells, bringing them into close proximity and activating the T cell, such that it destroys the lymphoblast. Both therapies have proven to be effective in some B-ALL patients who are refractory to conventional therapy.

The complicating factor of these therapies is that they lead to long-term complete elimination of CD19-expressing cells. Persistence or relapse of B-ALL in this setting will often be by lymphoblasts that have escaped therapy by down-regulating expression of CD19. All conventional MRD protocols use CD19 as the primary gating reagent by which B-lineage cells are detected. Thus, MRD may be difficult or even impossible to detect by these MFC techniques in the setting of anti-CD19 therapy. In the major anti-CD19 CAR-T trials for B-ALL, MRD detection was performed in some cases using conventional MFC based on gating for CD19[53] and in others by genetic methods based on detecting clonal rearrangements of the immunoglobulin heavy chain (IGH) gene.[54] Genetic studies looking for IGH rearrangement were also used as the method of MRD detection in the large studies evaluating the efficacy of blinatumomab.[50,55]

Alternative approaches are thus required to assess for MRD in patients on these therapies. These require the use of antibodies against other B-lineage antigens that are similarly expressed in early B-cell precursors, such as CD22, as the primary gating tools. Cherian and colleagues[56] have designed panels using these antibodies in combination with others against markers commonly aberrant in B-ALL. Using these panels, they were able to successfully detect both CD19-positive and CD19-negative B lymphoblast populations with performance comparable with conventional MRD panels.

REFERENCES

1. Rawstron AC, Böttcher S, Letestu R, et al. Improving efficiency and sensitivity: European Research Initiative in CLL (ERIC) update on the international harmonised approach for flow cytometric residual disease monitoring in CLL. Leukemia 2013;27(1):142–9.
2. Böttcher S, Ritgen M, Fischer K, et al. Minimal residual disease quantification is an independent predictor of progression-free and overall survival in chronic lymphocytic leukemia: a multivariate analysis from the randomized GCLLSG CLL8 trial. J Clin Oncol 2012;30(9):980–8.
3. Strati P, Keating MJ, Brien SMO, et al. Eradication of bone marrow minimal residual disease may prompt early treatment discontinuation in CLL. Blood 2014; 123(24):3727–32.
4. Loken MR, Alonzo TA, Pardo L, et al. Residual disease detected by multidimensional flow cytometry signifies high relapse risk in patients with de novo acute myeloid leukemia: a report from Children's Oncology Group. Blood 2012; 120(8):1581–8.
5. Hourigan CS, Karp JE. Minimal residual disease in acute myeloid leukaemia. Nat Rev Clin Oncol 2013;10(8):460–71.
6. Paiva B, Cedena M-T, Puig N, et al. Minimal residual disease monitoring and immune profiling in multiple myeloma in elderly patients. Blood 2016;127(25): 3165–74.
7. Rawstron AC, Paiva B, Stetler-Stevenson M. Assessment of minimal residual disease in myeloma and the need for a consensus approach. Cytometry B Clin Cytom 2016;90(1):21–5.
8. Teachey DT, Hunger SP. Predicting relapse risk in childhood acute lymphoblastic leukaemia. Br J Haematol 2013;162(5):606–20.
9. Wood BL. Principles of minimal residual disease detection for hematopoietic neoplasms by flow cytometry. Cytometry B Clin Cytom 2016;90(1):47–53.
10. Chen X, Wood BL. Monitoring minimal residual disease in acute leukemia: technical challenges and interpretive complexities. Blood Rev 2017;31(2):63–75.
11. Weir EG, Cowan K, LeBeau P, et al. A limited antibody panel can distinguish B-precursor acute lymphoblastic leukemia from normal B precursors with four color flow cytometry: implications for residual disease detection. Leukemia 1999; 13(4):558–67. Available at: http://www.ncbi.nlm.nih.gov/pubmed/10214862. Accessed May 6, 2014.
12. McKenna RW, Washington LT, Aquino DB, et al. Immunophenotypic analysis of hematogones (B-lymphocyte precursors) in 662 consecutive bone marrow specimens by 4-color flow cytometry. Blood 2001;98(8):2498–507. Available at: http://www.ncbi.nlm.nih.gov/pubmed/11588048.
13. McKenna RW, Asplund SL, Kroft SH. Immunophenotypic analysis of hematogones (B-lymphocyte precursors) and neoplastic lymphoblasts by 4-color flow cytometry. Leuk Lymphoma 2004;45(2):277–85. Available at: http://www.ncbi.nlm.nih.gov/pubmed/15101712. Accessed May 6, 2014.

14. Kroft SH, Asplund SL, McKenna RW, et al. Haematogones in the peripheral blood of adults: a four-colour flow cytometry study of 102 patients. Br J Haematol 2004; 126(2):209–12.
15. Seegmiller AC, Kroft SH, Karandikar NJ, et al. Characterization of immunopheno-typic aberrancies in 200 cases of B acute lymphoblastic leukemia. Am J Clin Pathol 2009;132(6):940–9.
16. Shaver AC, Greig BW, Mosse CA, et al. B-ALL minimal residual disease flow cytometry: an application of a novel method for optimization of a single-tube model. Am J Clin Pathol 2015;143(5):716–24.
17. Leitenberg D, Rappeport JM, Smith BR. B-cell precursor bone marrow reconstitution after bone marrow transplantation. Am J Clin Pathol 1994;102(2):231–6. Available at: http://www.ncbi.nlm.nih.gov/pubmed/8042594.
18. van Wering ER, van der Linden-Schrever BE, Szczepański T, et al. Regenerating normal B-cell precursors during and after treatment of acute lymphoblastic leukaemia: implications for monitoring of minimal residual disease. Br J Haematol 2000;110(1):139–46. Available at: http://www.ncbi.nlm.nih.gov/pubmed/10930991.
19. Borowitz MJ, Pullen DJ, Winick N, et al. Comparison of diagnostic and relapse flow cytometry phenotypes in childhood acute lymphoblastic leukemia: implications for residual disease detection: a report from the children's oncology group. Cytometry B Clin Cytom 2005;68(1):18–24.
20. Gaipa G, Basso G, Maglia O, et al. Drug-induced immunophenotypic modulation in childhood ALL: implications for minimal residual disease detection. Leukemia 2005;19(1):49–56.
21. Chen W, Karandikar NJ, McKenna RW, et al. Stability of leukemia-associated immunophenotypes in precursor B-lymphoblastic leukemia/lymphoma: a single institution experience. Am J Clin Pathol 2007;127(1):39–46.
22. Gaipa G, Basso G, Aliprandi S, et al. Prednisone induces immunophenotypic modulation of CD10 and CD34 in nonapoptotic B-cell precursor acute lymphoblastic leukemia cells. Cytometry B Clin Cytom 2008;74(4):150–5.
23. Dworzak MN, Gaipa G, Schumich A, et al. Modulation of antigen expression in B-cell precursor acute lymphoblastic leukemia during induction therapy is partly transient: evidence for a drug-induced regulatory phenomenon. Results of the AIEOP-BFM-ALL-FLOW-MRD-Study Group. Cytometry B Clin Cytom 2010; 78(3):147–53.
24. Wood BL. Flow cytometric monitoring of residual disease in acute leukemia. Methods Mol Biol 2013;999:123–36.
25. Rawstron AC, Fazi C, Agathangelidis A, et al. A complementary role of multiparameter flow cytometry and high-throughput sequencing for minimal residual disease detection in chronic lymphocytic leukemia: an European Research Initiative on CLL study. Leukemia 2016;30(4):929–36.
26. Theunissen P, Mejstrikova E, Sedek L, et al. Standardized flow cytometry for highly sensitive MRD measurements in B-cell acute lymphoblastic leukemia. Blood 2017;129(3):347–57.
27. Borowitz MJ, Pullen DJ, Shuster JJ, et al. Minimal residual disease detection in childhood precursor-B-cell acute lymphoblastic leukemia: relation to other risk factors. A Children's Oncology Group study. Leukemia 2003;17(8):1566–72.
28. Gaipa G, Basso G, Biondi A, et al. Detection of minimal residual disease in pediatric acute lymphoblastic leukemia. Cytometry B Clin Cytom 2013;84(6):359–69.
29. Muzzafar T, Medeiros LJ, Wang SA, et al. Aberrant underexpression of CD81 in precursor B-cell acute lymphoblastic leukemia: utility in detection of minimal residual disease by flow cytometry. Am J Clin Pathol 2009;132(5):692–8.

30. Orfao A, Ciudad J, Lopez-Berges MC, et al. Acute lymphoblastic leukemia (ALL): detection of minimal residual disease (MRD) at flow cytometry. Leuk Lymphoma 1994;13(Suppl 1):87–90.

31. Coustan-Smith E, Behm FG, Sanchez J, et al. Immunological detection of minimal residual disease in children with acute lymphoblastic leukaemia. Lancet 1998; 351(9102):550–4.

32. Coustan-Smith E, Sancho J, Hancock ML, et al. Use of peripheral blood instead of bone marrow to monitor residual disease in children with acute lymphoblastic leukemia. Blood 2002;100(7):2399–402.

33. Dworzak MN, Fröschl G, Printz D, et al. Prognostic significance and modalities of flow cytometric minimal residual disease detection in childhood acute lympho-blastic leukemia. Blood 2002;99(6):1952–8. Available at: http://www.ncbi.nlm.nih.gov/pubmed/11877265.

34. Björklund E, Mazur J, Söderhäll S, et al. Flow cytometric follow-up of minimal re-sidual disease in bone marrow gives prognostic information in children with acute lymphoblastic leukemia. Leukemia 2003;17(1):138–48.

35. Coustan-Smith E, Sancho J, Behm FG, et al. Prognostic importance of measuring early clearance of leukemic cells by flow cytometry in childhood acute lympho-blastic leukemia. Blood 2002;100(1):52–8.

36. Borowitz MJ, Devidas M, Hunger SP, et al. Clinical significance of minimal resid-ual disease in childhood acute lymphoblastic leukemia and its relationship to other prognostic factors: a Children's Oncology Group study. Blood 2008; 111(12):5477–85.

37. Bowman WP, Larsen EL, Devidas M, et al. Augmented therapy improves outcome for pediatric high risk acute lymphocytic leukemia: results of Children's Oncology Group trial P9906. Pediatr Blood Cancer 2011;57(4):569–77.

38. Borowitz MJ, Wood BL, Devidas M, et al. Prognostic significance of minimal re-sidual disease in high risk B-ALL: a report from Children's Oncology Group study AALL0232. Blood 2015;126(8):964–71.

39. Coustan-Smith E, Gajjar A, Hijiya N, et al. Clinical significance of minimal residual disease in childhood acute lymphoblastic leukemia after first relapse. Leukemia 2004;18(3):499–504.

40. Raetz EA, Borowitz MJ, Devidas M, et al. Reinduction platform for children with first marrow relapse of acute lymphoblastic leukemia: a Children's Oncology Group Study. J Clin Oncol 2008;26(24):3971–8.

41. Pui C-H, Pei D, Coustan-Smith E, et al. Clinical utility of sequential minimal resid-ual disease measurements in the context of risk-based therapy in childhood acute lymphoblastic leukaemia: a prospective study. Lancet Oncol 2015;16(4): 465–74.

42. Mullighan CG, Jeha S, Pei D, et al. Outcome of children with hypodiploid ALL treated with risk-directed therapy based on MRD levels. Blood 2015;126(26): 2896–9.

43. Leung W, Campana D, Yang J, et al. High success rate of hematopoietic cell transplantation regardless of donor source in children with very high-risk leuke-mia. Blood 2011;118(2):223–30.

44. Zhao X-S, Liu Y-R, Zhu H-H, et al. Monitoring MRD with flow cytometry: an effec-tive method to predict relapse for ALL patients after allogeneic hematopoietic stem cell transplantation. Ann Hematol 2012;91(2):183–92.

45. Leung W, Pui C-H, Coustan-Smith E, et al. Detectable minimal residual disease before hematopoietic cell transplantation is prognostic but does not preclude cure for children with very-high-risk leukemia. Blood 2012;120(2):468–72.

46. Ribera J-M, Oriol A, Morgades M, et al. Treatment of high-risk Philadelphia chromosome-negative acute lymphoblastic leukemia in adolescents and adults according to early cytologic response and minimal residual disease after consolidation assessed by flow cytometry: final results of the PETHEMA. J Clin Oncol 2014;32(15):1595–604.

47. Keeney M, Wood BL, Hedley B, et al. Experience with MRD testing in B-ALL by flow cytometry does not prevent interpretative discordance. Blood 2016;128: 2907.

48. Maude SL, Frey N, Shaw PA, et al. Chimeric antigen receptor T cells for sustained remissions in leukemia. N Engl J Med 2014;371(16):1507–17.

49. Maude SL, Teachey DT, Porter DL, et al. CD19-targeted chimeric antigen receptor T-cell therapy for acute lymphoblastic leukemia. Blood 2015;125(26):4017–23.

50. Topp MS, Gökbuget N, Stein AS, et al. Safety and activity of blinatumomab for adult patients with relapsed or refractory B-precursor acute lymphoblastic leukaemia: a multicentre, single-arm, phase 2 study. Lancet Oncol 2015;16(1): 57–66.

51. Zugmaier G, Gökbuget N, Klinger M, et al. Long-term survival and T-cell kinetics in relapsed/refractory ALL patients who achieved MRD response after blinatumomab treatment. Blood 2015;126(24):2578–84.

52. Kantarjian HM, Stein AS, Bargou RC, et al. Blinatumomab treatment of older adults with relapsed/refractory B-precursor acute lymphoblastic leukemia: results from 2 phase 2 studies. Cancer 2016;122(14):2178–85.

53. Lee DW, Kochenderfer JN, Stetler-Stevenson M, et al. T cells expressing CD19 chimeric antigen receptors for acute lymphoblastic leukaemia in children and young adults: a phase 1 dose-escalation trial. Lancet 2015;385(9967):517–28.

54. Davila ML, Riviere I, Wang X, et al. Efficacy and toxicity management of 19-28z CAR T cell therapy in B cell acute lymphoblastic leukemia. Sci Transl Med 2014;6(224):224ra25.

55. Topp MS, Gökbuget N, Zugmaier G, et al. Phase II trial of the anti-CD19 bispecific T cell-engager blinatumomab shows hematologic and molecular remissions in patients with relapsed or refractory B-precursor acute lymphoblastic leukemia. J Clin Oncol 2014;32(36):4134–40.

56. Cherian S, Miller V, McCullouch V, et al. A novel flow cytometric assay for detection of residual disease in patients with B-lymphoblastic leukemia/lymphoma post anti-CD19 therapy. Cytometry B Clin Cytom 2016. http://dx.doi.org/10.1002/cyto.b.21482.

How Do We Use Multicolor Flow Cytometry to Detect Minimal Residual Disease in Acute Myeloid Leukemia?

 CrossMark

Jie Xu, MD, PhD, Jeffrey L. Jorgensen, MD, PhD, Sa A. Wang, MD*

KEYWORDS

• Multicolor flow cytometry • Acute myeloid leukemia • Minimal residual disease

KEY POINTS

• Minimal residual disease (MRD) measurement has become an important component of acute myeloid leukemia (AML) management.

• Multicolor flow cytometry is a useful tool for MRD detection that can be used in most AML patients and is a powerful tool for risk stratification and clinical decision-making.

• AML MRD testing by flow cytometry is a complex assay but can be learned by diagnosticians and implemented at major laboratories.

• As use of this method increases, most likely in combination with molecular genetic methods of MRD measurement, understanding of the mechanisms of relapse will also increase.

• This information will assist with achievement of the ultimate goal of improved patient outcomes.

INTRODUCTION

With the current treatment regimens, many patients with acute myeloid leukemia (AML) will achieve a morphologic complete remission (CR) with the morphologic bone marrow (BM) blast count less than 5% (absolute neutrophil count greater than 1.0×10^9/L), with or without platelet recovery. However, many patients who achieve a morphologic CR after initial therapy eventually relapse.[1,2] In recent years, it has been recognized that morphologic assessment by conventional microscopy is neither sensitive nor specific in the detection of residual leukemic cells

The authors have nothing to disclose.
Department of Hematopathology, The University of Texas, MD Anderson Cancer Center, 1515 Holcombe Boulevard, Houston, TX 77030, USA
* Corresponding author. Department of Hematopathology, MD Anderson Cancer Center, 1515 Holcombe Boulevard, Unit 72, Houston, TX 77030.
E-mail address: swang5@mdanderson.org

Clin Lab Med 37 (2017) 787–802
http://dx.doi.org/10.1016/j.cll.2017.07.004
0272-2712/17/© 2017 Elsevier Inc. All rights reserved.

labmed.theclinics.com

after therapy. The presence of submicroscopic leukemic cells in the setting of morphologic CR, so-called minimal residual disease (MRD), contributes to ultimate leukemia relapse.

DETECTION OF MINIMAL RESIDUAL DISEASE IN ACUTE MYELOID LEUKEMIA BY MULTICOLOR FLOW CYTOMETRY

The morphologic blast count correlates poorly with multicolor flow cytometry (MFC) study,[3–5] indicating that reliance on morphology alone may result in a significant number of patients receiving chemotherapy that might not be necessary and, conversely, a significant number of patients with incomplete response to therapy being withheld further treatment. MFC, in conjunction with molecular and cytogenetic studies, is the most commonly used method to detect MRD in AML. MRD detection by MFC has a sensitivity of approximately 10^{-3} to 10^{-4} (0.1%–0.01%).[6] Many studies have shown a positive MFC MRD after induction and/or consolidation is correlated with an increased risk of relapse and worse survival.[7–15] Also, the presence of MRD before allogeneic hematopoietic stem cell transplantation (HSCT) is an important predictor of relapse and survival.[16–19] These studies indicate that MFC MRD can be used for risk stratification and clinical decision-making for patients with AML.

Detection of MRD by MFC is achieved by detection of immunophenotypic aberrancies on leukemic blasts (myeloblasts and/or monoblasts, or promonocytes) by using 2 major, partially overlapping analysis strategies: the first focuses on leukemia-associated immunophenotypes (LAIPs) detected at the time of diagnosis and the second is based on identifying any immunophenotypes that are different-from-normal in specimens submitted for MRD analysis. In approximately 90% of AML patients, leukemic blasts at diagnosis express a unique and specific individual or a combination of antigens, termed LAIPs, which differentiate them from normal myeloid precursors and other marrow cells. LAIPs can be categorized as (1) over or under expression of lineage and maturation stage-appropriate markers; (2) cross-lineage antigen expression, such as aberrant expression of lymphoid markers; and (3) asynchronous antigen expression (aberrant expression of antigens across maturation stages in the same lineage). In addition, abnormal forward scatter (FSC) patterns and side scatter (SSC) patterns are commonly observed in leukemic cells, further assisting in AML MRD detection. AML is a complex disease and intraleukemic immunophenotypic heterogeneity is a common finding. As a result, LAIPs in AML can be heterogeneous, with several blast populations each showing different LAIPs in a given case.[20,21]

Detecting MRD only based on LAIPs identified at the time of diagnosis can lead to some problems. LAIPs undergoing immunophenotypic shift at relapse occur in around 90% of AML.[22] A complete change in LAIPs is found in 24% of AML.[23] Antigenic drift or immunophenotypic switch may be attributed to several reasons: (1) antigenic instability in the original leukemic clone, (2) expansion of a pre-existing small subclone, or (3) emergence of a new leukemic clone. The frequent antigenic drift or immunophenotypic switch in the course of AML treatment makes LAIPs a moving target for MRD detection.[24] Furthermore, the original, pretreatment LAIPs may not be available for comparison with the post-treatment specimen, which is particularly problematic at tertiary referral centers. To circumvent these problems, a second MFC MRD analysis approach, so-called different-from-normal, can be used to distinguish abnormal leukemic blasts from normal myeloid precursors irrespective of diagnostic LAIPs. Normal hematopoietic precursors show a predictable sequential maturation pattern that can be visualized by MFC. The knowledge of normal expression must be obtained with a comprehensive control group of normal and regenerating BMs, run in the same laboratory with the same MRD panel. In most cases, it is possible to identify aberrant myeloblasts by their immunophenotypic deviation from normal expression patterns.

MD ANDERSON CANCER CENTER EXPERIENCE

MFC shows several advantages in MRD detection. It is easily accessible, relatively economical, applicable to most AML patients regardless of underlying molecular genetic alterations, and has short turn-around time. Despite these benefits, MFC in MRD detection is yet to be universally adopted due to several reasons, including the lack of standardization across different laboratories, high technical demand, and requirement of expertise and training in data analysis and interpretation. Available publications in the literature have been largely focused on the clinical impact of MFC MRD, with relatively little information on technical and analytical details. The authors have implemented an AML MRD MFC assay in their laboratory since 2012. Over the last 4 to 5 years, we have performed more than 12,000 AML MRD tests. Our results have been correlated in many cases with molecular tests, such as real-time quantitative polymerase chain reaction (PCR) or next-generation sequencing (NGS), as well as clinical outcomes, and are summarized in several publications.[1,5,15,19,25,26] The following sections illustrate the panel design, data analysis, and result interpretation, and summarize the diagnostic pearls and pitfalls. The aim is to provide practical information for pathologists or hematologists who are interested in bringing the test to their practice.

AML MRD analyses at the authors' institution are performed by pathologists who have received additional training and have demonstrated proficiency in the analysis and interpretation. FACS Canto II 8-color instruments (BD Biosciences, San Diego, CA, USA) are standardized daily using cytometer setup and tracking (CS&T) beads. In adequate specimens, a minimum of 200,000 events are acquired to achieve a potential sensitivity of 1 in 10^4 (0.01%). The sensitivity of the test varies from case to case depending on (1) the quality of the samples, (2) how distinctively the leukemic cells are different from normal (the number of aberrancies and the degree of aberrancies), and (3) if there is a large number of regenerating myeloid precursors in the background. Practically, the sensitivity ranges from 0.01% to 0.1%. The panel combinations for AML MRD by MFC are shown in **Table 1**. The fluorochrome choices have taken into account the intensity of each fluorochrome and the importance of each marker, as

Table 1
The 8-color minimal residual disease flow cytometry panel used at MD Anderson Cancer Center

FITC	PE	PerCP-Cy5.5	PE-Cy7	APC	APC-Vio770 or APC-Alexa –fluor780*	BV421/ V450**/ PacBlue***	V500
CD7	CD33	CD19	CD34	CD13	CD2	CD38	CD45
HLA-DR	CD117	CD4	CD34	CD123	CD19*	CD38	CD45
HLA-DR	CD36	CD56	CD34	CD64	CD19*	CD14**	CD45
CD5	CD25	CD22	CD34	CD38	CD19*	CD15***	CD45

* APC-Alexa-fluor780 is used as the fluorochrome.
** V450 is used as the fluorochrome.
*** PacBlue is used as the fluorochrome.

well as reducing spillover of bright signals into adjacent channels. For example, alterations in the expression levels of CD13, CD38, CD117, and CD123 are very important in identifying aberrancies; therefore, PE and APC, bright and stable colors, are chosen for these markers. CD38 is frequently the most critical marker to identify leukemic blasts; it is included in 3 of the 4 tubes, except the third tube, which focuses on monocytes. The panel is constructed based on the relationship of various markers and closely mirrors the original diagnostic acute leukemia panel. The latter approach facilitates the detection of LAIPs.

In each tube, after excluding debris and doublets, an initial wide gate (CD45dim gate) is drawn around the CD45dim blast and monocyte regions on a traditional CD45/SSC display (**Fig. 1**A), followed by back-gating to identify the CD34+ population (see **Fig. 1**B), as well as CD117+ cells on the CD45/SSC plot. Of note, CD117+ cells in normal BM include myeloid precursors, a subset of promyelocytes, early erythroid precursors, mast cells, and a subset of immature natural killer cells; therefore, CD117+ cells should not be all taken as myeloid precursors or blasts. Among the CD34+ cells, CD19 is used as an exclusion gate on most plots, to separate out normal immature precursor B cells (hematogones) and plasma cells from the CD45dim gate (see **Fig. 1**C). In cases of myeloblasts with aberrant CD19 expression, such as in AML with t(8;21) (q22;q22) (often a continuous expression pattern), this CD19 gate will be moved aside to display all blasts on all of the analysis plots. Data from each tube are evaluated for cells in the CD34+ myeloblast gate, as well as the CD45dim

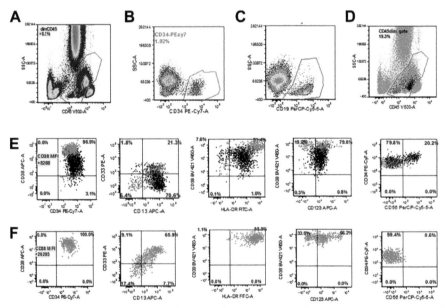

Fig. 1. Decreased CD38 allows identification of leukemic blasts. (*A*) A generous gate (so-called CD45dim gate) to include CD45dim+ cells and monocytes. (*B*) CD34+ cells are 1.02% of total events. (*C*) CD19+ hematogones are excluded from gates A and B (NOT gate). (*D*) Abnormal CD34+ myeloblasts (*black dots*) show an increased CD45 expression, whereas normal myeloid precursors and stage I hematogones (*red dots*) show a normal CD45 expression. (*E*) A subset of the CD34+ myeloblasts shows decreased CD38 (*black dots*). Other aberrancies are seen, from left to right: increased CD13, decreased HLA-DR, and aberrant CD56, together diagnostic for positive AML MRD. The remaining CD34+ cells are apparently normal myeloid precursors (*red dots*). (*F*) An example of normal CD34+ myeloid precursors is shown for comparison.

gate (see **Table 1**). The rationale behind the 2-gate analytical approach is that (1) CD34+ myeloblasts are the more resistant cells in AML post-therapy and they are the most reliable population of cells for examining aberrancies, (2) the sensitivity will drop significantly if CD34+ cells are simply colored and shown together with other cells, (3) this facilitates quantitation of the expression levels of important markers on CD34+ myeloblasts by median fluorescence intensity (MFI), and (4) examination of CD45dim+ gate is essential for the assessment of CD34-negative or partially positive AML (see later discussion of AML with monocytic differentiation). Anything unusual in the CD45dim+ gate should prompt further investigation.

Note that we do not set quadrant markers on negative control stains. Rather, markers are prepositioned and generally not shifted during analysis, thus serving as reference points for comparison with the position of benign BM elements on normal control plots. In some cases, the quads are positioned to facilitate quantitation of antigen expression levels on blasts.

Specimen Quality and Reporting

The sensitivity of AML MRD detection and, therefore, the level of robustness of a negative result depends critically on specimen quality. BM aspirates obtained after induction or consolidation therapy may be paucicellular, with too few cells available for acquisition of the 200,000 or more events per tube required for full sensitivity.

Positive for aberrant myeloblasts
A diagnosis of positive for aberrant myeloblasts will be established when the following are detected: (1) greater than or equal to 20 clustered events with greater than or equal to 2 aberrant markers, whether present in the original, diagnostic, pretreatment sample or not; (2) greater than or equal to 20 clustered events with only 1 aberrant marker markedly deviated from normal; or (3) less than 20 events that show multiple, highly distinctive aberrations. The levels of aberrant myeloblasts are reported as an approximate percentage of total events, after exclusion of unlysed red blood cells with low FSC. Note that a positive diagnosis may be obtained even from a limited, paucicellular specimen.

The interpretation of these aberrant myeloblasts as AML MRD, a preleukemic clone, or a subclone of the pretreatment AML can be challenging. In general, if the residual blasts are immunophenotypically similar to the original blasts, or at least share some similarity, a case may be considered to be positive for AML MRD. On the other hand, if an immunophenotype is significantly different from the original AML blasts, these cells may represent preleukemic cells, a subclone of the original AML, or complete antigen drift. To differentiate preleukemic cells from therapy selection of an AML subclone or complete antigen drift carries significant uncertainty; however, in an elderly patient with a preexisting MDS, MPN, or myelodysplastic syndrome (MDS)-myeloproliferative neoplasm (MPN), or a patient with a history of chronic cytopenia, the former interpretation is favored.

Negative for aberrant myeloblasts
In an adequate specimen, it seems reasonable to assert that, at the present time, no detection of MRD by MFC can be considered negative, given the heterogeneity of AML in general, as well as within an individual patient. A report on a negative result should include information on the level of sensitivity of the assay. This is now a requirement for laboratories certified in the United States by the College of American Pathologists (Flow Cytometry Checklist under the College of American Pathologists CAP Laboratory Accreditation Program Checklists; August 2016; Northfield, IL,

USA, College of American Pathologists; 2016). In a limited specimen, the sensitivity of MRD detection by MFC is decreased significantly and a negative result may not be appropriate for clinical decision-making or for correlation with outcome in a clinical trial. If there are 50,000 to 200,000 events per tube, we report it as no AML MRD identified by flow cytometry, in a limited specimen. If the total events are less than 50,000 in each tube, we report it as a markedly limited specimen, insufficient for assessment for AML MRD by flow cytometry.

Indeterminate for aberrant myeloblasts

Occasional specimens will contain a myeloid precursor population with mild or borderline phenotypic alterations that appear different from normal but also different from the original blast immunophenotype and, overall, do not meet the criteria for the positive described previously. In this situation, we report it as an atypical phenotype of uncertain significance, indeterminate for AML MRD, and add a comment stating the differential diagnosis includes an atypical recovery phenotype, an underlying dysplastic or preleukemic clone, or residual AML with phenotypic shifts. The clinical significance of these blast populations is as yet uncertain, but their presence may suggest closer follow-up of these patients. In the authors' experience, in some patients, these phenotypes may persist in subsequent specimens, compatible with a persistent dysplastic or preleukemic clone.

Analysis Strategy I: Focusing on CD34+ Cells

Patterns and expression levels of antigens on normal CD34+ myeloid precursors

AML MRD detection relies on the detection of changes on CD34+ myeloblasts that are not normal or do not appear to be consistent with reactive or regenerative changes. As a result, before implementation of this assay, the AML MRD panel and markers should be assessed in several normal BM samples to establish their normal patterns and the ranges of expression levels. Some atypical changes can be seen in the BMs of patients who have received chemotherapy or growth factors, are status or post-HSCT, or who have comorbid conditions. These may appear different from normal compared with an unperturbed marrow; therefore, the normal BM testing should include a reasonable array of BM samples from patients who do not have a hematopoietic myeloid neoplasm but have various medical conditions, or are recovering from treatment. Specimens that are negative by a molecular diagnostic test, particularly by reverse-transcription–PCR for a recurrent translocation, are particularly useful as normal controls. Archived normal control data plots (from unperturbed and recovering marrow specimens) can be used for side-by-side comparison to new MRD specimens. The normal ranges should allow some changes to fall into a borderline (indeterminate) category, in addition to abnormal and normal. Borderline values overlap with a neoplastic or a regenerating or reactive condition, and should be handled with caution (see later discussion).

Based on the established normal patterns and ranges, CD34+ cells in an MRD specimen are assessed for abnormalities. It can be particularly helpful to use archived analyses from normal controls for side-by-side comparison, especially for beginners. For instance, maturation of normal CD34+ myeloid precursors is accompanied by a gradual decline in CD13 and CD33 expression. When CD13 and CD33 are plotted against each other, a characteristic diagonal or slightly curved toward CD33 pattern is formed (see **Fig. 1**E, F). Leukemic blasts may show abnormal CD13 versus CD33 pattern outside of the normal area, allowing for their identification (see **Fig. 1**E). The normal ranges for expression levels (MFI) of certain important antigens, such as CD13, CD34, CD38, CD117, CD123, and HLA-DR, are established based on control

BM samples, providing objective numbers in addition to eyeballing (visual) inspection. Altered expression levels, such as increased CD13, CD34, CD117, and/or CD123 expression or decreased CD38 and/or HLA-DR expression, occur frequently on CD34+ AML blasts. Among these alterations, decreased CD38 is especially useful in identifying small numbers of leukemic blasts (see **Fig.** 1D, E; CD34+, CD38dimmer+ leukemic blasts with an abnormal CD13 versus CD33 pattern, increased CD45, partial CD123, decreased HLA-DR, and partial CD56) in a background of normal CD34+ myeloid precursors (see **Fig.** 1D, E). Simultaneously, one needs to be aware that CD34+ cells with decreased CD38 can also be normal early stage CD34+ myeloid precursors, frequently seen as a subset in a regenerating BM. The immunophenotype of this subset of early CD34+ myeloid precursors is highly predictable[27] and usually shows brighter expression of CD34 and CD45 (**Fig. 2**A); dimmer expression of CD13, CD33, CD117, CD123, and HLA-DR; and a low level of CD4 (see **Fig. 2**B). Antigenic alterations that are often observed on CD34+ leukemic blasts are listed in **Table 2**.

Regenerating bone marrow, negative for minimal residual disease

Normal CD34+ myeloid precursors can be significantly increased in an actively regenerating BM. By conventional criteria, greater than or equal to 5% blasts by microscopic counting in a postinduction BM would be considered to be positive for residual AML. However, it has been shown that, in children, up to 50% patients who had greater than or equal to 5% blasts in the postinduction BMs did not have residual AML.[3] In adult AML, this occurs less frequently, but at the authors' institution, approximately 1% to 5% BMs with greater than or equal to 5% blasts by morphologic examination have an immunophenotype consistent with regenerating BM.[5] These patients may be able to avoid unnecessary additional induction chemotherapy. The regenerating blasts show normal patterns and expression levels of CD13, CD38 (bright), CD117, CD123, and HLA-DR (**Fig. 3**B, C). Extra caution is needed for the interpretation of aberrant lymphoid antigen expression

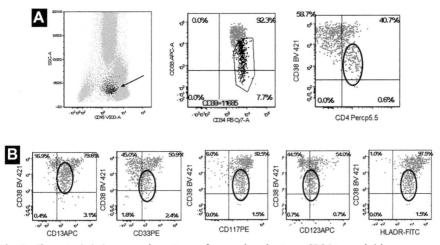

Fig. 2. Characteristic immunophenotype of normal early stage CD34+ myeloid precursors. Normal early-stage CD34+ myeloid precursors (*black dots* and *black circle*) are characterized by (*A*) increased expression of CD45 (*black arrow*), CD34 (*black dots*), and CD4 (*black circle*) and (*B*) dimmer expression of CD13, CD33, CD117, CD123, and HLA-DR.

Table 2
Alterations frequently observed in CD34+ acute myeloid leukemia blasts

Alterations by Categories	Markers
Antigen expression levels	
Decreased	CD38, HLA-DR, CD33
Increased	CD117, CD123, CD13, CD34
Increased or decreased	CD45, SSC
Cross-lineage antigen expression (eg, expression of lymphoid-associated antigens on myeloblasts or monocytes)	CD2, CD5, CD7, CD19, CD22, CD56
Asynchronous antigen expression (eg, expression of markers associated with maturity with markers associated with immaturity)	CD4, CD64, CD15

on myeloid precursors. CD2 and CD22 can be expressed in a subset of normal CD34+ CD38+ bright cells, likely corresponding to normal plasmacytoid dendritic cell precursors within the normal myeloid precursor compartment (see **Fig. 3**B). Low levels of CD7 expression can be seen on a subset of normal myeloid precursors, and the expression of CD7 may be increased in a regenerating marrow (see **Fig. 3**C). A useful tip to differentiate normal or regenerating changes from aberrant expression is that on benign myeloid precursors, CD2 and CD7 are often partially expressed on CD38 brighter+, CD13 and CD33 low or negative cells (see **Fig. 3**C); whereas on aberrant blasts they are often expressed on CD38 dimmer+, CD13 and CD33 brighter+ cells. Unlike CD2, CD7, and CD22, in the authors' experience, no expression of CD5, CD19, or CD56 should be seen on normal CD34+ myeloid precursors.

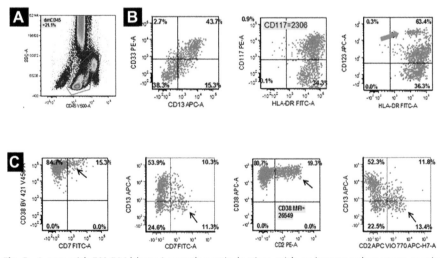

Fig. 3. A case with 5% BM blasts 1-month postinduction, with an immunophenotype consistent with benign regenerating myeloid precursors. (A) CD45dim gate to include CD45dim+ cells and monocytes. (B) Normal patterns and levels of antigen expressions on CD34+ myeloid precursors in regenerating marrow. Green arrow shows plasmacytoid dendritic cell precursors. (C) Black arrows show, from left to right: partial CD7 expression and partial CD2 expression on CD38 brighter+, CD13 low or negative cells.

Positive acute myeloid leukemia minimal residual disease, with
leukemia-associated immunophenotypes similar to original blasts

Although LAIPs undergo immunophenotypic shift at relapse in 91% of AML,[22] in the first post-treatment BM, residual leukemic blasts are often immunophenotypically similar to the pretreatment AML blasts. The original blasts (**Fig. 4**A) were positive for CD34, CD38 (decreased), CD123 (increased), HLA-DR, CD7 (very small subset), CD56, and CD5 (very small subset). The post-treatment CD34+ myeloblasts (see **Fig. 4**B) showed multiple aberrancies, including decreased CD38, increased CD123, increased CD7 (partial), and aberrant expression of CD56 (partial) and CD5 (partial). The post-treatment leukemic blasts were immunophenotypically similar to the original blasts, except that a subset of the original blasts had bright CD123 expression, but this population was not seen in the post-treatment BM. Of note, for alterations falling into borderline ranges, such as borderline increases in the expression of CD13, CD117, and/or CD123, if they are similar to the pretreatment AML blasts, they can be used as additional evidence in confirming the presence of residual AML. In contrast, if they are completely different from original AML, these borderline changes would be considered atypical but not diagnostic for residual AML.

Positive for aberrant myeloblasts, with a phenotype completely different
from original blasts

As noted previously, a complete change in LAIPs is found in 24% of AMLs post-therapy.[23] The immunophenotypic change can be due to several reasons:

1. A minor subclone of the leukemic cells, with an immunophenotype different from the predominant population of blasts, may survive therapy and appear to be a different myeloblast population at AML MRD detection.[28]
2. AML in the elderly is an extremely complex disease and leukemogenesis is a multi-step process with sequential acquisition of molecular genetic events, which more

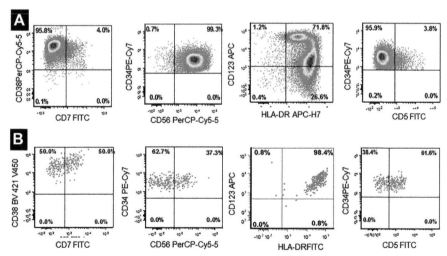

Fig. 4. A case positive for AML MRD showing therapy selection of a subset of original blasts. (A) The original blasts are, from left to right: CD38+ (decreased), CD7+ (very small subset), CD34+, CD56+ (bright and uniform), CD123+ (2 populations), and CD5 (very small subset). (B) Post-treatment CD34+ myeloblasts show an immunophenotype, indicating the selection of a subset of original blasts with CD7+ (large subset), CD56+ (partial), CD123+ (bright), CD5+ (large subset).

commonly evolves from an antecedent hematological disorder.[29–34] Preleukemic cells,[35,36] often present at a small number of cells at the time of AML diagnosis, may be more resistant to chemotherapy that targets actively proliferating cells.

3. AML cells may undergo clonal evolution, clonal regression, or both simultaneously. The latter occurs less frequently in the first BM after high-dose induction chemotherapy. However, with recent modifications of AML therapy in the elderly, such as the use of hypomethylating agents with or without various small molecule inhibitors,[26,29,37] the induction treatment course may take much longer than the standard induction chemotherapy. As a result, clonal evolution or regression may occur more frequently.

4. Treatment may alter the expression levels of some markers.[25]

Due to these reasons, the strategy of different-from-normal method should be used, in combination with the knowledge of the diagnostic LAIPs, if available. An example is shown in **Fig. 5**. The original blasts were negative for CD34 and HLA-DR, and positive for CD38, CD123, and CD117 (see **Fig. 5**A), with a normal karyotype and mutations of *DNMT3A*, *NPM1*, and *TET2* by NGS. At the time of diagnosis, the CD34+ myeloblasts were too few to be characterized properly. After therapy, no cells with the original LAIPs were identified (see **Fig. 5**B). However, a population of CD34+ CD117+ blasts were detected in the CD45dim gate, and they were positive for CD38 (bright), CD117 (increased), CD123 (increased), and HLA-DR (bright) (see **Fig. 5**B), and immunophenotypically completely different from the original blasts but aberrant. The diagnosis of positive for aberrant myeloblasts by MFC was supported by persistent mutations of *DNMT3A* and *TET2* (negative for *NPM1* mutation). Given that the blasts with complete different phenotype appear in a short time (2–3 months) and carry persistent *DNMT3A* and *TET2* mutations, this likely represents the underlying dysplastic or preleukemic clone. It is arguable that these cells are not really AML MRD per se, and molecular studies have shown that they

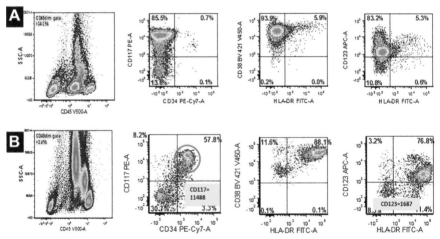

Fig. 5. A case positive for aberrant myeloblasts with a phenotype completely different from the original blasts. (*A*) The original myeloblasts are, from left to right: CD45dim+, CD34-, CD117+, HLA-DR- (markedly decreased), CD38+ (slightly decreased), and CD123+ (increased). (*B*) After treatment, CD45dim gate includes a small population of CD34+ CD117+ HLA-DR+ cells (*red circle*) with abnormally increased CD117 and CD123 expression. No cells with the original LAIPs are identified.

may persist through long clinical remissions.[35,36] However, the presence of these cells in some cases may be responsible for ultimate AML recurrence and further disease-modifying therapy may be considered. The patient in **Fig. 5** received hematopoietic stem cell transplantation (HSCT) shortly, and his BM 35 days status post SCT was negative for AML MRD by MFC and negative for *NPM1* mutation by qualitative PCR (*DNMT3A* and *TET2* mutations were not tested).

Acute myeloid leukemia with monocytic differentiation

It can be very challenging to analyze MRD for AML with monocytic differentiation, such as acute myelomonocytic leukemia (AMML; aka FAB AML, M4), acute monoblastic and monocytic leukemia (AMoL; aka FAB AML, M5a and M5b), and AML arising from chronic myelomonocytic leukemia. Distinguishing immature monocytes (monoblasts or promonocytes) from mature ones is very difficult and, in many cases, not possible by immunophenotyping. First, there are no highly specific immunophenotypic markers for immature monocytes. Complete loss of CD14 expression often indicates immaturity; however, this occurs in only a small subset of cases. Other markers, such as decreased CD13, CD36, and/or HLA-DR, and increased CD15 expression, are often observed in immature monocytes; however, these alterations are less specific as they can also be seen in reactive or dysplastic monocytes. Secondly, after therapy, neoplastic immature monocytes may show further immunophenotypic maturation or differentiation. On the other hand, after chemotherapy or HSCT, there are often many reactive monocytes that can show immunophenotypic atypia, such as increased expression of CD56 and decreased HLADR and CD45. Furthermore, it is not uncommon to have a small subset of neoplastic monocytes mixed with background reactive monocytes, making it nearly impossible for detection. Therefore, for AML with monocytic differentiation, it is not reliable to evaluate MRD based only on comparing the pretreatment and post-treatment monocytes. In the authors' experience, it is often more useful to focus the analysis of CD34+ myeloblasts in the post-treatment BM samples.

At diagnosis, AMML usually has both myeloblasts (CD34+ CD117+) and monoblasts or promonocytes. After therapy, the detection of aberrant CD34+ myeloblasts, regardless of the presence or absence of abnormal monocytes, is diagnostic for a positive MRD. An example of AML, M4 is shown in **Fig. 6**. The original myeloblast component was positive for CD13 (increased), CD33 (abnormal CD13 versus CD33 pattern), CD34, CD38 (decreased), CD123 (increased), and HLA-DR (decreased) (**see Fig. 6A**). The monocytic component (see **Fig. 6C**) was positive for CD64, CD14 (decreased), CD36 (decreased), and negative for CD34 and CD117. This case was positive for inv16 (p13.1q22) by chromosomal analysis and *CBFB-MYH11* by fluorescence in situ hybridization (FISH); therefore, the final diagnosis was AML with inv16(p13.1q22). The post-treatment monocytic elements (see **Fig. 6D**) appeared to be normal and mature (positive for CD64, CD14, CD36 [bright], and negative for CD34 and CD117). However, CD34+ myeloblasts show persistent immunophenotypic aberrancies (see **Fig. 6B**), similar to the original AML. The diagnosis of a positive MRD by MFC in this specimen was supported by chromosomal analysis and a FISH study. If MRD assessment of this case was based on monocytes only, it would be falsely called negative for MRD. In AMoL (both M5a and M5b), typically at the time of diagnosis, there are very few CD34+ myeloblasts, often too few to be properly characterized; the blasts seem to be exclusively of monocytic cells (monoblasts, promonocytes, and monocytes). Post-treatment, if it is a CR and recovering BM, normal CD34+ myeloid precursors should emerge and exhibit a normal phenotype. Conversely, in a BM with residual disease, the CD34+ myeloblasts, which are likely to be the precursor to monocytic blasts,

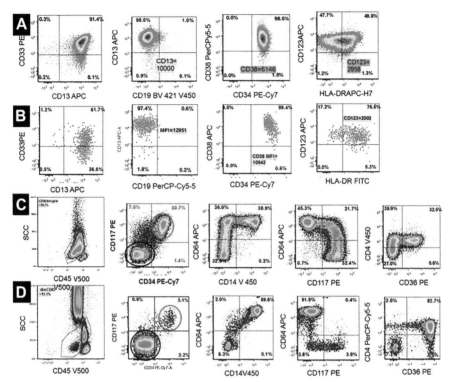

Fig. 6. A case of AML with myelomonocytic differentiation. (*A*) At diagnosis, the CD34+ myeloblasts show, from left to right: an abnormal CD13/33 pattern (uniform cluster), increased CD13, decreased CD38, increased CD123, and decreased (partial) HLA-DR expression. (*B*) The post-treatment CD34+ myeloblasts are immunophenotypically similar to the original blasts, positive for MRD. (*C*) At diagnosis, the CD45dim gate contains almost equal numbers of CD34+ blasts (*red circle*) and monocytes (*black circle*). The monocytes are, from left to right: CD34-, CD117-, CD14+ partial (decreased in a large subset), CD64 bright+, CD36+ partial (decreased in a large subset), and CD4+ (dim). (*D*) After treatment, the CD45dim gate contains predominantly monocytes (*black circle*), with a minor population of CD34+ blasts (*red circle*). The monocytes are, from left to right: CD34-, CD117-, CD64+, CD14+, CD36+, and CD4+, overall immunophenotypically unremarkable.

would appear to be relatively expanded and demonstrate immunophenotypic aberrancies. Therefore, focusing on CD34+ myeloblasts is still the best approach in AMoL cases. Overall, for AML with monocytic differentiation, if post-treatment monocytes are immunophenotypically abnormal, it is usually not diagnostic but may help support a diagnosis of a positive MRD in conjunction with the detection of abnormal CD34+ myeloblasts. If monocytes are normal, it does not equate to a negative MRD. The authors' recommendation when assessing MRD for AML with monocytic differentiation is to focus on CD34+ myeloblasts.

Analysis Strategy II: Assessing CD45dim Gate to Identify CD34-Negative, Nonmonocytic Blasts

Due to the heterogeneous nature of AML blasts, it is also important to carefully evaluate the CD45dim gate for CD34-negative myeloblasts. This is especially important for

AML with CD34-negative myeloblasts that are not monocytic because these blasts tend to retain the same immunophenotype at the time of MRD detection. On the other hand, for the previously mentioned reasons (ie, immunophenotypic switch or drift, subclone selection, or clonal evolution or regression may occur), examination of CD34-negative CD45dim+ cells is essential for AML MRD detection. An example is shown in **Fig. 7**. At diagnosis, the blasts were positive for CD33, CD13 (partial), CD117, CD123 (increased), and negative for CD34 and HLA-DR (see **Fig. 7A**), with a normal karyotype and positive for *DNMT3A*, *IDH2*, and *NPM1* mutations by NGS. The pretreatment CD34+ blasts were too few to assess for their immunophenotype. After therapy, CD34+ myeloblasts appeared as a discrete population with increased CD123 expression, aberrant but different from the original AML blasts (see **Fig. 7B**). A close examination of CD45dim gate identified abnormal CD34-negative blasts (see **Fig. 7C**), immunophenotypically similar to the original blasts. This case was positive for MRD by MFC, supported by the presence of very low level of *NPM1* (<5%) mutation, as well as persistent *IDH2* mutation, but negative for *DNMT3A* mutation. After further therapy, the CD34-negative myeloblasts were no longer detectable, but the abnormal CD34+ myeloblasts remained. NGS studies were negative for *NPM1* and *DNMT3a* mutations but showed persistent *IDH2* mutation, indicating preleukemic cells or an underlying MDS clone.

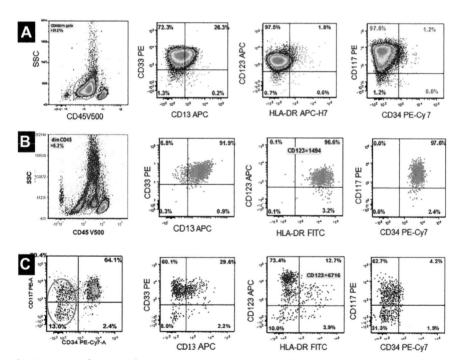

Fig. 7. A case of AML with CD34-negative, nonmonocytic blasts. (A) The original blasts are, from left to right: CD13+ (decreased, dim or partial), CD33+, HLA-DR- (markedly decreased), CD123+ (increased), CD34-, and CD117+. (B) Post-treatment CD34+ myeloblasts are, from left to right: CD13+, CD33+, HLA-DR+, CD123+ (increased), CD117+, CD38+ (bright), immunophenotypically abnormal. (C) Examination of the CD45dim gate (post-treatment specimen) shows CD34-negative blasts (*red circle*): from left to right: they are CD13+ (dim or partial), CD33+, HLA-DR-, CD123+ (increased), CD34-, and CD117+, immunophenotypically similar to the original blasts.

SUMMARY

MRD measurement has become an important component of AML management. It should ideally be assessed in any post-treatment marrow samples. MFC is a useful tool for MRD detection, which can be used in most AML patients, and is a powerful tool for risk stratification and clinical decision-making. AML MRD testing by flow cytometry is a complex assay but can be learned by diagnosticians and implemented at major laboratories. As use of this method increases, most likely in combination with molecular genetic methods of MRD measurement, understanding of the mechanisms of relapse will also increase. This information will assist with achievement of the ultimate goal of improved patient outcomes.

REFERENCES

1. Ravandi F. Relapsed acute myeloid leukemia: why is there no standard of care? Best Pract Res Clin Haematol 2013;26(3):253–9.
2. Bachas C, Schuurhuis GJ, Assaraf YG, et al. The role of minor subpopulations within the leukemic blast compartment of AML patients at initial diagnosis in the development of relapse. Leukemia 2012;26(6):1313–20.
3. Inaba H, Coustan-Smith E, Cao X, et al. Comparative analysis of different approaches to measure treatment response in acute myeloid leukemia. J Clin Oncol 2012;30(29):3625–32.
4. Loken MR, Alonzo TA, Pardo L, et al. Residual disease detected by multidimensional flow cytometry signifies high relapse risk in patients with de novo acute myeloid leukemia: a report from Children's Oncology Group. Blood 2012; 120(8):1581–8.
5. Ouyang J, Goswami M, Peng J, et al. Comparison of multiparameter flow cytometry immunophenotypic analysis and quantitative RT-PCR for the detection of minimal residual disease of core binding factor acute myeloid leukemia. Am J Clin Pathol 2016;145(6):769–77.
6. Buccisano F, Maurillo L, Del Principe MI, et al. Prognostic and therapeutic implications of minimal residual disease detection in acute myeloid leukemia. Blood 2012;119(2):332–41.
7. Venditti A, Buccisano F, Del Poeta G, et al. Level of minimal residual disease after consolidation therapy predicts outcome in acute myeloid leukemia. Blood 2000; 96(12):3948–52.
8. Kern W, Voskova D, Schoch C, et al. Determination of relapse risk based on assessment of minimal residual disease during complete remission by multiparameter flow cytometry in unselected patients with acute myeloid leukemia. Blood 2004;104(10):3078–85.
9. Sievers EL, Lange BJ, Alonzo TA, et al. Immunophenotypic evidence of leukemia after induction therapy predicts relapse: results from a prospective Children's Cancer Group study of 252 patients with acute myeloid leukemia. Blood 2003; 101(9):3398–406.
10. San Miguel JF, Martinez A, Macedo A, et al. Immunophenotyping investigation of minimal residual disease is a useful approach for predicting relapse in acute myeloid leukemia patients. Blood 1997;90(6):2465–70.
11. Feller N, van der Pol MA, van Stijn A, et al. MRD parameters using immunophenotypic detection methods are highly reliable in predicting survival in acute myeloid leukaemia. Leukemia 2004;18(8):1380–90.
12. San Miguel JF, Vidriales MB, Lopez-Berges C, et al. Early immunophenotypical evaluation of minimal residual disease in acute myeloid leukemia identifies

different patient risk groups and may contribute to postinduction treatment stratification. Blood 2001;98(6):1746–51.

13. Buccisano F, Maurillo L, Gattei V, et al. The kinetics of reduction of minimal residual disease impacts on duration of response and survival of patients with acute myeloid leukemia. Leukemia 2006;20(10):1783–9.

14. Freeman SD, Virgo P, Couzens S, et al. Prognostic relevance of treatment response measured by flow cytometric residual disease detection in older patients with acute myeloid leukemia. J Clin Oncol 2013;31(32):4123–31.

15. Ravandi F, Jorgensen J, Borthakur G, et al. Persistence of minimal residual disease assessed by multiparameter flow cytometry is highly prognostic in younger patients with acute myeloid leukemia. Cancer 2017;123(3):426–35.

16. Walter RB, Buckley SA, Pagel JM, et al. Significance of minimal residual disease before myeloablative allogeneic hematopoietic cell transplantation for AML in first and second complete remission. Blood 2013;122(10):1813–21.

17. Walter RB, Gooley TA, Wood BL, et al. Impact of pretransplantation minimal residual disease, as detected by multiparametric flow cytometry, on outcome of myeloablative hematopoietic cell transplantation for acute myeloid leukemia. J Clin Oncol 2011;29(9):1190–7.

18. Appelbaum FR. Measurement of minimal residual disease before and after myeloablative hematopoietic cell transplantation for acute leukemia. Best Pract Res Clin Haematol 2013;26(3):279–84.

19. Oran B, Jorgensen JL, Marin D, et al. Pre-transplantation minimal residual disease with cytogenetic and molecular diagnostic features improves risk stratification in acute myeloid leukemia. Haematologica 2017;102(1):110–7.

20. Kern W, Haferlach C, Haferlach T, et al. Monitoring of minimal residual disease in acute myeloid leukemia. Cancer 2008;112(1):4–16.

21. Kern W, Bacher U, Haferlach C, et al. The role of multiparameter flow cytometry for disease monitoring in AML. Best Pract Res Clin Haematol 2010;23(3):379–90.

22. Baer MR, Stewart CC, Dodge RK, et al. High frequency of immunophenotype changes in acute myeloid leukemia at relapse: implications for residual disease detection (Cancer and Leukemia Group B Study 8361). Blood 2001;97(11): 3574–80.

23. Voskova D, Schoch C, Schnittger S, et al. Stability of leukemia-associated aberrant immunophenotypes in patients with acute myeloid leukemia between diagnosis and relapse: comparison with cytomorphologic, cytogenetic, and molecular genetic findings. Cytometry B Clin Cytom 2004;62(1):25–38.

24. Zeijlemaker W, Gratama JW, Schuurhuis GJ. Tumor heterogeneity makes AML a "moving target" for detection of residual disease. Cytometry B Clin Cytom 2014; 86(1):3–14.

25. Huang L, Garcia-Manero G, Jabbour E, et al. Persistence of immunophenotypically aberrant CD34+ myeloid progenitors is frequent in bone marrow of patients with myelodysplastic syndromes and myelodysplastic/myeloproliferative neoplasms treated with hypomethylating agents. J Clin Pathol 2016;69:1001–8.

26. Quintas-Cardama A, Ravandi F, Liu-Dumlao T, et al. Epigenetic therapy is associated with similar survival compared with intensive chemotherapy in older patients with newly diagnosed acute myeloid leukemia. Blood 2012;120(24): 4840–5.

27. van Rhenen A, Moshaver B, Kelder A, et al. Aberrant marker expression patterns on the CD34+CD38- stem cell compartment in acute myeloid leukemia allows to distinguish the malignant from the normal stem cell compartment both at diagnosis and in remission. Leukemia 2007;21(8):1700–7.

28. Ding L, Ley TJ, Larson DE, et al. Clonal evolution in relapsed acute myeloid leukaemia revealed by whole-genome sequencing. Nature 2012;481(7382): 506–10.

29. Pollyea DA, Kohrt HE, Medeiros BC. Acute myeloid leukaemia in the elderly: a review. Br J Haematol 2011;152(5):524–42.

30. Heinemann V, Jehn U. Acute myeloid leukemia in the elderly: biological features and search for adequate treatment. Ann Hematol 1991;63(4):179–88.

31. Medeiros BC, Othus M, Fang M, et al. Prognostic impact of monosomal karyotype in young adult and elderly acute myeloid leukemia: the Southwest Oncology Group (SWOG) experience. Blood 2010;116(13):2224–8.

32. Wilson CS, Davidson GS, Martin SB, et al. Gene expression profiling of adult acute myeloid leukemia identifies novel biologic clusters for risk classification and outcome prediction. Blood 2006;108(2):685–96.

33. de Jonge HJ, de Bont ES, Valk PJ, et al. AML at older age: age-related gene expression profiles reveal a paradoxical down-regulation of p16INK4A mRNA with prognostic significance. Blood 2009;114(14):2869–77.

34. Rao AV, Valk PJ, Metzeler KH, et al. Age-specific differences in oncogenic pathway dysregulation and anthracycline sensitivity in patients with acute myeloid leukemia. J Clin Oncol 2009;27(33):5580–6.

35. Majeti R. Clonal evolution of pre-leukemic hematopoietic stem cells precedes human acute myeloid leukemia. Best Pract Res Clin Haematol 2014;27(3–4): 229–34.

36. Majeti R, Weissman IL. Human acute myelogenous leukemia stem cells revisited: there's more than meets the eye. Cancer Cell 2011;19(1):9–10.

37. Al-Ali HK, Jaekel N, Niederwieser D. The role of hypomethylating agents in the treatment of elderly patients with AML. J Geriatr Oncol 2014;5(1):89–105.

Flow Cytometric Assessment of Chronic Myeloid Neoplasms

Min Shi, MD, PhD, Phuong Nguyen, MD,
Dragan Jevremovic, MD, PhD*

KEYWORDS

- Flow cytometry • Myelodysplastic syndrome • Myeloid neoplasm • Diagnosis

KEY POINTS

- Flow cytometry immunophenotyping of the cells from the bone marrow can be used to help with diagnosis, prognosis, and therapy of chronic myeloid neoplasms.
- The number of abnormalities detected by flow cytometry correlates with disease severity and cytogenetic complexity.
- Scoring systems have been developed to quantify aberrancies for diagnostic and prognostic purposes.
- Flow cytometry remains only an adjunct diagnostic modality, which has to be correlated with clinical, morphologic, and genetic findings.

INTRODUCTION

Chronic myeloid neoplasms, including myelodysplastic syndrome (MDS), myeloproliferative neoplasms (MPN), and MDS/MPN, are clonal disorders of hematopoietic stem cells. They manifest as aberrancies of number, morphology and/or function in one or multiple lineages of hematopoietic elements. The World Health Organization classification of myeloid neoplasms is based on a mixture of clinical, morphologic, and genetic criteria.[1–3] The role of flow cytometry immunophenotyping (FCIP) in the diagnosis, classification, prognosis, and management of chronic myeloid neoplasms remains controversial, mainly owing to the lack of established standardized criteria. Nevertheless, an increasing number of mostly academic health care centers incorporate FCIP in the routine workup of patients with myeloid malignancies. This review is primarily centered on FCIP in MDS because that is the focus of the vast majority of studies so

Disclosure Statement: The authors have nothing to disclose.
Division of Hematopathology, Mayo Clinic, 200 1st Street Southwest, Hilton 8, Rochester, MN 55905, USA
* Corresponding author.
E-mail address: Jevremovic.dragan@mayo.edu

Clin Lab Med 37 (2017) 803–819
http://dx.doi.org/10.1016/j.cll.2017.07.006
0272-2712/17/© 2017 Elsevier Inc. All rights reserved.

labmed.theclinics.com

far. Because the number and extent of phenotypic changes are correlated with the degree of dysplasia, the changes are less prevalent, and not as applicable in MPN.

HISTORY AND RATIONALE FOR MYELOID FLOW CYTOMETRY IMMUNOPHENOTYPING

The history of FCIP in the diagnosis of chronic myeloid neoplasms can be roughly divided in 3 phases. In the first phase, from the mid 1980s to the mid 1990s, a scarcity of antibodies for hematopoietic cells resulted in rare published observations, most of which focused on apoptotic features, ploidy assessment, and proliferative index of cells in MDS.[4–10] From the mid 1990s to the mid 2000s, there was an increasing number of reported changes in myelopoiesis that could be detected by FCIP. Most of these studies were qualitative and correlative in nature, identifying FCIP aberrancies that correspond with the diagnosis of MDS.[11–17] Finally, since about the mid 2000s, there has been a stronger advocacy within the flow cytometry community for a quantitative approach and standardization among different laboratories.[18–21] The newly published studies have become more rigorous in determining the predictive value of FCIP changes in MDS, with longer clinical follow-up, and potential therapeutic impact.[22,23]

The basis of FCIP in the diagnosis of myeloid neoplasms is the ability to distinguish normal from abnormal myeloid cells. If we think of genetic and epigenetic changes as a root cause of abnormal hematopoiesis (or any other carcinogenesis), and the defect in number and function of cells as a final result of this process, then both morphology and immunophenotype fall somewhere in between. Unlike with FCIP, we have had tens or even hundreds of years of experience in using morphologic findings for diagnostic and therapeutic guidance. Knowledge in medicine is built on previous knowledge, and therein lies the challenge with incorporating any new approach: if a previous study to evaluate treatment for a myeloid malignancy used morphologic criteria to define a disease, then we cannot be sure that the results would have been the same had we defined it in a different way (ie, immunophenotypically). This leads to an ever-increasing number of correlative retrospective studies, but no truly prospective, therapy-guiding endeavors.

IMMUNOPHENOTYPING OF BLASTS (IMMATURE MYELOID PRECURSORS)

Blasts are a particularly appealing target for FCIP evaluation of myelopoiesis. First, because chronic myeloid neoplasms are clinical disorders of hematopoietic stem cells, blasts are likely to be affected in all cases, regardless of the number of lineages with morphologic dysplasia. Second, blast phenotype may be more stable than that of mature granulocytic cells. Third, FCIP can help with blast enumeration, which is an essential component of MDS and MDS/MPN stratification. Finally, morphologic assessment of blasts is limited mostly to enumeration (particularly at low blast percentages) because there are no definitive morphologic criteria for "abnormal blasts." In contrast, FCIP can identify phenotypically aberrant blasts. Because "blasts" are defined morphologically, the flow cytometry community started using the term "immature myeloid precursors" to avoid confusion with morphologic findings. However, it is uncertain whether this distinction is clear to hematologists in a routine clinical practice.

To date, for the purpose of diagnosis, subclassification, and prognostication, the gold standard for blast enumeration remains a morphologic assessment of the bone marrow aspirate. Blast definition by FCIP varies from study to study. The most commonly used definition is $CD34^+CD45^{dim}$, which tends to slightly underestimate the percentage of blasts. The best correlation with morphologic counts was obtained using CD34[24] and/or CD117[+]HLA-DR[+] cells out of all nucleated bone marrow cells.[24] Of note, immature monocytic precursors are often negative for both CD34 and CD117. Additional confounding factors for enumerating blasts by FCIP include hemodilution and lysis procedure. Hemodilution is a frequent problem with any routine FCIP applications, because the first bone marrow aspirate draw is usually reserved for cytomorphology. Several ways to quantify aspirate adequacy have been proposed,[25,26] but their value has not been tested independently. The lysis procedure can affect nucleated red blood cell precursors and change the denominator for blast percentage calculations.[27] Despite such limitations, FCIP can still be useful for blast enumeration, particularly when morphologic features are ambiguous. Importantly, the percentage of blasts as determined by FCIP has been shown to be of prognostic value for stratifying MDS.[28] Furthermore, an evaluation of bone marrow biopsy specimens by CD34 immunohistochemistry is an accepted way of blast quantification in clinical practice.

Phenotypic aberrancies in blasts can be separated into (a) aberrant brightness of markers that are normally expressed (CD38, CD117, HLA-DR), (b) asynchronous expression of mature markers (CD15), and (c) aberrant expression of nonlineage (lymphoid) markers (CD2, CD5, CD7). In addition, several other FCIP characteristics can be taken into account, including the side scatter of blasts (SSC), and the percentage of immature B-lymphoid cells (hematogones). CD34[+] blasts in normal marrow are a heterogeneous cell population; this heterogeneity is frequently lost in CMN.[29] CD34[+]CD19[+] hematogones are characteristically decreased in bone marrows from patients with myelodysplasia.[18,30–32] However, it is necessary to establish age-dependent normal ranges to use quantitative assessment of the percentage of hematogones.[33] A more detailed list of phenotypic abnormalities detected on blasts is shown in **Table 1**.

IMMUNOPHENOTYPING OF MATURING GRANULOCYTIC CELLS

Maturing granulocytic cells are a heterogeneous population, with a complex pattern of antigen gains and losses, from promyelocytes to mature neutrophils. Hypogranularity is considered one of the cardinal dysplastic features by morphology, and can be detected by FCIP, by comparing SSC between granulocyte and lymphocyte populations.[34] For SSC to be an accurate reflection of hypogranularity, exclusion of eosinophils from the granulocyte gates is necessary. Common single antigen abnormalities include gain of CD56 and CD36, and loss of CD16 and CD33 expression (see **Table 1**). However, none of these individual abnormalities are specific: gain of CD56 is present on activated granulocytes,[21] and loss of CD16 can be seen in paroxysmal nocturnal hemoglobinuria,[35] which should be excluded by examining other lineages. Therefore, a more common approach in evaluating maturing granulocytic cells is to assess for visual patterns of differentiation. For example, normal plot of CD13/CD16 expression shows a characteristic shape from immature to mature cells; this shape is lost in dysgranulopoiesis (**Fig. 1**). Of particular note is that FCIP of maturing granulocytic precursors requires a fresh specimen (ideally <24 hours from the draw), because CD11b and granularity are highly sensitive to storage effect.[27]

IMMUNOPHENOTYPING OF MONOCYTIC CELLS

Monocytes are evaluated by FCIP less frequently than blasts and granulocytes, for the diagnosis of MDS. In contrast, phenotypic abnormalities in monocytic lineage are of importance in distinguishing chronic myelomonocytic leukemia from reactive monocytosis.[36,37] The most common abnormalities detected in monocytes include their

Table 1
Most frequent FCIP abnormalities in immature myeloid progenitors, maturing granulocytic cells

Markers	Progenitor Myeloid	Neutrophils	Monocytes	Erythroid
SSC	Increased SSC	Low ratio to lymphocytes	Decreased SSC	
CD5	Abnormal expression on CD34$^+$ and/or CD117$^+$ cells	Abnormal expression	Abnormal expression	
CD7	Abnormal expression on CD34$^+$ and/or CD117$^+$ cells	Abnormal expression	Abnormal expression	
CD11b	Increased expression on CD34$^+$ cells		Decreased expression	
CD14			Decreased expression	
CD15	Asynchronous expression on progenitors	Asynchronous expression together with CD34		
CD19	Decreased CD34$^+$/CD19$^+$lymphoid progenitors	Abnormal expression		
CD34	Increased frequency of CD34$^+$/CD19$^-$ (>2%) Increased proportion of CD38$^{-/dim}$/CD34$^+$	Asynchronous expression	Asynchronous expression	
CD36		Increased expression	Abnormal Expression	Abnormal heterogeneous and/or low expression
CD45	Decreased expression	Decreased expression	Decreased expression	
CD56	Abnormal expression on CD34$^+$ and/or CD117$^+$ cells	Abnormal expression	Abnormal expression	
CD71				Abnormal heterogeneous and/or low expression
CD117	Decreased frequency	Increased expression		Increased frequency of positive precursors
HLA-DR	Increased proportion of HLA-DR$^{-/dim}$/CD34$^+$ cells	Increased expression	Decreased expression	
CD11b/ HLA-DR		Aberrant pattern	Aberrant pattern	
CD11b/CD16		Aberrant pattern (most often owing to low CD16)	Abnormal expression of CD16 on CD11b$^+$ monocytes	

(continued on next page)

Markers	Progenitor Myeloid	Neutrophils	Monocytes	Erythroid
Table 1 *(continued)*				
CD13/ HLA-DR	Aberrant pattern	Aberrant maturation pattern		
CD13/CD16		Aberrant maturation pattern		
CD13/CD33	Increased number of CD33$^+$/CD13$^-$ or CD33$^-$/CD13$^+$ cells	Increased number of CD33$^+$/CD13$^-$ or CD33$^-$/ CD13$^+$ cells	Increased number of CD33$^+$/CD13$^-$ or CD33$^-$/ CD13$^+$ cells	
CD15/CD10		Aberrant pattern, lack of CD10 on mature neutrophil granulocytes		
CD19/CD10				
CD36/CD14			Aberrant pattern	
CD71/CD235				Aberrant pattern

Items in boldface have been reported to have strong value in supporting MDS diagnosis.

Abbreviations: FCIP, flow cytometry immunophenotyping; MDS, myelodysplastic syndrome; SSC, side scatter of blasts.

Modified from Porwit A, van de Loosdrecht AA, Bettelheim P, et al. Revisiting guidelines for integration of flow cytometry results in the WHO classification of myelodysplastic syndromes-proposal from the International/European LeukemiaNet Working Group for flow cytometry in MDS. Leukemia 2014;28(9):1793; with permission.

number/percentage and aberrancies in expression of CD13, CD33, CD5, CD7, HLA-DR, CD11c, CD14, CD38, and CD56 (see **Table 1**). In addition, similar to the granulocytic precursors, patterns of antigen gain and loss are important in determining whether maturation occurs in an orderly fashion. A recent study showed that FCIP of

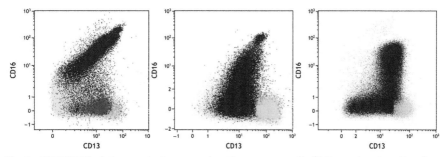

Fig. 1. CD13/CD16 plot on maturing granulocytic precursors. (*Left*) Normal maturation from promyelocytes (*teal*) through immature granulocytes (*yellow*) to mature neutrophils (*blue*). (*Middle*) Atypical maturation with some shape preservation. (*Right*) Abnormal maturation in a case of myelodysplastic syndrome.

mature monocytes in the peripheral blood can potentially distinguish reactive monocytosis from chronic myelomonocytic leukemia by a simple evaluation of CD14 and CD16 expression.[38] However, additional markers were necessary for accurate gating of monocytic cells. The most recent guidelines on the diagnosis, prognosis, and treatment of MDS/MPN focus on the molecular genetic findings, and do not address the use of FCIP.[2,39]

IMMUNOPHENOTYPING OF RED BLOOD CELL PRECURSORS

Erythroid precursors are morphologically most sensitive, but least specific, in the diagnosis of MDS. From an FCIP perspective, maturation of erythroid precursors was somewhat neglected, partly because of the lack of available reagents, partly because red blood cell lysis of the bone marrow aspirate specimens made quantification of different stages of maturation difficult. Recently, however, several studies showed that red blood cell maturation can be a useful addition to FCIP assessment of dysplasia.[40,41] The most common antigenic aberrancies were in the expression of CD36 and CD71, including the cell-to-cell variability (coefficient of variation of mean fluorescence intensity [MFI]). Abnormalities of CD235a, CD117, and CD105 were also correlated with the presence of dyserythropoiesis (see **Table 1**). A multicenter, mostly European, study showed a high specificity (90%) of the approach using coefficient of variation of CD36 and CD71 expression, together with CD71 MFI and percent CD117[+] erythroid progenitors, in a weighted point-based approach.[42]

QUANTITATIVE VERSUS QUALITATIVE ANALYSIS

There are 2 ways FCIP data can be assessed in evaluating chronic myeloid neoplasms (and other hematologic diseases). A quantitative approach expresses results as numbers (percentages, MFIs, ratios).[13,23,31,43–45] Intuitively, this approach can offer greater precision and reproducibility of results. It is also more amenable for automated software analysis and modeling. However, a quantitative approach depends on stringent instrument and specimen settings, which is difficult to standardize among different laboratories. In addition, quantitative reports require a much more extensive validation process for establishing normal ranges and cutoffs.[46] A qualitative approach relies on visualization of FCIP data on 2-dimensional dot plots.[11,12,16,29,34,39,47–50] It is less stringent in definition of normal versus abnormal for individual antigen expression; most commonly 0.5 log difference has been used as "significant," although 0.3 and 0.25 log differences are also present in the literature.[12,39,47] Importantly, a qualitative approach is particularly valuable in assessing complex patterns of maturation, with loss of normal antigen expression sequence in dyspoietic cells (see **Fig. 1**). Although a qualitative approach is easier to set up in the laboratory, its use requires significant training to achieve and maintain operator competency in interpretation.

It is important to recognize that these 2 approaches, quantitative and qualitative, are not mutually exclusive, and that they in fact almost invariably coexist. For example, even in very stringent quantitative studies, the raw data have been visually/qualitatively gated to isolate "pure" cell populations (the exception to this is the use of automated gating software(s), which still suffer from suboptimal reliability). Furthermore, every quantitative variable could be shown as a dot plot or a histogram for visual decision making, and vice versa, every complex plot could be described as a set of numbers. So this distinction is mostly useful in validating FCIP in terms of statistical analysis, coefficients of variation, and number of specimens needed to establish a reproducible test.

SCORING SYSTEMS

All the studies performed so far indicate that a single FCIP abnormality is unlikely to have sufficient sensitivity and specificity in distinguishing normal from dysplastic hematopoiesis. As a result, scoring systems have been developed as an attempt to quantify both the number of abnormalities across the different lineages, as well as the extent of any individual abnormality ("difference from normal"). Scoring systems can be used to either help distinguishing MDS from nonneoplastic cytopenias, or to provide prognostic value in patients with recognized MDS. In most studies, however, this distinction is blurred; the number of FCIP abnormalities correlates with both likelihood of having MDS, and the grade or severity of MDS.

One of the most commonly cited scoring system was developed by Ogata and colleagues.[18,51,52] It incorporates 4 cardinal quantitative parameters: (1) percent of CD34$^+$ myeloblasts, (2) percent of CD34$^+$ hematogones, (3) ratio of CD45 expression on lymphocytes/myeloblasts, and (4) ratio of SSC on granulocytes/lymphocytes (**Fig. 2**). In some variants of this scoring system, there were adjunct parameters that included expression of CD11b, CD15, and CD56 on myeloblasts.[18] Giving each abnormality 1 point, the authors were able to establish that progression to acute leukemia and overall survival were correlated with the flow cytometric score, with the score

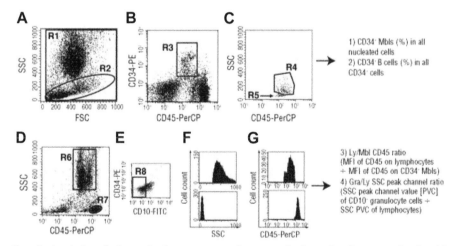

Fig. 2. Analysis of 4 cardinal parameters from a single cell aliquot stained with CD10-fluorescein isothiocyanate (FITC), CD34-PE, and CD45-PerCP antibodies. (*A*) All nucleated cells (R1) and cells with relatively low side scatter of blasts (SSC) (R2). (*B*) Cells in R2 in A were displayed on a CD34-versus-CD45 plot. CD34$^+$ cells with intermediate CD45 expression were gated (R3). (*C*) Cells in R3 in B were displayed on a CD45-versus-SSC plot. A cluster of CD34$^+$ B-cell progenitors was identified in the lower left region of CD34$^+$ cells (R5, *arrow*). The reliability of the R5 region was confirmed based on CD10 positivity. Cells in R4 were composed mainly of myeloblasts (Mbls). (*D*) Granulocytic cells other than Mbls (R6) and lymphocytes (R7) were gated on a CD45-versus-SSC plot. (*E*) Cells in R6 in D were displayed, and the CD10$^-$ fraction was gated (R8). (*F*) SSC of CD10$^-$ granulocytic cells (*top*) and lymphocytes (*bottom*). SSC peak channel values (SSC channel number where the maximum number of cells occurs) of both fractions were computed using the software. (*G*) CD45 expression of CD34$^+$ Mbls (*top*) and lymphocytes (*bottom*). Mean fluorescence intensity (MFI, GeoMean) of CD45 of both fractions was computed. (*From* Ogata K, Della Porta MG, Malcovati L, et al. Diagnostic utility of flow cytometry in low-grade myelodysplastic syndromes: a prospective validation study. Haematologica 2009;94(8):1066; with permission.)

of 0 to 1 showing low likelihood of progression and high survival rate, and a score of 3 to 4 showing high likelihood of progression and low survival rate[53] (**Fig. 3**). Importantly, the Ogata score was validated by independent patient sets and laboratories in Japan and Italy.

Wells and colleagues[54] designed a flow cytometric scoring system (FCSS) composed of qualitative and semiquantitative visual assessment of antigenic

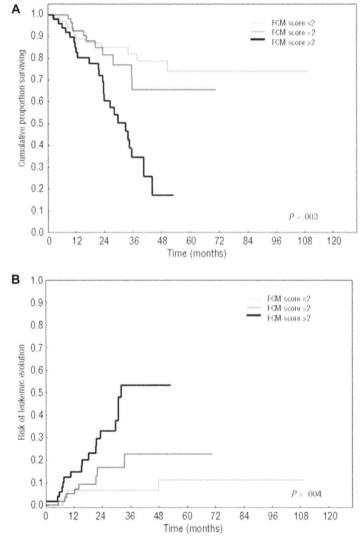

Fig. 3. (*A*) Overall survival and (*B*) risk of leukemic evolution of low-grade myelodysplastic syndrome patients stratified according to flow cytometry (FCM)-score. The 5-year overall survival was 74% in patients with an FCM score of less than 2, 65% in patients with an FCM score of 2, and 17% in patients with an FCM score of greater than 2 (*P* = .003). The 5-year risk of leukemic evolution was 11%, 22%, and 53%, respectively (*P* = .004). (*From* Della Porta MG, Picone C, Tenore A, et al. Prognostic significance of reproducible immunophenotypic markers of marrow dysplasia. Haematologica 2014;99(1):e9; with permission.)

aberrancies in myeloblasts and maturing granulocytic and monocytic cells (SSC, CD5, CD7, CD11b, CD19, CD33, CD45, CD56, HLA-DR, CD13/CD16 coexpression, and CD33/CD14 coexpression). For single antigens, an 0.5-log difference in brightness was used, and aberrant visual pattern observed by multiple operators was necessary to establish an abnormality. FCSS ranged between 0 and 3, depending on the number of abnormalities detected. Higher score correlated with the International Prognostic Scoring System (IPSS) for risk of progression and shorter overall survival in patients with MDS. Moreover, in a subpopulation of patients (IPSS-intermediate 1 risk), FCSS has been shown to provide also an added and independent prognostic value.[32,55]

Kern and colleagues[56] and Stachurski and colleagues[50] used a strategy similar to FCSS, with qualitative assessment of multiple antigenic abnormalities. They showed a correlation between a total number of FCIP abnormalities and IPSS[56] or cytogenetic and morphologic severity of MDS,[50] as well as a potentially predictive value of FCIP in patients without a definitive diagnosis of MDS.[48,57,58] The approach used for MDS diagnosis and prognosis was also shown to be useful in evaluating MPN and MDS/MPN.[50,59]

Recently, Van de Loosdrecht's group attempted to integrate Ogata score (diagnostic score) and FCSS into an integrated flow cytometric score for distinguishing MDS-related cytopenia from nonneoplastic causes in patients with unexplained cytopenias.[60] In parallel with this diagnostic approach, the same group developed a prognostic 3-parameter flow scoring system using only SSC and CD117 expression on myeloid progenitors and CD13 expression on monocytes (the MDS flow cytometry score).[61] Patients with high scores had worse overall survival than patients with low or intermediate scores, and this observation was able to further substratify patients within the revised IPSS (IPSS-R) low-risk category.

There are few available data on independent comparison of the usefulness of different scoring systems. Brodersen and colleagues[62] compared the Wells FCCS with the Ogata score in a limited study and found that the Wells FCCS outperformed the Ogata score in sensitivity and specificity, based on accordance with single nucleotide polymorphisms, comparative genomic hybridization, and conventional karyotype abnormalities (Wells FCCS showed sensitivity and specificity of 90% and 86%, respectively, compared with 65% and 81% by the Ogata score). This is not surprising, because the Wells FCCS incorporates many more parameters for defining and grading antigenic abnormalities. The addition of an erythroid progenitor evaluation by FCIP increased sensitivity for both the Ogata score and the integrated flow cytometric score.[49]

STANDARDIZATION OF FLOW CYTOMETRY IMMUNOPHENOTYPING IN MYELOID NEOPLASMS

There is an ongoing effort to standardize FCIP for myeloid neoplasms, predominantly led by the European LeukemiaNet group.[19–21] In the most recent update,[19] the group made several recommendations, which are now cited in the clinical practice guidelines.[63] Some of the highlights of the recommendations include the following:

- Strict guidelines for specimen processing, lysing, and staining.
- Usefulness of the Ogata score for limited screening and by smaller laboratories.
- Usefulness of comprehensive panels if available and incorporating FCIP findings for selective prognostic purposes.
- Not relying solely on FCIP for the diagnosis of MDS, but using an integrated approach and avoiding diagnosing MDS in standalone FCIP reports.

CURRENT STATE OF FLOW CYTOMETRY IMMUNOPHENOTYPING IN CHRONIC MYELOID NEOPLASMS AND FUTURE DIRECTIONS

It is difficult to accurately estimate the additive value of FCIP for chronic myeloid neoplasms in the current clinical practice. There are multiple reasons for this uncertainty.

First, standardization among laboratories is still far from optimal. It is questionable how quickly and to what extent can FCIP be truly standardized, at least in the United States. FCIP is a laboratory-developed test, which implies that every laboratory has to perform independent validation of its panels, including both technical components and clinical validation. This is expensive and time consuming. The laboratory practice (and medicine in the United States in general) is under scrutiny for financial perfor-mance. Therefore, each laboratory may have its own incentive for using its antibody panels and instruments of choice. Furthermore, there is an ever-changing list of anti-bodies to be used, which makes it difficult for clinical laboratories to follow the cutting edge research studies, because each change requires a new validation study.

Second, qualitative assessment of dyspoiesis by FCIP relies on visual evaluation of data in 2-dimensional dot plots, which are subjectively interpreted, similar to the morphologic assessment of dysplasia. **Fig. 1** shows how difficult it can be to assess dysplasia without proper training (many possible variations between an obviously normal and an obviously aberrant pattern). If FCIP is to become the standard of care for MDS diagnosis, visual interpretation of myeloid maturation has to be included in the training programs by governing bodies (ie, American Board of Pathology for United States). A consensus from the flow cytometry community regarding minimal FCIP criteria for MDS diagnosis is necessary. In the future, quantitative assessment of dyspoiesis may be automated by software applications, but this will introduce another level of regulatory complexity.

Third, as discussed in a recent review,[64] there has to be a clear separation of the diagnostic versus prognostic versus therapy-guiding use of FCIP. Prognostic data are easier to obtain retrospectively, with larger patient cohorts. It is clear that the higher number of abnormalities is associated with worse prognosis, measured by time to treatment, progression to acute leukemia, and/or overall survival.[28,34,49,61,65,66] However, the overall value of FCIP for prognostic stratification of patients is limited, mostly because there are already many other prognostic markers that are able to provide excellent stratification. For example, of the information extracted from the blood and bone marrow specimens, IPSS-R does not even take into consideration morphologic subtype of MDS, but requires only blast percentage and cytogenetic findings for stratification.[67] There has been an attempt at merging the World Health Organization classification with the IPSS-R,[68] but the gains in stratification seem to be minimal (**Fig. 4**). FCIP may have a role for MDS prognosis in future, but at this point it seems to be of limited usefulness, and therefore difficult to justify added cost to the patient.

Where FCIP could have the most clinical impact is in the diagnostic evaluation of MDS and premyeloid conditions (idiopathic cytopenia of uncertain significance, clonal cytopenia of uncertain significance, clonal hematopoiesis of indeterminate potential). As with prognostic use, there is an observation that the more FCIP abnormalities detected, the higher likelihood of a myeloid neoplasm. There is, however, scarcity of studies with proper assessment of the predictive value of FCIP. Cremers and colleagues[60] examined additive value of FCIP in cases of unexplained cytopenia. Of 164 patients without a definitive diagnosis by morphology, cytogenetics or molecular genetics, the additive value of diagnosing MDS or myeloid neoplasm by FCIP was

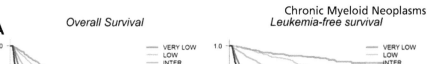

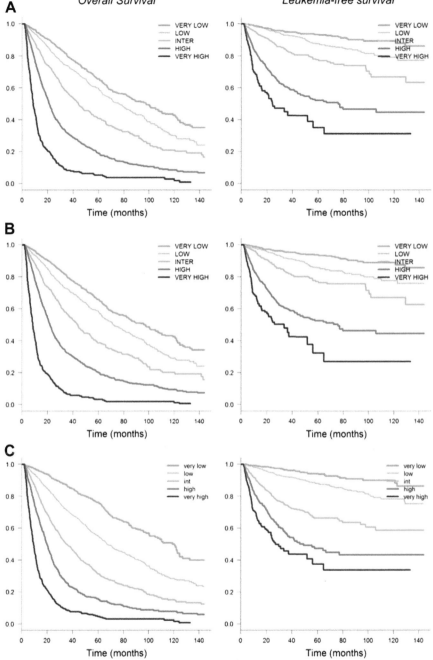

Fig. 4. Overall and leukemia-free survival of patients with myelodysplastic syndrome stratified according to different prognostic scores. (*A*) The WHO Classification-based Prognostic Scoring System (WPSS). (*B*) WPSS with new cytogenetic features. (*C*) Revised International Prognostic Scoring System. (*From* Della Porta MG, Tuechler H, Malcovati L, et al. Validation of WHO classification-based Prognostic Scoring System (WPSS) for myelodysplastic syndromes and comparison with the revised International Prognostic Scoring System (IPSS-R). A study of the International Working Group for Prognosis in Myelodysplasia (IWG-PM). Leukemia 2015;29(7):1502; with permission.)

seen in only 2 of 8 patients (positive predictive value of 25%). In contrast, the negative predictive value was high as 72 of 79 patients (91%) with normal FCIP findings were found not to have MDS after a relatively short median follow-up of 381 days (patient with intermediate/indeterminate FCIP score were excluded from this calculation). Another study by Hoffmann and Kim[69] showed an even higher negative predictive value using a limited FCIP approach in a community health care setting, with a lower incidence of MDS. Importantly, FCIP-negative patients were very unlikely to have cytogenetic abnormalities (98% negative predictive value), which could lead to a decrease in chromosomal studies and significantly reduce the cost of the MDS diagnostic approach. Similar data were obtained by Truong and colleagues.[48] More studies are needed, with an honest approach to establishing a true additive value of FCIP to current diagnostic algorithms. Additionally, many patients with early MDS are initially being only closely observed. Therefore, establishing a firm diagnosis at an early stage of MDS does not necessarily indicate a different therapeutic approach. It is important to recognize that test use is becoming more scrutinized by governmental agencies and private insurers.

Finally, a different, more radical approach to FCIP implementation would involve changing the definition of diseases. The World Health Organization 2016 update on the classification of myeloid neoplasms maintained a predominantly morphologic and cytogenetic framework of chronic myeloid neoplasms.[2] Although single mutations are slowly finding their way in the disease definitions (SF3B1, JAK2, CALR, MPL, and CSF3R), phenotypic aberrancies are still not represented. The only exception is the aberrant CD25 and CD2 expression on mast cells for the diagnosis of systemic mastocytosis.[2] At present, the hematology community accepts that morphologic findings are often subtle and equivocal, yet there is a requirement that immunophenotypic results be clear and definitive. Studies have shown that FCIP can reliably establish a clinically relevant percentage of $CD34^+$ cells if adjusted for hemodilution.[32,58,70] The additional value of identifying phenotypically abnormal progenitors would justify the replacement of morphology with FCIP approach. However, defining myeloid disease by phenotype would be a radical change, with potential case volume redistribution, from smaller and morphology-oriented practices, to large laboratories with FCIP expertise, and eventually to informatics-based groups, using statistical and computational, rather than morphologic, expertise. Whether the diagnostics market is ready for this shift remains uncertain.

SUMMARY

FCIP can be a valuable addition to diagnostic work-up of patients with chronic myeloid neoplasms, particularly MDS. However, its usefulness is not well-established yet, owing to (i) lack of standardization, (ii) complexity and cost of the panels, and (iii) scarcity of studies showing predictive value in a general patient population. Efforts are under way to bridge these gaps and introduce FCIP into routine diagnostic algorithms.

REFERENCES

1. Arber DA, Hasserjian RP. Reclassifying myelodysplastic syndromes: what's where in the new WHO and why. Hematol Am Soc Hematol Educ Program 2015;2015:294–8.

2. Arber DA, Orazi A, Hasserjian R, et al. The 2016 revision to the World Health Organization classification of myeloid neoplasms and acute leukemia. Blood 2016;127(20):2391–405.

3. Brunning RD, Orazi A, Germing U, et al. Myelodysplastic syndromes/neoplasms, overview. In: Swerdlow SH, Campo E, Harris NL, et al, editors. WHO classification of tumours of haematopoietic and lymphoid tissues. Lyon (France): IARC; 2008. p. 88–93.

4. Clark RE, Smith SA, Jacobs A. Myeloid surface antigen abnormalities in myelo-dysplasia: relation to prognosis and modification by 13-cis retinoic acid. J Clin Pathol 1987;40(6):652–6.

5. Jensen IM. Myelopoiesis in myelodysplasia evaluated by multiparameter flow cytometry. Leuk Lymphoma 1995;20(1–2):17–25.

6. Jensen IM, Hokland M, Hokland P. A quantitative evaluation of erythropoiesis in myelodysplastic syndromes using multiparameter flow cytometry. Leuk Res 1993;17(10):839–46.

7. Ohsaka A, Saionji K, Watanabe N, et al. Complement receptor type 1 (CR1) deficiency on neutrophils in myelodysplastic syndrome. Br J Haematol 1994; 88(2):409–12.

8. Peters SW, Clark RE, Hoy TG, et al. DNA content and cell cycle analysis of bone marrow cells in myelodysplastic syndromes (MDS). Br J Haematol 1986;62(2): 239–45.

9. Riccardi A, Montecucco CM, Danova M, et al. Flow cytometric evaluation of proliferative activity and ploidy in myelodysplastic syndromes and acute leuke-mias. Basic Appl Histochem 1986;30(2):181–92.

10. Baumann MA, Keller RH, McFadden PW, et al. Myeloid cell surface phenotype in myelodysplasia: evidence for abnormal persistence of an early myeloid differen-tiation antigen. Am J Hematol 1986;22(3):251–7.

11. Kussick SJ, Fromm JR, Rossini A, et al. Four-color flow cytometry shows strong concordance with bone marrow morphology and cytogenetics in the evaluation for myelodysplasia. Am J Clin Pathol 2005;124(2):170–81.

12. Kussick SJ, Wood BL. Four-color flow cytometry identifies virtually all cytogenet-ically abnormal bone marrow samples in the workup of non-CML myeloprolifera-tive disorders. Am J Clin Pathol 2003;120(6):854–65.

13. Ogata K, Nakamura K, Yokose N, et al. Clinical significance of phenotypic fea-tures of blasts in patients with myelodysplastic syndrome. Blood 2002;100(12): 3887–96.

14. Ogata K, Yoshida Y. Clinical implications of blast immunophenotypes in myelo-dysplastic syndromes. Leuk Lymphoma 2005;46(9):1269–74.

15. Otawa M, Kawanishi Y, Iwase O, et al. Comparative multi-color flow cytometric analysis of cell surface antigens in bone marrow hematopoietic progenitors between refractory anemia and aplastic anemia. Leuk Res 2000;24(4):359–66.

16. Pirruccello SJ, Young KH, Aoun P. Myeloblast phenotypic changes in myelodys-plasia. CD34 and CD117 expression abnormalities are common. Am J Clin Pathol 2006;125(6):884–94.

17. Stetler-Stevenson M, Arthur DC, Jabbour N, et al. Diagnostic utility of flow cyto-metric immunophenotyping in myelodysplastic syndrome. Blood 2001;98(4): 979–87.

18. Ogata K, Della Porta MG, Malcovati L, et al. Diagnostic utility of flow cytometry in low-grade myelodysplastic syndromes: a prospective validation study. Haemato-logica 2009;94(8):1066–74.

19. Porwit A, van de Loosdrecht AA, Bettelheim P, et al. Revisiting guidelines for integration of flow cytometry results in the WHO classification of myelodysplastic syndromes-proposal from the International/European LeukemiaNet Working Group for Flow Cytometry in MDS. Leukemia 2014;28(9):1793–8.

20. van de Loosdrecht AA, Alhan C, Béné MC, et al. Standardization of flow cytometry in myelodysplastic syndromes: report from the first European LeukemiaNet working conference on flow cytometry in myelodysplastic syndromes. Haematologica 2009;94(8):1124–34.

21. Westers TM, Ireland R, Kern W, et al. Standardization of flow cytometry in myelodysplastic syndromes: a report from an international consortium and the European LeukemiaNet Working Group. Leukemia 2012;26(7):1730–41.

22. Alhan C, Westers TM, van der Helm LH, et al. Absence of aberrant myeloid progenitors by flow cytometry is associated with favorable response to azacitidine in higher risk myelodysplastic syndromes. Cytometry B Clin Cytom 2014;86(3): 207–15.

23. Westers TM, Alhan C, Chamuleau ME, et al. Aberrant immunophenotype of blasts in myelodysplastic syndromes is a clinically relevant biomarker in predicting response to growth factor treatment. Blood 2010;115(9):1779–84.

24. Sandes AF, Kerbauy DM, Matarraz S, et al. Combined flow cytometric assessment of CD45, HLA-DR, CD34, and CD117 expression is a useful approach for reliable quantification of blast cells in myelodysplastic syndromes. Cytometry B Clin Cytom 2013;84(3):157–66.

25. Brooimans RA, Kraan J, van Putten W, et al. Flow cytometric differential of leukocyte populations in normal bone marrow: influence of peripheral blood contamination. Cytometry B Clin Cytom 2009;76(1):18–26.

26. Loken MR, Chu SC, Fritschle W, et al. Normalization of bone marrow aspirates for hemodilution in flow cytometric analyses. Cytometry B Clin Cytom 2009;76(1): 27–36.

27. Alhan C, Westers TM, Cremers EM, et al. Application of flow cytometry for myelodysplastic syndromes: pitfalls and technical considerations. Cytometry B Clin Cytom 2016;90(4):358–67.

28. Falco P, Levis A, Stacchini A, et al. Prognostic relevance of cytometric quantitative assessment in patients with myelodysplastic syndromes. Eur J Haematol 2011;87(5):409–18.

29. Jevremovic D, Timm MM, Reichard KK, et al. Loss of blast heterogeneity in myelodysplastic syndrome and other chronic myeloid neoplasms. Am J Clin Pathol 2014;142(3):292–8.

30. Maftoun-Banankhah S, Maleki A, Karandikar NJ, et al. Multiparameter flow cytometric analysis reveals low percentage of bone marrow hematogones in myelodysplastic syndromes. Am J Clin Pathol 2008;129(2):300–8.

31. Matarraz S, López A, Barrena S, et al. The immunophenotype of different immature, myeloid and B-cell lineage-committed CD34+ hematopoietic cells allows discrimination between normal/reactive and myelodysplastic syndrome precursors. Leukemia 2008;22(6):1175–83.

32. van de Loosdrecht AA, Westers TM, Westra AH, et al. Identification of distinct prognostic subgroups in low- and intermediate-1-risk myelodysplastic syndromes by flow cytometry. Blood 2008;111(3):1067–77.

33. McKenna RW, Washington LT, Aquino DB, et al. Immunophenotypic analysis of hematogones (B-lymphocyte precursors) in 662 consecutive bone marrow specimens by 4-color flow cytometry. Blood 2001;98(8):2498–507.

34. Della Porta MG, Picone C, Pascutto C, et al. Multicenter validation of a reproducible flow cytometric score for the diagnosis of low-grade myelodysplastic syndromes: results of a European LeukemiaNET study. Haematologica 2012; 97(8):1209–17.

35. Sutherland DR, Illingworth A, Keeney M, et al. High-sensitivity detection of PNH Red blood cells, red cell precursors, and white blood cells. Curr Protoc Cytom 2015;72:6.37.1-30.

36. Harrington AM, Schelling LA, Ordobazari A, et al. Immunophenotypes of chronic myelomonocytic leukemia (CMML) subtypes by flow cytometry: a comparison of CMML-1 vs CMML-2, myeloproliferative vs dysplastic, De Novo vs therapy-related, and CMML-specific cytogenetic risk subtypes. Am J Clin Pathol 2016; 146(2):170–81.

37. Sojitra P, Gandhi P, Fitting P, et al. Chronic myelomonocytic leukemia monocytes uniformly display a population of monocytes with CD11c underexpression. Am J Clin Pathol 2013;140(5):686–92.

38. Selimoglu-Buet D, Wagner-Ballon O, Saada V, et al. Characteristic repartition of monocyte subsets as a diagnostic signature of chronic myelomonocytic leukemia. Blood 2015;125(23):3618–26.

39. Mughal TI, Cross NC, Padron E, et al. An International MDS/MPN Working Group's perspective and recommendations on molecular pathogenesis, diagnosis and clinical characterization of myelodysplastic/myeloproliferative neoplasms. Haematologica 2015;100(9):1117–30.

40. Eidenschink Brodersen L, Menssen AJ, Wangen JR, et al. Assessment of erythroid dysplasia by "difference from normal" in routine clinical flow cytometry workup. Cytometry B Clin Cytom 2015;88(2):125–35.

41. Mathis S, Chapuis N, Debord C, et al. Flow cytometric detection of dyserythropoiesis: a sensitive and powerful diagnostic tool for myelodysplastic syndromes. Leukemia 2013;27(10):1981–7.

42. Westers TM, Cremers EM, Oelschlaegel U, et al. Immunophenotypic analysis of erythroid dysplasia in myelodysplastic syndromes. A report from the IMDSFlow working group. Haematologica 2017;102(2):308–19.

43. De Smet D, Trullemans F, Jochmans K, et al. Diagnostic potential of CD34+ cell antigen expression in myelodysplastic syndromes. Am J Clin Pathol 2012;138(5): 732–43.

44. Goardon N, Nikolousis E, Sternberg A, et al. Reduced CD38 expression on CD34+ cells as a diagnostic test in myelodysplastic syndromes. Haematologica 2009;94(8):1160–3.

45. Maynadie M, Picard F, Husson B, et al. Immunophenotypic clustering of myelodysplastic syndromes. Blood 2002;100(7):2349–56.

46. Wood B, Jevremovic D, Béné MC, et al. Validation of cell-based fluorescence assays: practice guidelines from the ICSH and ICCS - part V - assay performance criteria. Cytometry B Clin Cytom 2013;84(5):315–23.

47. Harrington A, Olteanu H, Kroft S. The specificity of immunophenotypic alterations in blasts in nonacute myeloid disorders. Am J Clin Pathol 2010;134(5):749–61.

48. Truong F, Smith BR, Stachurski D, et al. The utility of flow cytometric immunophenotyping in cytopenic patients with a non-diagnostic bone marrow: a prospective study. Leuk Res 2009;33(8):1039–46.

49. Cremers EM, Westers TM, Alhan C, et al. Implementation of erythroid lineage analysis by flow cytometry in diagnostic models for myelodysplastic syndromes. Haematologica 2017;102(2):320–6.

50. Stachurski D, Smith BR, Pozdnyakova O, et al. Flow cytometric analysis of myelomonocytic cells by a pattern recognition approach is sensitive and specific in diagnosing myelodysplastic syndrome and related marrow diseases: emphasis on a global evaluation and recognition of diagnostic pitfalls. Leuk Res 2008; 32(2):215–24.

51. Ogata K, Kishikawa Y, Satoh C, et al. Diagnostic application of flow cytometric characteristics of CD34+ cells in low-grade myelodysplastic syndromes. Blood 2006;108(3):1037–44.
52. Satoh C, Dan K, Yamashita T, et al. Flow cytometric parameters with little interexaminer variability for diagnosing low-grade myelodysplastic syndromes. Leuk Res 2008;32(5):699–707.
53. Della Porta MG, Picone C, Tenore A, et al. Prognostic significance of reproducible immunophenotypic markers of marrow dysplasia. Haematologica 2014;99(1): e8-10.
54. Wells DA, Benesch M, Loken MR, et al. Myeloid and monocytic dyspoiesis as determined by flow cytometric scoring in myelodysplastic syndrome correlates with the IPSS and with outcome after hematopoietic stem cell transplantation. Blood 2003;102(1):394–403.
55. Scott BL, Wells DA, Loken MR, et al. Validation of a flow cytometric scoring system as a prognostic indicator for posttransplantation outcome in patients with myelodysplastic syndrome. Blood 2008;112(7):2681–6.
56. Kern W, Haferlach C, Schnittger S, et al. Clinical utility of multiparameter flow cytometry in the diagnosis of 1013 patients with suspected myelodysplastic syndrome: correlation to cytomorphology, cytogenetics, and clinical data. Cancer 2010;116(19):4549–63.
57. Kern W, Bacher U, Haferlach C, et al. Multiparameter flow cytometry provides independent prognostic information in patients with suspected myelodysplastic syndromes: a study on 804 patients. Cytometry B Clin Cytom 2015;88(3):154–64.
58. Kern W, Haferlach C, Schnittger S, et al. Serial assessment of suspected myelodysplastic syndromes: significance of flow cytometric findings validated by cytomorphology, cytogenetics, and molecular genetics. Haematologica 2013;98(2): 201–7.
59. Kern W, Bacher U, Schnittger S, et al. Multiparameter flow cytometry reveals myelodysplasia-related aberrant antigen expression in myelodysplastic/myeloproliferative neoplasms. Cytometry B Clin Cytom 2013;84(3):194–7.
60. Cremers EM, Westers TM, Alhan C, et al. Multiparameter flow cytometry is instrumental to distinguish myelodysplastic syndromes from non-neoplastic cytopenias. Eur J Cancer 2016;54:49–56.
61. Alhan C, Westers TM, Cremers EM, et al. The myelodysplastic syndromes flow cytometric score: a three-parameter prognostic flow cytometric scoring system. Leukemia 2016;30(3):658–65.
62. Brodersen LE, Menssen A, Zehentner BK, et al. A comparative assessment of flow cytometric scoring systems in MDS, in ASH. Blood 2014;124:5589.
63. Aster JC. Clinical manifestations and diagnosis of the myelodysplastic syndromes. Waltham (MA): UpToDate; 2016. Version 37.0.
64. Aanei CM, Picot T, Tavernier E, et al. Diagnostic utility of flow cytometry in myelodysplastic syndromes. Front Oncol 2016;6:161.
65. Alhan C, Westers TM, Cremers EM, et al. High flow cytometric scores identify adverse prognostic subgroups within the revised International Prognostic Scoring System for myelodysplastic syndromes. Br J Haematol 2014;167(1): 100–9.
66. Matarraz S, López A, Barrena S, et al. Bone marrow cells from myelodysplastic syndromes show altered immunophenotypic profiles that may contribute to the diagnosis and prognostic stratification of the disease: a pilot study on a series of 56 patients. Cytometry B Clin Cytom 2010;78(3):154–68.

67. Greenberg PL, Tuechler H, Schanz J, et al. Revised International Prognostic Scoring System for myelodysplastic syndromes. Blood 2012;120(12):2454–65.
68. Della Porta MG, Tuechler H, Malcovati L, et al. Validation of WHO classification-based prognostic scoring system (WPSS) for myelodysplastic syndromes and comparison with the revised International Prognostic Scoring System (IPSS-R). A study of the International Working Group for prognosis in myelodysplasia (IWG-PM). Leukemia 2015;29(7):1502–13.
69. Hoffmann DG, Kim BH. Limited flow cytometry panels on bone marrow specimens reduce costs and predict negative cytogenetics. Am J Clin Pathol 2014; 141(1):94–101.
70. Della Porta MG, Lanza F, Del Vecchio L. Flow cytometry immunophenotyping for the evaluation of bone marrow dysplasia. Cytometry B Clin Cytom 2011;80(4): 201–11.

Diagnosis of Plasma Cell Dyscrasias and Monitoring of Minimal Residual Disease by Multiparametric Flow Cytometry

CrossMark

Kah Teong Soh, MS*, Joseph D. Tario Jr, PhD, Paul K. Wallace, PhD

KEYWORDS

- Plasma cell dyscrasia • Plasma cell neoplasm • Multiparametric flow cytometry
- Multiple myeloma • Minimal residual disease • MRD • Panel optimization
- High-sensitivity assay

KEY POINTS

- Plasma cell dyscrasia is a hematological disorder in which normal plasma cells become transformed in the bone marrow and soft tissues.
- Multiparametric flow cytometry is a reliable tool to evaluate plasma cell dyscrasias.
- Flow cytometry is a high-sensitivity assay that can be used to detect minimal residual disease, which has been shown to correlate with progression-free survival and overall survival.

INTRODUCTION

Plasma cells (PC) are terminally differentiated and nondividing immune cells arising from B cells whose primary function is to secrete antibodies to fight infection.[1–3] PCs can live for a long period, even a lifetime, in the bone marrow if survival signals, such as interleukin (IL)-6, A proliferation-inducing ligand, and B-cell activating factor are provided by stromal cells and various hematopoietic cells, such as eosinophil.[4–9] PCs can produce only a single kind of antibody in a single class of immunoglobulin, but each cell can produce several thousand antibodies per second, making it an integral

Disclosure Statement: The authors have no commercial or financial conflicts of interest to disclose.
Flow cytometry services were provided by the Flow and Image Cytometry Core facility at the Roswell Park Cancer Institute, which is supported in part by the NCI Cancer Center Support Grant 5P30 CA016056.
Department of Flow and Image Cytometry, Roswell Park Cancer Institute, Elm and Carlton Streets, Buffalo, NY 14263, USA
* Corresponding author.
E-mail address: kahteong.soh@roswellpark.org

Clin Lab Med 37 (2017) 821–853
http://dx.doi.org/10.1016/j.cll.2017.08.001
0272-2712/17/© 2017 Elsevier Inc. All rights reserved.

labmed.theclinics.com

part of the humoral immune response.[10] PCs, like all other leukocytes, are susceptible to transformation. Most plasma cell dyscrasias (PCDs) develop after affinity maturation has occurred in the germinal center, as the gene sequence of most myeloma cells are hypermutated, exhibit phenotypic features similar to those of long-lived PCs, and are usually distributed in multiple compartments of the bone marrow.[1,11–13] Once a clonal PC population is established, it has the potential to behave in many ways, not all of which will require treatment. Currently, there are several subtypes of PCDs, including (1) monoclonal gammopathy of undetermined significance (MGUS), (2) asymptomatic myeloma, (3) multiple myeloma, (4) PC leukemia, (5) plasmacytoma, and (6) amyloidosis.[14,15]

PLASMA CELL DISORDERS

Normal PCs generate a spectrum of antibodies with different heavy chain (immunoglobulin [Ig]M, IgG, IgA, IgD, and IgE) and light chain (kappa and lambda) characteristics. With the exception of a very few nonsecreting cases, a common early finding in early PCDs is the presence of a monoclonal heavy and light chain restricted antibody, referred to as an a paraprotein or M protein. These often appear before any relevant clinical symptoms are discerned. A monoclonal gammopathy is defined as any situation in which a clonal M protein is present in the blood or urine and is reflective of a clonal plasma or lymphoid cell proliferation. Purely reactive proliferations will often generate a polyclonal immunoglobulin response, but these are by definition not monoclonal M proteins. Because both PC and lymphoproliferative disorders can produce M proteins, making the distinction between which type of disorder is responsible for the M protein is critically important and flow cytometry can assist in this process. Diseases of PCs include MGUS, multiple myeloma, and PC leukemia.

Monoclonal Gammopathy of Undetermined Significance

MGUS is the most-common PC disorder. Its incidence rises rapidly with age and affects 3% of individuals 50 years or older and 10% of individuals older than 70.[16–19] Increasingly more sensitive assays and more frequent testing have resulted in increased diagnosis. MGUS is characterized by a serum M protein of less than 30 g/L with fewer than 10% PCs in the bone marrow and no evidence of bone or organ damage.[14] Although it reflects the presence of an expanded clone of immunoglobulin-secreting cells, it is not considered a malignancy and no immediate therapeutic intervention is required. Only approximately 1% of patients with MGUS will progress to myeloma each year.[20] The immunophenotype of MGUS frequently shows 2 populations of $CD38^{br}$, $CD138^{br}$ PCs, one with a normal $CD19^+$, $CD56^-$ phenotype that is polyclonal and a second that is either $CD19^-$ and $CD56^+$ or $CD56^-$ and monoclonal.[21]

Asymptomatic Plasma Cell Myeloma

Asymptomatic myeloma is characterized by an M protein concentration of greater than 30 g/L, with more than 10% PCs in the bone marrow, but with no related tissue or end-organ damage or clinical sequelae, such as hypercalcemia, renal failure, anemia, and bone lesions.[14,22] The presence of radiographically detected bone lesions, even if not symptomatic, would exclude a patient from this category because these are an indication for treatment. Approximately 10% of patients with asymptomatic myeloma will progress to multiple myeloma each year.[23,24] Because smoldering and indolent PC myeloma are a continuum, neither can be reliably diagnosed prospectively, and both are asymptomatic, thus the term asymptomatic PC myeloma is preferred to describe both.

Multiple Myeloma

Multiple myeloma is characterized by an M protein concentration of greater than 30 g/L, greater than 10% PCs in the bone marrow, and evidence of organ and tissue damage.[14] It is also characterized by calcium elevation, renal insufficiency, anemia, and bone lesions due to the accumulation of clonal PCs in the bone marrow. Unlike PC leukemia, the PCs in multiple myeloma circulate in the blood at such a low frequency they cannot be readily detected morphologically. Each year in the United States, nearly 27,000 people are diagnosed with multiple myeloma, which accounts for 1% of all malignancies and 10% of all hematological neoplasms.[25] Normally, PCs make up fewer than 5% of leukocytes in the bone marrow, but if they transform, PCs can fill up the bone marrow, and also cause damage to the bone through the release of osteoclast-activating factors.[26] Over time, they collect and form tumors in multiple areas of the bones, giving rise to the term "multiple" myeloma.

Plasma Cell Leukemia

PC leukemia is similar to multiple myeloma but differs in presentation due to the presence of PCs in the peripheral blood circulation. It is defined as a population of at least 2×10^3 PCs/μL or representing more than 20% of circulating leukocytes.[16] PC leukemia may be present at the time of initial diagnosis but more commonly evolves as a late feature of multiple myeloma (secondary PC leukemia). Primary PC leukemia is found in 2% to 5% of myeloma cases and has a poor prognosis.[27–29] PC leukemias are usually associated with hypercalcemia, renal failure, and anemia, but not bone lesions. Phenotypically, it is more often CD56$^-$ than multiple myelomas.

Plasmacytoma

Plasmacytoma is a discrete solid PC tumor found either in the bone (solitary bone plasmacytoma) or soft tissues (extramedullary plasmacytoma). Approximately 80% of extramedullary plasmacytomas occur in the upper respiratory tract, including the oropharynx, nasopharynx, sinuses, or larynx, although they can occur in any soft tissue. Approximately 20% of cases have a small M protein, most typically IgA. Symptoms are generally related to the tumor mass and compression of adjacent tissues. Plasmacytomas are characterized by a similar range of immunophenotypic and genotypic abnormalities to those encountered in multiple myeloma.[30]

Primary Amyloidosis

Primary amyloidosis is a rare disorder caused by a PC that produces intact immunoglobulins or most commonly immunoglobulin light chain fragments and rarely heavy chain fragments. These build up in tissues and organs forming β-amyloid sheets. Renal and cardiac amyloid deposition can cause serious organ impairment and death. The immunophenotype of PCs causing primary amyloidosis, like myeloma, are typically light chain restricted, CD38 and CD138 positive, CD45 negative or dim, with most being CD56$^+$, CD117$^+$, and CD19$^-$.[31,32]

DIAGNOSIS

The diagnosis of PCD is challenging. For instance, studies have reported similar genetic alteration between premalignant MGUS and multiple myeloma.[11] Accordingly, diagnosis is usually based on several factors. A standard workup includes total serum protein, serum and urine protein electrophoresis, immunofixation in serum and urine, detection of serum-free light chains (sFLCs), and the following additional parameters: complete blood count, serum creatinine, electrolytes (including calcium), lactate dehydrogenase, and β2 microglobulin. In a patient with suspected multiple myeloma, a bone marrow biopsy is normally obtained.

Multiparametric flow cytometry (MFC) is a powerful technique that has been routinely used in clinical settings to characterize, diagnose, and monitor hematological malignancies.[33–39] Although the assessment of myeloma cells in the bone marrow compartment by flow cytometry has been conducted since the 1990s, the technology has only recently been widely accepted as a routine clinical test for multiple myeloma.[40–44] This delayed acceptance was due primarily to the unavailability of specific markers that could be used for reliable detection of PCs and selective loss of PCs while making a single-cell suspension from bone marrow.[45,46] Technical variables, including PC baseline autofluorescence levels, inconsistent staining profiles, and the use of different monoclonal antibody (mAb) clones and fluorochromes all contributed to the slow adoption of MFC for the detection of PCDs.[42,45–50]

With the increased understanding of human cell biology and the expansion of mAb choices, recent reports published by independent investigators have shown that the expression of several markers can be used to distinguish normal from abnormal PCs.[37,43–45,48,51–54] As such, more than 95% of patients with multiple myeloma are found to have an aberrant phenotype associated with their neoplastic PCs. The remainder of this article focuses on the utilization of MFC immunophenotyping and how it can be helpful in the diagnosis, prognosis, and disease monitoring of PCDs. Specifically, the methodological considerations involved during panel design, including the selection and validation of informative mAbs, and data analysis is elaborated.

Methodological Considerations for Evaluating Abnormal Plasma Cells

MFC is a reliable technique that enables concurrent and correlated detection and analysis of multiple parameters at the single-cell level. It permits the study of large number of cells within a relatively short period, storage of that information for further evaluation, quantitative evaluation of antigen expression levels, and combined detection of surface and intracellular antigens.[36,45,55,56] Before flow cytometry can be applied to clinical diagnosis of PCDs, optimizing sample preparation, panel configuration, and analysis and gating strategies is critical.[57–63] This topic has been previously addressed in detail and the reader is referred to the Cytometry B Special Issue dedicated to the validation of cell-based fluorescence assays from the International Council for Standardization of Haematology and the International Clinical Cytometry Society.[57,59–61,64] Major efforts over the past couple of years have also been invested into reaching a consensus over which mAb panels should be run on bone marrow samples from newly diagnosed patients with multiple myeloma and when testing them for minimal residual disease (MRD).[58,65,66] Presently, the lack of External Quality Assessment (EQA)/Proficiency Testing (PT) programs for PCD testing constrains the evaluation of interlaboratory reproducibility and concordance.[55,67] At the time of this writing, the UK NEQAS (United Kingdom National External Quality Assessment Service) group had begun a prototype EQA/PT program that evaluated the reproducibility of multiple myeloma MRD detection among 8 participating laboratories. Before such programs become widely available, the optimization and validation of a flow cytometry-based PCD assay should be taken with care, using current published consensus protocols as a guideline and validated by comparing results with a laboratory that has a well-established assay. This section describes in detail sample handling, mAb and fluorochrome selection, panel design, sample staining, data analysis, evaluation of sample quality, and reporting.

Panel Selection

In clinical flow cytometry, cell populations are considered as abnormal if they have an atypical differentiation pattern, increased or decreased expression of normal antigens, asynchronous maturational patterns, or the expression of aberrant antigens. Currently, the most commonly used markers for the discrimination of normal plasma and myeloma cells from other leukocytes include CD38, CD138, CD45, CD19, CD56, and cytoplasmic immunoglobulin light chains in combination with light scatter.[37,41] Practically, an assay for detecting PCD should be able to identify disease in all tested patients, which is a strength of flow cytometry when compared with other technologies. It does not necessarily have to fully characterize the disease but should retain the capability of detecting the presence of diseased cells with appropriate specificity and sensitivity. The minimum mAbs recommended for initial assessment of PCDs are CD38, CD138, CD45, CD19, and CD56, with the expression of secondary antigens considered to be informative when added as necessary.[58] The expression patterns of CD38, CD138, and CD45 antigens are recommended by the European Myeloma Network to be used as the backbone markers for the identification and enumeration of PCs in all tubes.[66,68] The unique expression patterns of CD19, CD20, CD27, CD28, CD56, CD81, CD117, and cytoplasmic immunoglobulin light chains have all been used for the discrimination between normal or reactive versus clonal PCs (**Table 1**).[45,48,68,69]

An effective panel that has been proposed and validated by the International Clinical Cytometry Society (ICCS) multiple myeloma MRD consensus group and the EuroFlow consortium consists of two 8-color tubes that measure a total of 10 specific antigens.[53,70] The final panel used by these groups has 8 surface markers in the first tube (tube 1), and the second tube (tube 2) is composed of 6 surface and 2 intracellular markers (**Table 2**). In our configuration, Tube 1 and Tube 2 have a backbone of CD38, CD138, and CD45, which in combination with light scatter provides the best approach for identification of PCs and their discrimination from

Table 1
Comparison of antigen expression patterns between normal and abnormal plasma cells

| Antigen(s) | Normal Plasma Cells | | Abnormal Plasma Cells | |
	Expression Level	Percentage	Expression Level	Percentage
a. Identification of normal and abnormal plasma cells in bone marrow				
CD45[a]	+++	94	−	73–80
CD38[a]	+++	100	+	80
CD138	++	98	++	98
b. Markers useful for the distinction of normal and abnormal plasma cells in bone marrow				
CD19	++	>70	−	95
CD56	−	>85	+++	60–75
CD117	−	100	++	30–32
CD27	+++	100	− to +	40–68
CD81	++	100	− to +	55
CD28	− to +	<15 dim cells	+++	15–45
CD20	−	>95	++	17–30
CD200	−	N/A	+++	70

+, Dimly Positive; ++, Moderately Positive; +++, Strongly Positive; −, Negative.
[a] Can be used to identify and distinguish normal and abnormal plasma cells.

Table 2
Composition of panel used for the characterization of plasma cells

Antigen	Fluorochrome	Clone	Source
a. Tube 1			
CD138	BV421	MI15	Becton Dickinson (San Jose, CA)
CD27	BV510	O323	BioLegend (San Diego, CA)
CD38	FITC	T16	Beckman Coulter (Brea, CA)
CD56	PE	C5.9	Cytognos (Salamanca, Spain)
CD45	PcPCy5.5	HI30	BioLegend (San Diego, CA)
CD19	PECy7	J3-119	Beckman Coulter (Brea, CA)
CD117	APC	104D2	Becton Dickinson (San Jose, CA)
CD81	APC-C750	M38	Cytognos (Salamanca, CA)
b. Tube 2			
CD138	BV421	MI15	Becton Dickinson (San Jose, CA)
CD27	BV510	O323	BioLegend (San Diego, CA)
CD38	FITC	T16	Beckman Coulter (Brea, CA)
CD56	PE	C5.9	Cytognos (Salamanca, Spain)
CD45	PcPCy5.5	HI30	BioLegend (San Diego, CA)
CD19	PECy7	J3-119	Beckman Coulter (Brea, CA)
cKappa	APC	poly	Dako (Carpinteria, CA)
cLambda	APC-C750	poly	Cytognos (Salamanca, Spain)
c. Tube 3			
CD138	BV421	MI15	Becton Dickinson (San Jose, CA)
Live Dead Aqua	—	—	Thermo Fisher Scientific (Grand Island, NY)
CD38	FITC	T16	Beckman Coulter (Brea, CA)
CD45	PcPCy5.5	H130	BioLegend (San Diego, CA)

Abbreviations: APC, allophycocyanin; APC-C750, Allophycocyanin Tandem 750; BV421, Brilliant Violet 421; BV510, Brilliant Violet 510; FITC, fluorescein isothiocyanate; PcPCy5.5, Peridinin Chlorophyll Cyanine 5.5; PE, phycoerythrin; PECy7, Phycoerythrin Cyanine 7.

all other cells in the sample. Both tubes also contain CD19, CD56, and CD27. In combination with CD38 and CD45, which can be aberrantly dim or absent, the lack of CD19 expression and/or strong CD56 expression and/or dim CD27 expression differentiates in most cases neoplastic PCs from their normal counterpart. Tube 1 also has CD81 and CD117, whereas in tube 2 these mAbs are substituted with cytoplasmic anti-kappa and anti-lambda polyclonal antibodies. The merit of using two 8-color tubes with redundancy in the design allows for the confirmation of the presence and number of abnormal PCs in acquired samples from a statistical and internal quality control standpoint. As the costs associated with the 2-tube approach are higher and the technical aspect of clinical flow cytometer continues to improve to accommodate more fluorescent parameters, a few laboratories have explored using a single 10-color tube.[71,72] Regardless, both approaches are in harmony. When directly compared, the single 10-color tube had a slight reduction in total cell number, although there was no apparent loss of either normal or abnormal PCs. To perform a viability assessment and to establish background autofluorescent levels, the authors' laboratory uses a third tube, which contains a Fixable Live Dead reagent with anti-CD38, anti-CD138, and anti-CD45.

The significance of CD19, CD20, CD27, CD28, CD38, CD45, CD56, CD81, CD117, and CD138 as they relate to PCDs is described as follows:

CD19

CD19 is normally expressed at all stages of B-cell development ranging from pro-B to PCs. In patients with MGUS, the expression of CD19 on PCs is normally high, whereas PCs in multiple myeloma are most often either negative or dim for CD19 expression.[24] The decreased expression of CD19 is usually caused by the altered expression of PAX-5.[63] The lack of expression of CD19 has been a facilitating feature when identifying malignant PCs, as more than 95% of abnormal PCs are negative for CD19, whereas it is noteworthy that CD19 is positively expressed only by approximately 70% of normal PCs.[62]

CD20

CD20 expression occurs later in early B-cell maturation while CD34 is concurrently downregulated. As B cells differentiate into normal PCs, they lose CD20, but it is expressed on roughly one-third of abnormal PCs. The CD20 antigen has been associated with shorter patient survival; however, the prognostic significance of CD20 expression is unclear.[73] CD20 is associated with a mature morphology and often with a small PC, lymphoplasmacytic morphology with the t(11:14) translocation.[69]

CD27

CD27 plays a role in helping B cells differentiate into PCs. In the B-cell lineage, CD27 is considered as a memory marker because its expression is limited to germinal center cells, memory B cells, and PCs.[69] In MGUS, the expression of CD27 on PCs is usually high. In patients with multiple myeloma, the expression of CD27 on abnormal PCs is often dimmer than normal PCs. When CD27 is expressed at normal intensities on abnormal PCs, it is usually correlated with a better prognosis, and loss of CD27 expression has been associated with shorter progression-free survival (PFS) and overall survival (OS).[74,75]

CD28

CD28 is normally not expressed on PCs and rarely in patients with MGUS, but in one-third of patients with multiple myeloma it is found on their abnormal PCs. The expression of CD28 is associated with an aggressive myeloma phenotype. When used concurrently with CD117, it has been found that CD28 can be used to stratify multiple myeloma cases into 3 risk categories[49]: (1) good prognosis CD28−/CD117+, (2) intermediate prognosis CD28−/CD117−, and (3) poor prognosis CD28+/CD117−. As the disease progresses, CD28 expression increases and it is often associated with relapse.[76] Interestingly, although the expression of CD28 can induce antigen-independent T-cell activation, it does not induce proliferation in neoplastic PCs; instead, it is speculated to act as a prosurvival signal to myeloma cells by ligating CD80/CD86 on myeloid DC facilitating the secretion of supportive cytokines such as IL-6 and IL-8,[69,77,78] as well as the immunosuppressive enzyme IDO.[79]

CD38

CD38 is present on many cells, including B-cell progenitors and germinal center B cells.[80,81] Both abnormal and normal PCs brightly express CD38, with neoplastic cells often expressing it at a slightly lower intensity than normal PC.[82] Antibodies to CD38 are currently being used therapeutically for the treatment of multiple myeloma, which can block the binding of many mAb clones used in flow cytometry, causing the myeloma in samples from these patients to appear CD38 negative.

CD45

CD45 is a well-known marker that is expressed at variable levels on leukocyte subsets. Normal PCs, although generally positive, also can be negative for CD45.[82] In patients with MGUS, heterogeneous distribution of CD45+ normal and CD45− abnormal PCs in bone marrow have been observed.[83] In patients with multiple myeloma, however, the expression of CD45 on neoplastic PCs is negative to dim in most cases. The expression of CD45 with other markers, such as CD19 or CD27, allows further refinement of the PC identification process.[84]

CD56

CD56, also known as the neural cell adhesion molecule (NCAM), is a common marker used for the identification of natural killer (NK) and NKT cells, as well as a valuable marker that can be used to define an abnormal phenotype of neoplastic PCs. It is an adhesion molecule involved in anchorage of myelomatous PC to the bone marrow stroma and its absence of expression is associated in some studies with extramedullary spreading and more aggressive disease.[49] Positive CD56 expression can be found on PCs in the bone marrow in most patients with multiple myeloma. Myeloma cells circulating into the peripheral blood usually lack CD56, whereas myeloma cells located in pleural or ascetic effusions are usually CD56+. The down-modulation of CD56 by a formerly positive myeloma may indicate extramedullary diffusion of the disease,[85] whereas its initial absence has been associated with the presence of extra-marrow involvement, a tendency to leukemization, a lower frequency of osteolytic lesions, and plasmablastic morphology.[86–88] When combined with CD19, the expression of CD56 can provide substantial diagnostic value.[69] Lack of CD19 expression and/or strong CD56 expression differentiates neoplastic PCs from their normal counterpart in most cases. However, it should be noted that with improving outcomes and increased sensitivity of flow-MRD methods, it is now well-established that a subset of normal PCs can be CD19− and/or CD56+.[69]

CD81

CD81 is a tetraspanin family member broadly expressed on hematopoietic cells with the exception of erythrocytes, platelets, and neutrophils.[89] It is expressed on all B cells, where it forms a multimolecular complex with CD19 and CD21, which together are involved in signaling of B-cell maturation and antibody production. The expression of CD81 on immature B cells is brighter than on mature B cells. In approximately half of the patients with multiple myeloma, the expression of CD81 is dim to negative in comparison with normal PCs.[37] It has been found that patients with CD81 expression on myeloma cells have shorter PFS and OS when compared with those who do not express it.[90]

CD117

CD117, also known as the proto-oncogene c-Kit, is commonly found on myeloid, erythroid, and megakaryocytic progenitors, and mast cells, whereas normal PCs are CD117−.[91–93] In MGUS, 50% of the cases express CD117; in multiple myeloma, approximately one-third of patients are CD117+.[93] The expression of CD117 on PCs predicted better outcome, and it can be used in combination with CD28 to allow for risk stratification (see CD28 described previously).

CD138

CD138, also known as syndecan-1, is a transmembrane heparin sulfate proteoglycan that is expressed during PC stage of B-cell maturation. CD138 functions as the alpha receptor for collagen, fibronectin, and thrombospondin.[94] In addition, CD138 also can be shed into the extracellular matrix to trap growth-promoting and proangiogenic cytokines.[95,96] Both abnormal and normal PCs in MGUS and multiple myeloma express high levels of CD138.[82] Currently, CD138 serves as a universal marker for PC detection and it can provide a basis to quantify or assess disease burden. The staining intensity of CD138 mAbs may be attenuated when samples are exposed to sodium heparin, stored for long periods, refrigerated, or frozen.[95,97,98]

Performance Evaluation of Fluorochrome-Conjugated Monoclonal Antibodies

When selecting the mAbs to be incorporated into a multiple myeloma panel, the cytometrist is presented with a variety of choices in clones, fluorochromes, and sources. **Table 2** presents a list of markers found to give the best resolution of PCs from other leukocytes with excellent discrimination between normal and abnormal PCs. This table should be used as a general guide for laboratories designing their own panels to diagnose and monitor PCDs. The strategies used to assess the performance of individual mAbs, such as fluorescence intensity, percentage of negative versus positive cells, signal-to-noise ratio, and stain index will vary from laboratory-to-laboratory; however, we have found signal-to-noise and stain index to be the most informative. Building on the experience of the EuroFlow group,[70] we evaluated several additional clones and fluorochromes to derive the panel described in **Table 2**. The most significant adjustment was to replace CD138 Pac Blue with BV421 and CD27 Pac Orange with BV510, changes that were also adopted by the EuroFlow group. We also found CD38 clone T16 from Beckman Coulter gave a slightly higher signal-to-noise ratio. The detection of CD38 is becoming problematic with the introduction and clinical use of daratumumab, a humanized IgG1 kappa mAb targeting CD38 and shown to significantly improve outcomes in refractory multiple myeloma. Daratumumab blocks the binding of most anti-CD38 mAbs used in flow cytometry interfering with the assessment of PCDs. To date, the only partial solution found has been to use a multi-epitope anti-CD38 containing a cocktail of mAbs. Other approaches under investigation have been to look at substituting or combining mAbs to CD38 with mAb to CD54, CD229, and CD319.[54]

In panel development, to confirm that the fluorochromes selected for each mAb do not have significant signal broadening or cross-laser excitation artifact that would compromise the resolution of important populations, we use a fluorescence minus one (FMO) approach.[99] This consists of an mAb cocktail in which the mAbs included are identical to those in the test article, except for the exclusion of the one fluorochrome that is being controlled. To completely validate the PCD tubes, we control for all fluorochromes. In the 8-color cocktails shown in **Table 2**, we set up 9 tubes for each cocktail; the first tube containing all the mAbs except for the fluorescein isothiocyanate–conjugated mAb, the second minus the phycoerythrin-conjugated mAb, continuing this process for all fluorochromes and finishing with a tube containing all the mAbs. Each FMO is compared with the fully stained panel ensuring that all populations of interest are well separated.

The panel in **Table 2** represents a consensus approach that can be readily adopted.[66,70] Laboratories desiring to modify the consensus approach should demonstrate that their panel is comparable or better than the consensus panel. A strategy to determine the performance of an alternative mAb is to evaluate its staining resolution in conjunction with all the other mAbs used in the panel, rather than using the mAb alone. This is best accomplished by defining a negatively and positively stained population and calculating their signal-to-noise ratio as first described by Rawston and colleagues.[100] As an example (**Fig. 1**), when evaluating the performance of CD81, the signal-to-noise ratio may be calculated by dividing the fluorescence intensity of an

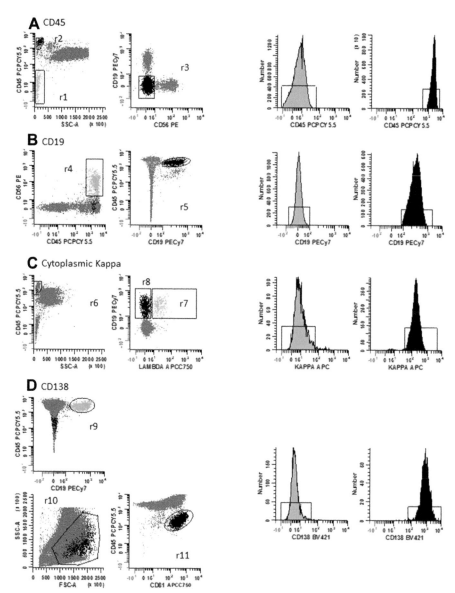

Fig. 1. Signal-to-noise ratio performance assessment strategy for mAbs. The strategy to assess the performance of each mAb in the PCD panel relies on defining a negatively and positively staining population for each mAb. These populations are defined in **Table 3**. Next, the median fluorescence intensity (MFI) is determined for each population and the signal-to-noise ratio calculated by dividing the positive population's MFI by the negative population's MFI. To qualify as an acceptable mAb, the calculated signal-to-noise value should be greater than the recommend value in **Table 4**. (*A*) For CD45, erythroid precursors are used as the negative population defined as SSC^{lo}/CD45$^-$ events (r1: *yellow dots* and corresponding histogram) and T cells as the positive population defined as CD45^{br}/SSC^{lo} (r2) and CD19$^-$/CD56$^-$ events (r3: *black dots* and corresponding histogram). (*B*) For CD19, NK cells are used as the negative population defined as CD45^{br}/CD56$^+$ events (r4: *yellow dots* and corresponding histogram) and B cells as the positive population defined as CD19+/CD45^{br} events

internal positive population (eg, T lymphocytes defined as CD19$^-$/CD56$^-$/CD45^{br}/SSC^{lo}) by the fluorescence intensity of an internal negative population (eg, granulocytes defined as CD45^{dim}/SSC^{hi}). This approach can be performed on both peripheral blood and bone marrow samples, but it should be noted that the specimen used should mimic the condition and type of the specimens to be tested. In **Tables 3** and **4**, the data for all mAbs from our analysis of 10 bone marrow samples with no hematological disease are provided. Laboratories initiating a validation of their PCD panel may use this table as a guideline to measure the performance of each mAb in their tube(s). CD138 was an exception. Due to the paucity of CD138-positive cells in normal bone marrow we used a CD-CHEX CD103 PLUS control reagent (Streck, Omaha, NE) that contains a CD138-positive control population and compared its fluorescence intensity with B cells defined as CD19$^+$/CD45^{br}/SSC^{lo}.

Sample Storage and Quality

Bone marrow aspirate, blood, and fine needle aspirate (FNA) are appropriate specimens for the routine detection of PCs. Multiple myeloma MRD testing has been established on bone marrow aspirates. The detection and assessment of abnormal PCs in peripheral blood at initial diagnosis and 2 weeks before an autologous stem cell collection may become a routine test as studies have demonstrated these can be clinically relevant.[101,102] Regardless of the types of specimen received for testing, the importance of having good-quality samples before processing cannot be overemphasized.

As the age of a specimen is a critical factor for any test carried out using flow cytometry, the sample tube should be labeled with the collection date and time. It is recommended that blood and bone marrow specimen be stored at room temperature.[103] Standard practice is to process specimens as soon as possible and preferably within 48 hours of collection. Samples may be collected in either an EDTA or sodium heparin vacutainer tube, although EDTA is preferable due to attenuation of CD138 signal when stored in heparin. Tissue samples may be placed in a small volume of RPMI as a holding medium and should be processed immediately.

A compromised specimen such as one that is excessively hemodilute, partially clotted, too warm or cold to the touch, or displays sign of hemolysis will not yield the same results as when optimal specimens are processed. For this reason, the quality and integrity of a bone marrow specimen should be qualitatively assessed on receipt via physical observations. Hemodilution can be determined by confirming the presence of normal PCs, B-cell progenitors, mast cells, and nucleated red blood cells in the bone marrow specimen.[65] The viability and the presence of PCs in a specimen can

---

(r5: *black dots* and corresponding histogram). (*C*) For cKappa light chain, cLambda light chain$^+$ B cells are used as the negative population defined as CD45^{br}/SSC-A^{lo} (r6) and CD19$^+$/cLambda light chain$^+$ events (r7: *yellow dots* and corresponding histogram) and cLambda light chain$^-$ cells as the positive population defined as CD45^{br}/SSC-A^{lo} (r6) and CD19$^+$/cLambda light chain$^-$ events (r8: *black dots* and corresponding histogram). (*D*) For CD138 a procedural control for immunophenotyping, CD-Chex CD103 Plus cells, which contains a CD138-positive population are spiked into a bone marrow sample. B cells are used as the negative population defined as CD45^{br}/CD19$^+$ events (r9: *yellow dots* and corresponding histogram) and spiked control cells as the positive population defined by FSC-A and SSC-A (r10) and as CD45^{dim}/CD81$^+$ events (r11: *black dots* and corresponding histogram). Note these data are all gated on R1 and R2 and R3, "Total Leukocytes" as defined in **Fig. 2**. In data not shown, for the CD19 negative and positive populations, and CD138 negative population an FSC-A versus SSC-A plot was used to define lymphocytes.

Table 3
Determination of internal negative and positive populations using bone marrow sample for the selection of optimal monoclonal antibody combination

Tested Markers	Negative Population		Positive Population	
	Phenotype	Generic Name	Phenotype	Generic Name
CD45	CD45$^-$/SSC^{lo}	Erythroid cells	CD19$^-$/CD56$^-$/CD45^{br}/SSC^{lo}	T cells
CD19	CD45^{br}/CD56$^+$/SSC^{lo}	Natural killer cells	CD19$^+$/CD45^{br}/SSC^{lo}	B cells
CD27	CD117$^+$/CD45^{dim}	Mast cells	CD19$^-$/CD56$^-$/CD45^{br}/SSC^{lo}	T cells
CD81	CD45^{dim}/SSC^{hi}	Granulocytes	CD19$^-$/CD56$^-$/CD45^{br}/SSC^{lo}	T cells
CD56	CD19$^+$/CD56$^-$/CD45^{br}/SSC^{lo}	B cells	CD19$^-$/CD56$^+$/CD45^{br}/SSC^{lo}	NK cells
CD117	CD19$^-$/CD56$^-$/CD45^{br}/SSC^{lo}	T cells	CD45^{dim}/CD117$^+$	Mast cells
CD138	CD19$^+$/CD45^{br}/SSC^{lo}	B cells	CD45^{dim}/CD81$^+$	Spiked control[a]
CD38	CD19$^+$/CD81$^-$	Mature B	CD19$^+$/CD81$^+$	B-progenitors
cKappa	CD19$^+$/CD45^{br}/cLambda$^+$/SSC^{lo}	cLambda$^+$ B cells	CD19$^+$/CD45^{br}/cLambda$^-$/SSC^{lo}	Lambda$^-$ B cells
cLambda	CD19$^+$/CD45^{br}/cKappa$^+$/SSC^{lo}	cKappa$^+$ B cells	CD19$^+$/CD45^{br}/cKappa$^-$/SSC^{lo}	Kappa$^-$ B cells

[a] A procedural control for immunophenotyping, CD-Chex CD103 Plus (Streck, Omaha, NE), which contains CD138, was spiked into the bone marrow sample and used as the positive population.

be checked using the staining tube 3. Samples with less than 85% viability are deemed suboptimal for flow cytometry testing. In such cases, it is recommended that each report include a statement about sample quality including a notation of hemodilution and viability. In the event an irreplaceable and rare specimen, such as bone

Table 4
Evaluation of staining performance of monoclonal antibody in the context of multicolor analysis

Tested Markers	Evaluated Sample, n[a]	Signal-to-Noise		
		Mean ± SD	Range	Recommended
CD45	10	323.7 ± 101.0	226.0–573.2	>100
CD19	10	134.5 ± 56.6	37.6–215.3	>10
CD27	10	20.7 ± 6.9	10.3–32.1	>5
CD81	10	25.3 ± 12.2	11.8–49.4	>5
CD56	10	50.1 ± 25.1	32.0–114.9	>10
CD117	10	46.1 ± 31.0	15.2–99.9	>10
CD138	10	83.9 ± 46.3	30.9–144.3	>10
CD38	10	19.5 ± 9.8	4.8–36.0	>3
cKappa	10	18 ± 13.2	4.9–45.2	>3
cLambda	10	13.5 ± 5.4	5.8–25.4	>3

[a] Ten random patient bone marrow samples received for flow cytometric evaluation that had no evidence of hematological disease by flow cytometry or histopathological assessment.

marrow, is compromised due to unforeseen circumstances, it should not be rejected for flow cytometry testing. Instead a notation must be included clearly stating that the result may have been compromised and why.

Staining Procedure to Label Leukocyte Subsets

Depending on the level of sensitivity required, there are 2 staining procedures that can be used for the assessment of PCDs, these are (1) the routine PCD test (eg, low-sensitivity assay) and (2) the MRD high-sensitivity test. The reason for 2 different staining procedures is due to the difference in frequency of abnormal cells that are present between overt disease (eg, at the time of diagnosis) and rare cell detection (eg, after the patients have undergone treatment). The routine test is less labor intensive but lacks the sensitivity of the MRD assay. This section discusses the procedure for routine PCD testing. High-sensitivity MRD testing is described in the section entitled "Minimal Residual Disease Testing." In both procedures, the panel described in **Table 2** is applicable. For routine testing, a less comprehensive panel consisting of at least CD38, CD138, CD45, CD19, and CD56 can be used with secondary mAbs to CD27, CD117, cytoplasmic light chain reagents, and other mAbs added as required.

Details of our routine testing procedures can be found elsewhere.[104] Briefly, bone marrow samples received for PCD testing are filtered through a 70-μm cell strainer (Corning, Manassas, VA) to exclude spicules from the samples. An absolute cell count on blood, bone marrow, and FNA is performed using an automated cell counter (eg, Sysmex XS-1000i, Lincolnshire, IL). The specimen is then transferred to a 15-mL conical tube and washed twice using flow cytometry (FCM) buffer (containing 0.5% bovine serum albumin, 0.1% sodium azide, 0.04 g/L and sodium EDTA in phosphate-buffered saline [PBS]) to remove plasma immunoglobulins. A second cell count is performed, and approximately 1×10^6 cells are transferred to 3 labeled 12×75-mm polystyrene tubes. Cocktails of fluorochrome-conjugated mAbs are added to each tube according to **Table 2** and the samples are incubated for 30 minutes at room temperate in the dark. After surface labeling, 2 mL FACS Lysing Solution (BD Biosciences, San Jose, CA) is added to each tube and allowed to stand at room temperature for 10 minutes. All the tubes are then centrifuged at 540g for 5 minutes and washed once using FCM buffer.

Tubes to be labeled with surface mAbs only (eg, Tube 1 and tube 3) are resuspended in 500 μL 0.5% methanol-free formaldehyde (Polysciences, Warrington, PA) in PBS. For intracellular staining with anti-kappa and anti-lambda reagents (eg, tube 2), following the first wash in FCM buffer, the cells are resuspended in 300 μL 2% formaldehyde and incubated in the dark for 20 minutes at room temperature. Fixed cells are then washed with 3 mL FCM buffer and resuspended in 50 μL Permeabilization Medium B (Thermo Fisher Scientific, Carlsbad, CA). Saturating amounts of kappa and lambda antibodies are added and the sample is incubated in the dark for 30 minutes at room temperature. Finally, this tube is washed once using FCM buffer and resuspended in 500 μL FCM buffer or 0.5% formaldehyde for data acquisition.

Data Analysis and Gating Strategy

The analysis approach recommended by the ICCS Consensus Group uses the expression of CD38, CD138, CD45, and light-scatter characteristics to define PCs, while excluding contaminant lymphocytes, doublets, and debris. Such "fit-for-purpose" gating strategy can be easily adapted to any multiple myeloma analysis, regardless of the instrument, panel, or type of flow cytometric analysis software package used. The recommended gating steps for an inclusive identification, enumeration, and characterization of PCs are as follows:

Identification of total plasma cells

a. Place a rectangular region (R1) on a bivariate plot (A) of time versus side scatter (SSC)-A to circumscribe all events collected in continuity (**Fig. 2**). This dot plot can be used to assess the chronologic heterogeneity of the acquisition by eliminating any invalid events, such as air bubbles, which may occur during the run.

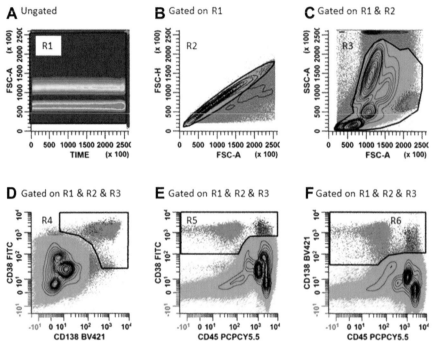

Fig. 2. Gating strategy used for the identification of normal and abnormal plasma cells. (A) A rectangular region (R1) is placed on the bivariate plot of time versus SSC-A to circumscribe all events collected in continuity. This dot plot can be used to assess the chronologic heterogeneity of the acquisition by eliminating any invalid events such as air bubbles that occur during the run. (B) Serial gating is performed by applying the region R1 to a bivariate plot of FSC-A versus FSC-H. A rhomboid region (R2) is then created to include the singlet cell population. Caution should be exercised not to exclude hyperdiploid or tetraploid plasma cells that may exhibit aberrantly high light-scatter characteristics. (C) Gate a bivariate plot of FSC-A versus SSC-A on (R1 and R2). An irregular region (R3) is created to circumscribe the cell population of interest and exclude aggregated events, debris, and dead and apoptotic events. Create 3 separate bivariate plots ([D] CD138 vs CD38), ([E] CD45 vs CD38), and ([F] CD45 vs CD138). Gate each of these bivariate plots on "Total Leukocytes" (R1 and R2 and R3). An irregular region (R4) is drawn on panel 2D circumscribing the CD138$^+$/CD38$^+$ events; another irregular region (R5) is drawn on panel 2E circumscribing the CD45$^{+/-}$/CD38$^+$ events; a third irregular region (R6) is drawn on panel 2F circumscribing the CD45$^{+/-}$/CD138$^+$ events. CD45 is helpful for defining PCs and identifying any CD38$^-$ or CD138$^-$ PC populations. The Boolean gate (R1 and R2 and R3 and R4 and R5 and R6) defines both normal (*blue*) and abnormal (*red*) PCs for subsequent immunophenotyping.

b. On a bivariate plot (B) of forward scatter (FSC)-A versus FSC-H, create a rectangular region (R2) to include the singlet cell population. Doublets will have more FSC-A than FSC-H. Gate this bivariate histogram on (R1).

c. On a bivariate plot (C) of FSC-A versus SSC-A, create an irregular region (R3) to circumscribe the cell population of interest and exclude aggregates, debris, and dead or apoptotic events. Gate this bivariate histogram on (R1 and R2). Cells gated on (R1 and R2 and R3) define "Total Leukocytes."

d. Create 3 separate bivariate plots (D: CD138 vs CD38), (E: CD45 vs CD38), and (F: CD45 vs CD138). Gate each of these bivariate plots on (R1 and R2 and R3). An irregular region (R4) is drawn on plot D circumscribing the $CD138^+/CD38^+$ events; another irregular region (R5) is drawn on plot E circumscribing the $CD45^{+/-}/CD38^+$ events; a third irregular region (R6) is drawn on plot F circumscribing the $CD45^{+/-}/CD138^+$ events. CD45 is helpful for gating but should not be used as a marker for cell exclusion because both normal and clonal PCs can exhibit variable CD45 expression. When setting regions consider that CD138 expression may be attenuated and/or that PCs from patients on anti-CD38 immunotherapy may appear to be CD38-negative by flow cytometry. Because CD45 on PCs is generally dim to negative, evaluating it in combination with CD38 and CD138 can help in these situations. The combined Boolean gate definition (R1 and R2 and R3 and R4 and R5 and R6) defines both normal and neoplastic PCs ("Total PCs") that are present in the sample for subsequent analysis.

Phenotypic characterization of normal and abnormal plasma cells
As PCD is a heterogeneous disease in which neoplastic PCs can express variable antigen levels, defining abnormal PCs can be challenging (**Fig. 3**). Currently, there is not a single marker that can be used alone to reliably distinguish abnormal PCs from normal PCs. However, provided that a sufficient number of events are acquired, the combination of markers used in both Tube 1 and Tube 2 are capable of resolving abnormal PCs in a high percentage of cases. For this reason, all permutation of bivariate plots should be created and gated on "Total PCs," which is identified previously as cells circumscribed using the aforementioned Boolean gate definition (R1 and R2 and R3 and R4 and R5 and R6).

An individual is considered to have a PCD if the PCs express 2 or more aberrant cell markers, which are often some combination of $CD38^{dim}$, $CD45^{-\ to\ dim}$, $CD19^-$, $CD56^+$, $CD27^{dim}$, $CD81^{dim}$, $CD117^+$ and clonally restricted. Non-neoplastic PCs exhibit heterogeneous expression of CD45 and CD19, are mostly negative for CD20 and CD117, and invariably show homogeneously bright expression of CD81. Moreover, dim or absent CD81 expression is observed only in abnormal PCs, with 95% sensitivity and 100% specificity. The expression of CD56 and CD27 is observed in a subset of non-neoplastic PCs (between 5% and 20% of all PCs) with the latter more frequently expressed in posttreatment bone marrow samples. Given the nature of clonal PCs, antigen expression is often more uniform in myeloma cells rather than present across a heterogeneous spectrum, as is seen in normal PCs. Neoplastic PCs will often show additional aberrancies, such as $CD117^+$ or $CD27^{dim}$ expression; and these aberrancies will be coexpressed within the same cell population, whereas immunophenotypic variations in normal PCs tend to be heterogeneous and/or distributed among different subsets. Finally, provided a sufficient number of PCs are acquired, analysis of cytoplasmic light chain expression within subsets showing a myeloma-like aberrant phenotypes (eg, $CD19^-$ or $CD56^+$ PCs), while not routinely required, can be a valuable additional step in confirming the diagnosis.

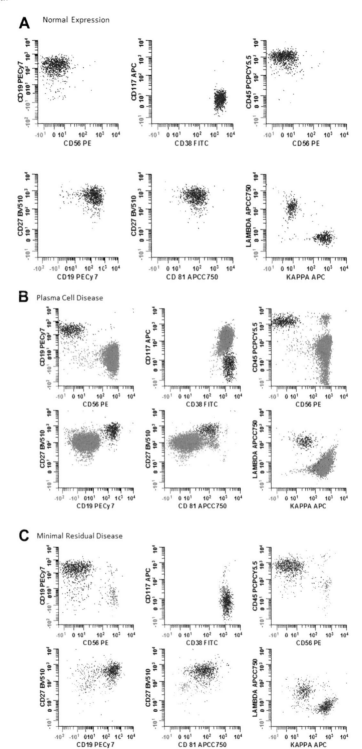

Fig. 3. Immunophenotypic profiles of normal and abnormal PCs. The immunophenotypic profiles of bone marrow from a patient (*A*) with no obvious hematological disease at

Representative cases to compare and contrast the immunophenotypic profile of PCs in bone marrow samples are illustrated in **Fig. 3**. Data from a patient with no hematological disease is presented in **Fig. 3A**. Note the positive expression of CD19, CD38, CD27, and CD81. The PCs are also polytypic for cytoplasmic light chains. In **Fig. 3B**, an obvious population of abnormal PCs (red) expresses CD56 and CD117; are dim for CD45 and CD27; negative for CD19 and CD81; and are cytoplasmic kappa light chain restricted. In **Fig. 3C**, an MRD population (red) is intermixed with normal PCs (blue) with a phenotype similar to that seem in **Fig. 3B** but note the slightly dimmer expression of CD38 on the abnormal cells.

Quality assessment of bone marrow aspirates

Tube 1 in the panel described here is designed to assess if the patient bone marrow aspirate is hemodilute by evaluating for the presence of erythroid precursors, mast cells, and hematogones **(Fig. 4)**. If abnormal PCs are found or these populations are present in the aspirate, then the sample should be reported as adequately representative of bone marrow based. Conversely, if no PCs are found and these populations are absent or reduced, then the sample should be reported out as hemodilute. The following gating parameters are used in the identification of mast cells, hematogones, and erythroblasts.

a. Using the bivariate plots shown in **Fig. 2**, total leukocytes are identified using the Boolean strategy R1 and R2 and R3.

b. As shown in **Fig. 4A**, draw a rectangular region (R7) to circumscribe the CD27$^-$/ CD117$^+$ events to identify the mast cells.

c. To define hematogones, B cells are first identified by creating a region (R8) on a bivariate plot of CD56 versus CD19 to circumscribe CD56$^-$/CD19$^+$ cells. This region (R8) is then applied to a bivariate plot of CD45 versus CD81, and the CD45^{dim}/CD81^{br} cells (R9) identify the hematogones.

d. As shown in **Fig. 4D**, erythroid precursors (R10) are identified as CD45^{dim}/SSC-A^{lo} events.

MINIMAL RESIDUAL DISEASE TESTING

In the routine diagnoses of PCDs the presence of monoclonal proteins are important for the evaluation of disease. They are measured in the urine and serum and can be identified by immunofixation electrophoresis (IFE) and quantified by protein electrophoresis (urine protein electrophoresis or serum protein electrophoresis [SPEP]). Changes in monoclonal protein concentrations are used to determine response to therapy or disease progression. Other assessments include the morphologic evaluation of PC concentration in the bone marrow and whether there is evidence of new lytic bone lesions or plasmacytomas.[105] A complete response (CR) before the use of novel agents was uncommon and responses were divided into several disease states, including stable, minimal, partial, very good partial, and complete responses. Improvements in therapy and methodologies to detect monoclonal proteins allows better

---

testing; (*B*) a patient with PCD; and (*C*) a patient with multiple myeloma MRD are shown. As PCD is a heterogeneous disease, no single marker can be reliably used to identify all abnormal cell populations. Instead the interpretation is based on all the markers included in the analysis. In this example, 6 different bivariate plots that were each separately gated on plasma cells using the strategy defined in **Fig. 2** are shown. Blue: normal plasma cells; Red: neoplastic plasma cells.

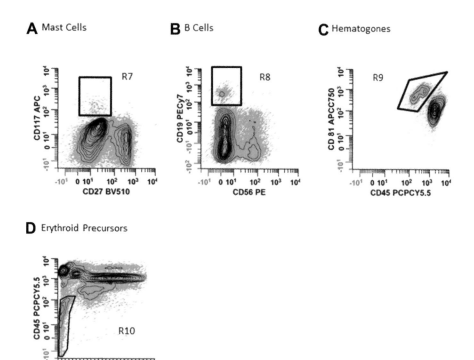

Fig. 4. Presence of mast cells, hematogones, and erythroid precursors can be used for quality assessment of bone marrow aspirates. (A) Mast cells are identified by drawing a rectangular region (R7) to circumscribe CD27$^-$/CD117$^+$ events. (B, C) B cells are first identified by creating a region (R8) on a bivariate plot of CD56 versus CD19 to circumscribe CD56$^-$/CD19$^+$ cells. Then a bivariate plot of CD45 versus CD81, gated on R8 and Total Leukocytes is used to define mature and immature B cells. Hematogones (immature B cells) are defined by R9 as the CD45^{dim}/CD81^{br} population. (D) Erythroid precursors are defined by R10 on a bivariate plot of SSC-A versus CD45, which circumscribes the CD45$^{-/dim}$/SSC^{lo} population. Note: these histograms are all gated on "Total Leukocytes:" identified using the Boolean strategy (R1 and R2 and R3) defined in **Fig. 2.**

stratification of good responses. Patients fulfilling the definition of CR may still have disease detected by IFE, which is defined as a near CR (nCR).[105,106] Similarly, utilization of sensitive sFLC assays may detect remaining imbalances of kappa and lambda concentrations suggestive of persistent disease in patients who were otherwise deemed to be in CR.[107] The rationale for adding the sFLC ratio to the multiple myeloma response criteria was to provide a more sensitive and precise indication of CR for use in comparative clinical trials by enabling the detection of small quantities of abnormal proteins in patients with little or no detectable monoclonal protein on SPEP and IFE. The International Myeloma Working Group defined a stringent CR as a patient who satisfied the criteria for a CR and was negative for sFLC.[108]

Achievement of stringent complete response (sCR) is associated with a significantly longer OS and PFS than CR or nCR are, regardless of the therapy used.[109–114] With novel therapeutics such as immunomodulatory drugs, proteasome inhibitors, and immunotherapy evolving at an unprecedented rate there is a need for even more sensitive methods to evaluation response to therapy. The development and testing of new therapeutics have been limited because almost all patients achieve an sCR and consequently randomized Phase 3 clinical trials take years to show benefits since PFS and OS are used as study endpoints.[55,115–118] Due to the long latency between drug development and approval to be considered as a therapeutic option, the measurement of MRD by MFC as an independent method to predict PFS and OS for patients diagnosed with PCD has been championed.[119,120] All flow cytometric studies to date have strongly correlated with PFS and OS at the day 100 time point, reducing the time required to reach meaningful clinical outcomes from years to months.[121–124]

There are currently 3 methods for detecting MRD that focus on the malignant multiple myeloma clone: immunophenotyping by flow cytometry, allele-specific oligonucleotide real time quantitative polymerase chain reaction (ASO-qPCR), and next-generation sequencing (NGS). Flow cytometry and ASO-qPCR have approximately the same sensitivity, whereas NGS is approximately 10 times more sensitive. Whereas flow cytometry is applicable for virtually all patients with multiple myeloma ($\geq$95% of cases), ASO-qPCR and NGS have a more restricted applicability (50%–90% of cases). This is mainly due to the high number of somatic hypermutations in the complementarity-determining regions (CDR) of the B-cell immunoglobulin gene that cause variable levels of primer annealing with unpredictable amplification and quantitation of results.

Two large studies have reported the correlation of immunophenotyping by flow cytometry with PFS and OS in uniformly treated patients. Paiva and colleagues[124] assessed MRD status at day 100 by MFC in 295 newly diagnosed patients with multiple myeloma treated with induction therapy followed by autologous hematopoietic stem cell transplantation in the GEM2000 protocol. Compared with patients who are MRD positive at day 100, those with MRD-negative status had longer PFS (median 71 vs 37 months; $P<.001$) and OS (median not reached vs 89 months; $P = .002$).[124] In multivariate analyses, MRD status by MFC at day 100 after transplantation was the most important independent prognostic factor for both PFS and OS. Rawstron and colleagues[122] evaluated the role of MFC in assessing MRD after induction therapy (n = 378) and at day 100 after transplantation (n = 397) in the MRC Myeloma IX Study. MRD status at day 100 after transplantation was highly predictive of PFS (28.6 vs 15.5 months; $P<.001$) and OS (80.6 vs 59 months; $P = .0183$) for MRD-negative and MRD-positive patients, respectively. In a smaller Phase 2 trial of 31 patients, the Intergroupe Francophone du Myélome reported 21 (68%) patients became MRD-negative by flow cytometry after treatment. After 39 months of follow-up, none of the flow-MRD negative patients had relapsed. Thus, from each of these studies it can be concluded that MRD testing by flow cytometry represents a sensitive, easily and quickly performed, surrogate method of predicting PFS and OS within months of therapy.

Measuring Minimal Residual Disease by Flow Cytometry

Previously, we described our routine or low-sensitivity flow cytometry method for detecting PCDs. The high-sensitivity assay discussed in this section is basically a modification of the lower sensitivity assay designed to acquire more cells. Because abnormal PCs are often present in very low numbers in posttreatment bone marrow aspirates, it is critical to acquire many events. The current recommendation of the ICCS Multiple Myeloma Consensus Group is acquire a minimum of 2×10^6 cells and preferably 5×10^6 cells. Obviously, using 100 μL bone marrow would be insufficient to achieve these numbers. Therefore, it is necessary to use high volumes of sample. Two methodologies have been used for this, namely the "Pre-lysis" and "Pooled-tube" approaches.

In the Pre-lysis approach, approximately 30×10^6 cells are treated with ammonium-chloride-potassium (ACK) lysing buffer (155 mM ammonium chloride, 10 mM potassium bicarbonate, and 0.2 mM EDTA) for 10 minutes at room temperature (at a 1–9 sample: ACK lysing buffer ratio).[125] The cells are then washed with FCM buffer and adjusted to approximately 5×10^7 cells/mL. To tubes containing the mAbs described in **Table 2**, 100 to 200 μL sample is added and the cells are incubated in the dark for 30 minutes at room temperature. After incubation, the residual erythrocytes are lysed a second time with saponin-based BD FACS Lysing Solution for 10 minutes and then washed with FCM buffer and processed as described previously for flow cytometric acquisition. Intracellular staining for tube 2 is performed as previously described.

In the Pooled-tube approach, the sample is washed, counted, and adjusted to 1×10^7 cells/mL. Six replicates for each of the mAb cocktails described in **Table 2** are set up. To each tube 200 μL of washed sample are added and the cells are incubated, lysed, and washed as described in the routine assay. During the last wash, the cells from replicate samples are combined for flow cytometric acquisition. Intracellular staining is separately performed on the pooled sample.

Either method is satisfactory and capable of staining a sufficient number of cells to easily acquire 5×10^6 events. The major advantage of the Pre-lysis approach is that although it requires more mAbs than conventional staining to achieve saturation of the cells, it does not require as many mAbs as the Pooled-tube approach. The advantage of the Pooled-tube method is that it more readily fits into the standard workflow of a laboratory. The Pre-lysis method can adversely impact surface staining of some antigens particularly CD138 and may facilitate the breakdown of some tandem dyes. Ficoll Hypaque enrichment must never be used, as it may significantly reduce PC numbers and it accelerates antigen loss from PCs, especially CD138[126]; in addition, it will compromise PC quantitation due to differential cell enrichment during gradient density centrifugation.

Assay Sensitivity Metrics and Reporting

We (submitted) and others[120] have clearly established that the more events that are acquired, the more sensitive the assay becomes, and the higher the predictive value for PFS. In most clinical laboratories, the detection sensitivity of MFC to identify neoplastic PCs in the bone marrow ranges from 10^{-4} (1 in 10,000 cells) to 10^{-5} (1 in 100,000 cells).[127] Even though multicenter data have demonstrated that a minimum detection sensitivity of 0.01% is of clear prognostic value for MRD monitoring by MFC, it is evident that as assay sensitivity has increased, so has the correlation between MRD status and clinical outcomes. Today a minimum sensitivity of 0.001% is the accepted norm, and the threshold for abnormal PCs used in the determination of MRD ranges from 20 to 100 cells.[121] There are numerous studies demonstrating that 20 events are a conservative value for the smallest number of a homogeneous and clustered population of cells that can be reliably detected by an experienced cytometrist.[128,129] Using this value, the limit of detection (LOD) is calculated as follows:

$$LOD = \left(\frac{20 \text{ Events}}{\text{Total Number of Events}} \right) \times 100\%$$

For example, if the minimum threshold for is 20 events and 5×10^6 "Total Leukocytes" are acquired, then the LOD is 0.0004%. It is generally accepted that between 50 and 100 events represent the minimum number of events required to accurately quantify a cell population.[130,131] Thus, the lower limit of quantification (LLOQ) is calculated as:

$$LLOQ = \left(\frac{50 \text{ Events}}{\text{Total Number of Events}} \right) \times 100\%$$

If 50 events represent the LLOQ threshold and 5×10^6 "Total Leukocytes" are collected, then the LLOQ is 0.001%. Regardless of the theoretic values for LOD and LLOQ, the College of American Pathologists requires that each laboratory experimentally confirm these values in their assay.

Finally, it is important that a PCD MRD report contain the following information:

- The number and percentage of normal and abnormal PCs
- The LOD, LLOQ, or both
- Optionally the total number of leukocytes evaluated after excluding doublets and debris
- The phenotype of the abnormal cells
- A statement about the quality of the bone marrow aspirate (ie, hemodilution and viability as necessary)

DISCUSSION

PCD is a heterogeneous disease with a spectrum of severities and clinical outcomes. Although overall it is not a prevalent form of cancer, PCDs represent the second most-common hematological disorder and the focal, anatomically isolated nature of the neoplasm constitutes a considerable challenge for medical practice. A relatively large percentage of patients with PCDs exhibit indolent forms of the disease (eg, MGUS); however, many suffer with aggressive malignancy (eg, multiple myeloma or plasma cell leukemia) that manifests with symptoms of organ failure, bone destruction, and perturbed hematopoiesis. Most types of PCD are developed after affinity maturation has already taken place, as the genetic sequences of myeloma cells have been found to be consistently hypermutated, and exhibit phenotypic features similar to those of long-lived PCs.[132–134] The oversecretion of M protein, the elevated percentage of PCs in the bone marrow, and the presence of organ damage are typically considered when determining the specific subtype of PCD.

The various manifestations of PCD require different treatment regiments. Historically, many patients respond to first-line agents; however, most become refractory to therapy and eventually relapse. The treatment of multiple myeloma has evolved significantly over time. Initial therapies developed in the 1960s involved the use of hematopoietic stem cell transplantation (HSCT) along with chemotherapeutic agents, such as melphalan, vincristine, doxorubicin, or cyclophosphamide in combination with prednisone. Although these treatments modestly improved patient survival, their efficacy was limited due to the low mitotic index of PCs.[135–137]

Based on these findings, alternative systemic approaches to the treatment of PCDs were explored; primarily involving the use of thalidomide, which functions as an inhibitor of angiogenesis and also acts as an immune modulator by opposing the activity of IL-6. This cytokine otherwise promotes the survival of malignant PCs by upregulating cell adhesion molecules, tumor promoting cytokines, and downregulating tumor suppressor proteins. Modest success with this approach eventually led to the development and implementation of the next generation of therapies. Such drugs include bortezomib (a selective proteosome inhibitor), dexamethasone (an anti-inflammatory agent), and the thalidomide analogue lenalidomide (an immune modulator and anti-angiogenic) which further extended OS in treated patients. When these medicines were used in concert with HSCT, OS increased to an unprecedented, but still grim 5 years for 45% of multiple myeloma cases.[138]

The conventional medical age has added targeted therapies to the armamentarium of drugs used to treat PCDs. Immunotherapeutic agents such as anti-PD-1 (CD279), anti-PD-L1 (CD274), and anti-CD38 (daratumumab) have been used; with their successes driving the development of additional immunotherapies.[139] These novel therapeutics are quickly advancing but their mainstream transition has been limited because randomized Phase 3 clinical trials take years to show benefits when PFS and OS are used as study endpoints.[55,115–118] Due to the long latency between drug development and the approval to be considered as therapeutic options, the measurement of MRD by MFC as an independent method to predict PFS and OS for patients diagnosed with PCD has been used.[119,120] All flow cytometric studies to date have strongly correlated the measurement of MRD with PFS and OS at the day 100 time point, reducing from years to months the time required to reach meaningful clinical outcomes.[121–124]

Although the use of mAbs to target cell surface molecules on PCs has expanded as an innovative therapeutic choice, their use can obstruct the detection of PCs by MFC. Daratumumab and isatuximab can impair the measurement of CD38,[70,139] likewise indatuximab ravtansine may interfere with CD138 detection.[139] Even though the discovery of these mAb therapies offer a new avenue by which we can approach the detection of multiple myeloma, they have made the search for alternative markers to identify both normal and neoplastic PCs by MFC a priority.[140] Independent investigators have reported the expression of CD54, CD229, CD269, and CD319 to be valuable for this purpose.[54,141,142] In particular, CD269 and CD319 were found to be more versatile markers and withstood storage longer than CD138.[141] It will be interesting to see how these markers can be integrated into the clinical test setting of MRD by MFC.

Besides MFC, alternatives for the detection of multiple myeloma MRD are ASO-qPCR and NGS whose assay performance characteristics are contrasted in **Table 5**. Before NGS, ASO-qPCR was regarded as one of the most sensitive assays to detect PCDs with a sensitivity limit of 10^{-5} to 10^{-6}.[127] ASO-qPCR involves the design of specific primers complementary to the clonal rearrangement in the CDR genes of mature B cells. Puig and colleagues[143] analyzed data from 3 consecutive myeloma trials that used both ASO-qPCR and 4-color MFC to evaluate the MRD-negativity and clinical outcome in 170 patients. The results showed both technologies correlated well with MRD-negativity to predict PFS and OS. However, 58% of the patients could not be evaluated by ASO-qPCR due to the failure of clonal detection, unsuccessful sequencing, or suboptimal performance of primer or probe sets. These technical shortcomings are due to the highly mutated CDR region, as well as the heterogeneous infiltration of disease into the marrow.[143,144] As a potential solution, personalized primer and probe sets are required to detect the somatic-mutated sequence for each patient. Therefore, this finding suggests that even though ASO-qPCR is sensitive and specific, it is only applicable to a subset of patients. Furthermore, it may be more laborious and time-consuming that MFC, indicating that MFC is probably a more practical and feasible tool for routine MRD assessment than ASO-qPCR.[34]

The other approach to MRD detection is NGS. When compared with ASO-qPCR, both technologies have a similar detection sensitivity of 10^{-5}, but under ideal circumstances, NGS may detect as few as 1 neoplastic cell in a million. NGS also has the advantage of being applicable to more patients, as it does not require patient-specific primers.[145,146] In a study conducted by Martinez-Lopez and colleagues,[147] patients who were MRD-negative by NGS had a longer PFS and increased OS. Summarily, the concordance rate between NGS and MFC, and also NGS and ASO-qPCR were 83% and 85%, respectively. As myeloma cells become rarer, NGS is better than

Table 5
Comparison of flow cytometry and molecular techniques for MRD analysis in multiple myeloma

Parameters	Flow Cytometry		Molecular Techniques	
	2008 EMN Consensus (4–6 Colors)	2016 ICCS Consensus (≥8 Colors)	ASO-qPCR	Next-Generation Sequencing
Applicability, %	>95	>99	50–90	80–90
LLOQ, %	0.01	>0.001	>0.001	>0.001
Number of cells/ Amount of DNA required for LLOQ	0.5×10^6 cells/ tube	$2–5 \times 10^6$ cells/ tube	500 ng (1,000,000 cells for triplicate analysis)	14 µg (2,000,000 cells for triplicate analysis)
LOD, %	0.0040	0.0004	0.0001	0.0001
Reproducibility	High	High	Low	High
Pretreatment evaluation	Required	Not required	Required	Required
Fresh sample	Required, <48 h old storage		Recommended, <48 h before DNA extraction	
Diagnostic sample	Useful, but not required		Required	
Quantitative	Yes		No	
Sample quality assurance	Not required		Additional tests are required	
Cost	Low		High (at diagnosis) Medium (follow-up)	High
Turnaround	Can take up to 1 d		Can take several days	
Availability	Widely available		Intermediare	Limited
Harmonization	Yes (EMN)	Yes (ICCS/ESCCA)	Yes	Ongoing (EuroMRD)

Abbreviations: ASO-qPCR, allele-specific oligonucleotide real time quantitative polymerase chain reaction; CCS, International Clinical Cytometry Society; EMN, European myeloma network; ESCCA, European Society for Clinical Cell Analysis; LLOQ, lower limit of quantification; LOD, limit of detection.
Data from Refs.[41,68,122,124,143,145,150–157]

MFC for detecting MRD but it has the disadvantage of being susceptible to the evolving heterogeneity of myeloma commensurate with therapy. A recent study published by Munshi and colleagues[148] suggested that several evolved clonotypes were measured in 37.6% of the posttreatment multiple myeloma samples, which could confound the ability of NGS but not MFC to detect MRD. NGS remains the least studied MRD testing modality and continued clinical correlations will be required before widespread adoption is possible.

Multiple MFC consensus panels have been proposed in the past 2 decades, but they typically included largely overlapping lists of CD markers for each disease category. Virtually all consensus proposals lack information about reference antibody clones for the proposed CD markers and they only provide limited information on the most appropriate combinations of relevant markers for multicolor mAb panels. In 2013, the ICCS Multiple Myeloma MRD Consensus Group was formed and tasked with the development of consensus documents for the detection of MRD by MFC. These documents were reviewed with the Food and Drug Administration (FDA) in March 2014 and published in January 2015. It was proposed that MRD testing by flow cytometry needs to be integrated now into the response criteria for multiple myeloma and determined that for regulatory approval, a surrogate must be shown to be reasonably likely to predict clinical benefit. This has already been accomplished by Paiva and colleagues[124] and Rawstron and colleagues.[68] Therefore, the FDA concluded that "MRD assessment in multiple myeloma has the potential to be a surrogate clinical endpoint that could be used to support regulatory purposes for drug review" with a standardized approach.[149] Therefore, there is an urgent need for adoption of consensus protocols within the multiple myeloma community for inclusion of MRD-negativity by MFC as a surrogate endpoint in clinical trials.

REFERENCES

1. Shapiro-Shelef M, Calame K. Plasma cell differentiation and multiple myeloma. Curr Opin Immunol 2004;16(2):226–34.
2. Shapiro-Shelef M, Calame K. Regulation of plasma-cell development. Nat Rev Immunol 2005;5(3):230–42.
3. Nutt SL, Hodgkin PD, Tarlinton DM, et al. The generation of antibody-secreting plasma cells. Nat Rev Immunol 2015;15(3):160–71.
4. Sze DM, Toellner KM, Garcia de Vinuesa C, et al. Intrinsic constraint on plasma-blast growth and extrinsic limits of plasma cell survival. J Exp Med 2000;192(6): 813–21.
5. Chu VT, Beller A, Nguyen TT, et al. The long-term survival of plasma cells. Scand J Immunol 2011;73(6):508–11.
6. Mackay F, Schneider P, Rennert P, et al. BAFF AND APRIL: a tutorial on B cell survival. Annu Rev Immunol 2003;21:231–64.
7. Moreaux J, Legouffe E, Jourdan E, et al. BAFF and APRIL protect myeloma cells from apoptosis induced by interleukin 6 deprivation and dexamethasone. Blood 2004;103(8):3148–57.
8. Belnoue E, Pihlgren M, McGaha TL, et al. APRIL is critical for plasmablast survival in the bone marrow and poorly expressed by early-life bone marrow stromal cells. Blood 2008;111(5):2755–64.
9. Minges Wols HA, Underhill GH, Kansas GS, et al. The role of bone marrow-derived stromal cells in the maintenance of plasma cell longevity. J Immunol 2002;169(8):4213–21.
10. Nutt SL, Hodgkin PD, Tarlinton DM, et al. The generation of antibody-secreting plasma cells. Nat Rev Immunol 2015;15(3):160–71.
11. Kuehl WM, Bergsagel PL. Multiple myeloma: evolving genetic events and host interactions. Nat Rev Cancer 2002;2(3):175–87.
12. Anderson KC, Carrasco RD. Pathogenesis of myeloma. Annu Rev Pathol 2011; 6:249–74.
13. Bakkus MH, Heirman C, Van Riet I, et al. Evidence that multiple myeloma Ig heavy chain VDJ genes contain somatic mutations but show no intraclonal variation. Blood 1992;80(9):2326.
14. Kyle RA, Rajkumar SV. Criteria for diagnosis, staging, risk stratification and response assessment of multiple myeloma. Leukemia 2009;23(1):3–9.
15. Slovak ML. Multiple myeloma: current perspectives. Clin Lab Med 2011;31(4): 699–724, x.

16. International Myeloma Working Group. Criteria for the classification of monoclonal gammopathies, multiple myeloma and related disorders: a report of the International Myeloma Working Group. Br J Haematol 2003;121(5):749–57.
17. Kyle RA, Finkelstein S, Elveback LR, et al. Incidence of monoclonal proteins in a Minnesota community with a cluster of multiple myeloma. Blood 1972;40(5):719–24.
18. Saleun JP, Vicariot M, Deroff P, et al. Monoclonal gammopathies in the adult population of Finistère, France. J Clin Pathol 1982;35(1):63–8.
19. Axelsson U, Bachmann R, Hallen J. Frequency of pathological proteins (M-components) on 6,995 sera from an adult population. Acta Med Scand 1966;179(2):235–47.
20. Bianchi G, Munshi NC. Pathogenesis beyond the cancer clone(s) in multiple myeloma. Blood 2015;125(20):3049–58.
21. Pittaluga S, Wlodarska I, Pulford K, et al. The monoclonal antibody ALK1 identifies a distinct morphological subtype of anaplastic large cell lymphoma associated with 2p23/ALK rearrangements. Am J Pathol 1997;151(2):343–51.
22. Rajkumar SV, Landgren O, Mateos M-V. Smoldering multiple myeloma. Blood 2015;125(20):3069.
23. Perez-Persona E, Vidriales MB, Mateo G, et al. New criteria to identify risk of progression in monoclonal gammopathy of uncertain significance and smoldering multiple myeloma based on multiparameter flow cytometry analysis of bone marrow plasma cells. Blood 2007;110(7):2586–92.
24. Campana D, Coustan-Smith E. Minimal residual disease studies by flow cytometry in acute leukemia. Acta Haematol 2004;112(1–2):8–15.
25. Siegel RL, Miller KD, Jemal A. Cancer statistics, 2016. CA Cancer J Clin 2016;66(1):7–30.
26. Noll JE, Williams SA, Tong CM, et al. Myeloma plasma cells alter the bone marrow microenvironment by stimulating the proliferation of mesenchymal stromal cells. Haematologica 2014;99(1):163–71.
27. Avet-Loiseau H, Daviet A, Brigaudeau C, et al. Cytogenetic, interphase, and multicolor fluorescence in situ hybridization analyses in primary plasma cell leukemia: a study of 40 patients at diagnosis, on behalf of the Intergroupe Francophone du Myelome and the Groupe Francais de Cytogenetique Hematologique. Blood 2001;97(3):822–5.
28. Dimopoulos MA, Palumbo A, Delasalle KB, et al. Primary plasma cell leukaemia. Br J Haematol 1994;88(4):754–9.
29. Garcia-Sanz R, Orfao A, Gonzalez M, et al. Primary plasma cell leukemia: clinical, immunophenotypic, DNA ploidy, and cytogenetic characteristics. Blood 1999;93(3):1032–7.
30. Boll M, Parkins E, O'Connor SJ, et al. Extramedullary plasmacytoma are characterized by a 'myeloma-like' immunophenotype and genotype and occult bone marrow involvement. Br J Haematol 2010;151(5):525–7.
31. Hu Y, Wang M, Chen Y, et al. Immunophenotypic analysis of abnormal plasma cell clones in bone marrow of primary systemic light chain amyloidosis patients. Chin Med J 2014;127(15):2765–70.
32. Paiva B, Vidriales MB, Perez JJ, et al. The clinical utility and prognostic value of multiparameter flow cytometry immunophenotyping in light-chain amyloidosis. Blood 2011;117(13):3613–6.
33. Ocqueteau M, Orfao A, Almeida J, et al. Immunophenotypic characterization of plasma cells from monoclonal gammopathy of undetermined significance

patients. Implications for the differential diagnosis between MGUS and multiple myeloma. Am J Pathol 1998;152(6):1655–65.

34. Sarasquete ME, Garcia-Sanz R, Gonzalez D, et al. Minimal residual disease monitoring in multiple myeloma: a comparison between allelic-specific oligonucleotide real-time quantitative polymerase chain reaction and flow cytometry. Haematologica 2005;90(10):1365–72.

35. Orfao A, Ortuno F, de Santiago M, et al. Immunophenotyping of acute leukemias and myelodysplastic syndromes. Cytometry A 2004;58(1):62–71.

36. Vidriales MB, San-Miguel JF, Orfao A, et al. Minimal residual disease monitoring by flow cytometry. Best Pract Res Clin Haematol 2003;16(4):599–612.

37. van Dongen JJ, Lhermitte L, Bottcher S, et al. EuroFlow antibody panels for standardized n-dimensional flow cytometric immunophenotyping of normal, reactive and malignant leukocytes. Leukemia 2012;26(9):1908–75.

38. Foon KA, Todd RF 3rd. Immunologic classification of leukemia and lymphoma. Blood 1986;68(1):1–31.

39. van Dongen JJ, Adriaansen HJ, Hooijkaas H. Immunophenotyping of leukaemias and non-Hodgkin's lymphomas. Immunological markers and their CD codes. Neth J Med 1988;33(5–6):298–314.

40. Terstappen LW, Johnsen S, Segers-Nolten IM, et al. Identification and characterization of plasma cells in normal human bone marrow by high-resolution flow cytometry. Blood 1990;76(9):1739–47.

41. Kumar S, Paiva B, Anderson KC, et al. International Myeloma Working Group consensus criteria for response and minimal residual disease assessment in multiple myeloma. Lancet Oncol 2016;17(8):e328–46.

42. San Miguel JF, Gonzalez M, Gascon A, et al. Immunophenotypic heterogeneity of multiple myeloma: influence on the biology and clinical course of the disease. Castellano-Leones (Spain) Cooperative Group for the Study of Monoclonal Gammopathies. Br J Haematol 1991;77(2):185–90.

43. Rawstron AC, Davies FE, DasGupta R, et al. Flow cytometric disease monitoring in multiple myeloma: the relationship between normal and neoplastic plasma cells predicts outcome after transplantation. Blood 2002;100(9):3095–100.

44. San Miguel JF, Almeida J, Mateo G, et al. Immunophenotypic evaluation of the plasma cell compartment in multiple myeloma: a tool for comparing the efficacy of different treatment strategies and predicting outcome. Blood 2002;99(5):1853–6.

45. Paiva B, Almeida J, Perez-Andres M, et al. Utility of flow cytometry immunophenotyping in multiple myeloma and other clonal plasma cell-related disorders. Cytometry B Clin Cytom 2010;78(4):239–52.

46. Nadav L, Katz BZ, Baron S, et al. Diverse niches within multiple myeloma bone marrow aspirates affect plasma cell enumeration. Br J Haematol 2006;133(5):530–2.

47. Ng AP, Wei A, Bhurani D, et al. The sensitivity of CD138 immunostaining of bone marrow trephine specimens for quantifying marrow involvement in MGUS and myeloma, including samples with a low percentage of plasma cells. Haematologica 2006;91(7):972–5.

48. Harada H, Kawano MM, Huang N, et al. Phenotypic difference of normal plasma cells from mature myeloma cells. Blood 1993;81(10):2658–63.

49. Mateo G, Montalban MA, Vidriales MB, et al. Prognostic value of immunophenotyping in multiple myeloma: a study by the PETHEMA/GEM cooperative study groups on patients uniformly treated with high-dose therapy. J Clin Oncol 2008;26(16):2737–44.

50. Mateo Manzanera G, San Miguel Izquierdo JF, Orfao de Matos A. Immunophenotyping of plasma cells in multiple myeloma. Methods Mol Med 2005;113:5–24.
51. Pellat-Deceunynck C, Bataille R. Normal and malignant human plasma cells: proliferation, differentiation, and expansions in relation to CD45 expression. Blood Cells Mol Dis 2004;32(2):293–301.
52. Cannizzo E, Bellio E, Sohani AR, et al. Multiparameter immunophenotyping by flow cytometry in multiple myeloma: the diagnostic utility of defining ranges of normal antigenic expression in comparison to histology. Cytometry B Clin Cytom 2010;78(4):231–8.
53. Flores-Montero J, de Tute R, Paiva B, et al. Immunophenotype of normal vs. myeloma plasma cells: toward antibody panel specifications for MRD detection in multiple myeloma. Cytometry B Clin Cytom 2016;90(1):61–72.
54. Pojero F, Flores-Montero J, Sanoja L, et al. Utility of CD54, CD229, and CD319 for the identification of plasma cells in patients with clonal plasma cell diseases. Cytometry B Clin Cytom 2016;90(1):91–100.
55. Oldaker TA, Wallace PK, Barnett D. Flow cytometry quality requirements for monitoring of minimal disease in plasma cell myeloma. Cytometry B Clin Cytom 2016;90(1):40–6.
56. San-Miguel JF, Vidriales MB, Orfao A. Immunological evaluation of minimal residual disease (MRD) in acute myeloid leukaemia (AML). Best Pract Res Clin Haematol 2002;15(1):105–18.
57. Wood B, Jevremovic D, Bene MC, et al. Validation of cell-based fluorescence assays: practice guidelines from the ICSH and ICCS—part V—assay performance criteria. Cytometry B Clin Cytom 2013;84(5):315–23.
58. Wood BL, Arroz M, Barnett D, et al. 2006 Bethesda International Consensus recommendations on the immunophenotypic analysis of hematolymphoid neoplasia by flow cytometry: optimal reagents and reporting for the flow cytometric diagnosis of hematopoietic neoplasia. Cytometry B Clin Cytom 2007; 72(Suppl 1):S14–22.
59. Davis BH, Dasgupta A, Kussick S, et al. Validation of cell-based fluorescence assays: practice guidelines from the ICSH and ICCS—part II—preanalytical issues. Cytometry B Clin Cytom 2013;84(5):286–90.
60. Davis B, Wood B, Oldaker T, et al. Validation of cell-based fluorescence assays: practice guidelines from the ICSH and ICCS—part I—rationale and aims. Cytometry B Clin Cytom 2013;84(5):282–5.
61. Barnett D, Louzao R, Gambell P, et al. Validation of cell-based fluorescence assays: practice guidelines from the ICSH and ICCS—part IV—postanalytic considerations. Cytometry B Clin Cytom 2013;84(5):309–14.
62. Stetler-Stevenson M, Davis B, Wood B, et al. 2006 Bethesda International Consensus Conference on flow cytometric immunophenotyping of hematolymphoid neoplasia. Cytometry B Clin Cytom 2007;72(Suppl 1):S3.
63. Purvis NB, Oldaker T. Validation and quality control in clinical flow cytometry. In: Kottke-Marchant K, Davis BH, editors. Laboratory Hematology Practice. Oxford: Wiley-Blackwell; 2012. p. 115–30.
64. Tanqri S, Vall H, Kaplan D, et al. Validation of cell-based fluorescence assays: practice guidelines from the ICSH and ICCS—part III—analytical issues. Cytometry B Clin Cytom 2013;84(5):291–308.
65. Arroz M, Came N, Lin P, et al. Consensus guidelines on plasma cell myeloma minimal residual disease analysis and reporting. Cytometry B Clin Cytom 2016;90(1):31–9.

66. Stetler-Stevenson M, Paiva B, Stoolman L, et al. Consensus guidelines for myeloma minimal residual disease sample staining and data acquisition. Cytometry B Clin Cytom 2016;90(1):26–30.

67. Kalina T, Flores-Montero J, Lecrevisse Q, et al. Quality assessment program for EuroFlow protocols: summary results of four-year (2010-2013) quality assurance rounds. Cytometry A 2015;87(2):145–56.

68. Rawstron AC, Orfao A, Beksac M, et al. Report of the European Myeloma Network on multiparametric flow cytometry in multiple myeloma and related disorders. Haematologica 2008;93(3):431–8.

69. Bataille R, Jego G, Robillard N, et al. The phenotype of normal, reactive and malignant plasma cells. Identification of "many and multiple myelomas" and of new targets for myeloma therapy. Haematologica 2006;91(9):1234–40.

70. Flores-Montero J, Sanoja-Flores L, Paiva B, et al. Next Generation Flow for highly sensitive and standardized detection of minimal residual disease in multiple myeloma. Leukemia 2017. [Epub ahead of print].

71. Royston DJ, Gao Q, Nguyen N, et al. Single-tube 10-fluorochrome analysis for efficient flow cytometric evaluation of minimal residual disease in plasma cell myeloma. Am J Clin Pathol 2016;146(1):41–9.

72. Roshal M, Flores-Montero JA, Gao Q, et al. MRD detection in multiple myeloma: comparison between MSKCC 10-color single-tube and EuroFlow 8-color 2-tube methods. Blood Adv 2017;1(12):728.

73. Ruiz-Arguelles GJ, San Miguel JF. Cell surface markers in multiple myeloma. Mayo Clin Proc 1994;69(7):684–90.

74. Guikema JE, Hovenga S, Vellenga E, et al. CD27 is heterogeneously expressed in multiple myeloma: low CD27 expression in patients with high-risk disease. Br J Haematol 2003;121(1):36–43.

75. Moreau P, Robillard N, Jégo G, et al. Lack of CD27 in myeloma delineates different presentation and outcome. Br J Haematol 2006;132(2):168–70.

76. Robillard N, Jego G, Pellat-Deceunynck C, et al. CD28, a marker associated with tumoral expansion in multiple myeloma. Clin Cancer Res 1998;4(6):1521–6.

77. Jackson N, Ling NR, Ball J, et al. An analysis of myeloma plasma cell phenotype using antibodies defined at the IIIrd International Workshop on Human Leucocyte Differentiation Antigens. Clin Exp Immunol 1988;72(3):351–6.

78. Shapiro VS, Mollenauer MN, Weiss A. Endogenous CD28 expressed on myeloma cells up-regulates interleukin-8 production: implications for multiple myeloma progression. Blood 2001;98(1):187–93.

79. Nair JR, Carlson LM, Koorella C, et al. CD28 expressed on malignant plasma cells induces a pro-survival and immunosuppressive microenvironment. J Immunol 2011;187(3):1243–53.

80. Reinherz EL, Kung PC, Goldstein G, et al. Discrete stages of human intrathymic differentiation: analysis of normal thymocytes and leukemic lymphoblasts of T-cell lineage. Proc Natl Acad Sci U S A 1980;77(3):1588–92.

81. Reinherz EL, Schlossman SF. The characterization and function of human immunoregulatory T lymphocyte subsets. Immunol Today 1981;2(4):69–75.

82. Bataille R, Robillard N, Pellat-Deceunynck C, et al. A cellular model for myeloma cell growth and maturation based on an intraclonal CD45 hierarchy. Immunol Rev 2003;194:105–11.

83. Kumar S, Rajkumar SV, Kyle RA, et al. Prognostic value of circulating plasma cells in monoclonal gammopathy of undetermined significance. J Clin Oncol 2005;23(24):5668–74.

84. Moreau P, Robillard N, Avet-Loiseau H, et al. Patients with CD45 negative multiple myeloma receiving high-dose therapy have a shorter survival than those with CD45 positive multiple myeloma. Haematologica 2004;89(5):547–51.

85. Pellatdeceunynck C, Barille S, Puthier D, et al. Adhesion molecules on human myeloma cells—significant changes in expression related to malignancy, tumor spreading, and immortalization. Cancer Res 1995;55(16):3647–53.

86. Pellat-Deceunynck C, Barille S, Jego G, et al. The absence of CD56 (NCAM) on malignant plasma cells is a hallmark of plasma cell leukemia and of a special subset of multiple myeloma. Leukemia 1998;12(12):1977–82.

87. Ely SA, Knowles DM. Expression of CD56/neural cell adhesion molecule correlates with the presence of lytic bone lesions in multiple myeloma and distinguishes myeloma from monoclonal gammopathy of undetermined significance and lymphomas with plasmacytoid differentiation. Am J Pathol 2002;160(4): 1293–9.

88. Sahara N, Takeshita A. Prognostic significance of surface markers expressed in multiple myeloma: CD56 and other antigens. Leuk Lymphoma 2004;45(1):61–5.

89. Langebrake C, Brinkmann I, Teigler-Schlegel A, et al. Immunophenotypic differences between diagnosis and relapse in childhood AML: implications for MRD monitoring. Cytometry B Clin Cytom 2005;63(1):1–9.

90. Paiva B, Gutierrez NC, Chen X, et al. Clinical significance of CD81 expression by clonal plasma cells in high-risk smoldering and symptomatic multiple myeloma patients. Leukemia 2012;26(8):1862–9.

91. Bataille R, Pellat-Deceunynck C, Robillard N, et al. CD117 (c-kit) is aberrantly expressed in a subset of MGUS and multiple myeloma with unexpectedly good prognosis. Leuk Res 2008;32(3):379–82.

92. Schmidt-Hieber M, Pérez-Andrés M, Paiva B, et al. CD117 expression in gammopathies is associated with an altered maturation of the myeloid and lymphoid hematopoietic cell compartments and favorable disease features. Haematologica 2011;96(2):328–32.

93. Kraj M, Poglod R, Kopec-Szlezak J, et al. C-kit receptor (CD117) expression on plasma cells in monoclonal gammopathies. Leuk Lymphoma 2004;45(11): 2281–9.

94. Ridley RC, Xiao H, Hata H, et al. Expression of syndecan regulates human myeloma plasma cell adhesion to type I collagen. Blood 1993;81(3):767–74.

95. Yang Y, Borset M, Langford JK, et al. Heparan sulfate regulates targeting of syndecan-1 to a functional domain on the cell surface. J Biol Chem 2003; 278(15):12888–93.

96. Dhodapkar MV, Kelly T, Theus A, et al. Elevated levels of shed syndecan-1 correlate with tumour mass and decreased matrix metalloproteinase-9 activity in the serum of patients with multiple myeloma. Br J Haematol 1997;99(2): 368–71.

97. Jourdan M, Ferlin M, Legouffe E, et al. The myeloma cell antigen syndecan-1 is lost by apoptotic myeloma cells. Br J Haematol 1998;100(4):637–46.

98. San Antonio JD, Karnovsky MJ, Gay S, et al. Interactions of syndecan-1 and heparin with human collagens. Glycobiology 1994;4(3):327–32.

99. Mahnke YD, Roederer M. Optimizing a multi-colour immunophenotyping assay. Clin Lab Med 2007;27(3):469, v.

100. Rawstron AC, Fazi C, Agathangelidis A, et al. A complementary role of multiparameter flow cytometry and high-throughput sequencing for minimal residual disease detection in chronic lymphocytic leukemia: an European Research Initiative on CLL study. Leukemia 2016;30(4):929–36.

101. Nowakowski GS, Witzig TE, Dingli D, et al. Circulating plasma cells detected by flow cytometry as a predictor of survival in 302 patients with newly diagnosed multiple myeloma. Blood 2005;106(7):2276–9.

102. Dingli D, Nowakowski GS, Dispenzieri A, et al. Flow cytometric detection of circulating myeloma cells before transplantation in patients with multiple myeloma: a simple risk stratification system. Blood 2006;107(8):3384–8.

103. Lin P, Owens R, Tricot G, et al. Flow cytometric immunophenotypic analysis of 306 cases of multiple myeloma. Am J Clin Pathol 2004;121(4):482–8.

104. Tario JD, Wallace PK. Reagents and cell staining for immunophenotyping by flow cytometry. In: McManus LM, Mitchell RN, editors. Pathobiology of human disease. San Diego (CA): Elsevier; 2014. p. 3678–701.

105. Lahuerta JJ, Martinez-Lopez J, Serna JD, et al. Remission status defined by immunofixation vs. electrophoresis after autologous transplantation has a major impact on the outcome of multiple myeloma patients. Br J Haematol 2000; 109(2):438–46.

106. Richardson PG, Barlogie B, Berenson J, et al. A phase 2 study of bortezomib in relapsed, refractory myeloma. N Engl J Med 2003;348(26):2609–17.

107. Bradwell AR, Carr-Smith HD, Mead GP, et al. Highly sensitive, automated immunoassay for immunoglobulin free light chains in serum and urine. Clin Chem 2001;47(4):673–80.

108. Blade J, Rosinol L, Cibeira MT, et al. Hematopoietic stem cell transplantation for multiple myeloma beyond 2010. Blood 2010;115(18):3655–63.

109. Attal M, Harousseau J-L, Stoppa A-M, et al. A prospective, randomized trial of autologous bone marrow transplantation and chemotherapy in multiple myeloma. N Engl J Med 1996;335(2):91–7.

110. Barlogie B, Jagannath S, Vesole DH, et al. Superiority of tandem autologous transplantation over standard therapy for previously untreated multiple myeloma. Blood 1997;89(3):789–93.

111. Kyle RA, Leong T, Li S, et al. Complete response in multiple myeloma: clinical trial E9486, an Eastern Cooperative Oncology Group study not involving stem cell transplantation. Cancer 2006;106(9):1958–66.

112. Lahuerta JJ, Mateos MV, Martinez-Lopez J, et al. Influence of pre- and posttransplantation responses on outcome of patients with multiple myeloma: sequential improvement of response and achievement of complete response are associated with longer survival. J Clin Oncol 2008;26(35):5775–82.

113. Niesvizky R, Richardson PG, Rajkumar SV, et al. The relationship between quality of response and clinical benefit for patients treated on the bortezomib arm of the international, randomized, phase 3 APEX trial in relapsed multiple myeloma. Br J Haematol 2008;143(1):46–53.

114. Hoering A, Crowley J, Shaughnessy JD Jr, et al. Complete remission in multiple myeloma examined as time-dependent variable in terms of both onset and duration in Total Therapy protocols. Blood 2009;114(7):1299–305.

115. Chou T. Multiple myeloma: recent progress in diagnosis and treatment. J Clin Exp Hematop 2012;52(3):149–59.

116. Laubach J, Hideshima T, Richardson P, et al. Clinical translation in multiple myeloma: from bench to bedside. Semin Oncol 2013;40(5):549–53.

117. Laubach JP, Voorhees PM, Hassoun H, et al. Current strategies for treatment of relapsed/refractory multiple myeloma. Expert Rev Hematol 2014;7(1):97–111.

118. Kocoglu M, Badros A. The role of immunotherapy in multiple myeloma. Pharmaceuticals 2016;9(1):3.

119. Landgren O, Gormley N, Turley D, et al. Flow cytometry detection of minimal residual disease in multiple myeloma: lessons learned at FDA-NCI roundtable symposium. Am J Hematol 2014;89(12):1159–60.
120. Paiva B, Cedena M-T, Puig N, et al. Minimal residual disease monitoring and immune profiling in multiple myeloma in elderly patients. Blood 2016;127(25):3165.
121. Roschewski M, Stetler-Stevenson M, Yuan C, et al. Minimal residual disease: what are the minimum requirements? J Clin Oncol 2014;32(5):475–6.
122. Rawstron AC, Child JA, de Tute RM, et al. Minimal residual disease assessed by multiparameter flow cytometry in multiple myeloma: impact on outcome in the Medical Research Council Myeloma IX Study. J Clin Oncol 2013;31(20):2540–7.
123. Landgren O, Devlin S, Boulad M, et al. Role of MRD status in relation to clinical outcomes in newly diagnosed multiple myeloma patients: a meta-analysis. Bone Marrow Transplant 2016;51(12):1565–8.
124. Paiva B, Vidriales MB, Cervero J, et al. Multiparameter flow cytometric remission is the most relevant prognostic factor for multiple myeloma patients who undergo autologous stem cell transplantation. Blood 2008;112(10):4017–23.
125. Jasper GA, Arun I, Venzon D, et al. Variables affecting the quantitation of CD22 in neoplastic B cells. Cytometry B Clin Cytom 2011;80(2):83–90.
126. Morice WG, Hanson CA, Kumar S, et al. Novel multi-parameter flow cytometry sensitively detects phenotypically distinct plasma cell subsets in plasma cell proliferative disorders. Leukemia 2007;21(9):2043–6.
127. Nishihori T, Song J, Shain KH. Minimal residual disease assessment in the context of multiple myeloma treatment. Curr Hematol Malig Rep 2016;11:118–26.
128. Hedley BD, Keeney M. Technical issues: flow cytometry and rare event analysis. Int J Lab Hematol 2013;35(3):344–50.
129. Subira D, Castanon S, Aceituno E, et al. Flow cytometric analysis of cerebrospinal fluid samples and its usefulness in routine clinical practice. Am J Clin Pathol 2002;117(6):952–8.
130. Rawstron AC, Bottcher S, Letestu R, et al. Improving efficiency and sensitivity: European Research Initiative in CLL (ERIC) update on the international harmonised approach for flow cytometric residual disease monitoring in CLL. Leukemia 2013;27(1):142–9.
131. Nieto WG, Almeida J, Romero A, et al. Increased frequency (12%) of circulating chronic lymphocytic leukemia-like B-cell clones in healthy subjects using a highly sensitive multicolor flow cytometry approach. Blood 2009;114(1):33–7.
132. Hallett WH, Jing W, Drobyski WR, et al. Immunosuppressive effects of multiple myeloma are overcome by PD-L1 blockade. Biol Blood Marrow Transplant 2011;17(8):1133–45.
133. Walker BA, Wardell CP, Johnson DC, et al. Characterization of IGH locus breakpoints in multiple myeloma indicates a subset of translocations appear to occur in pregerminal center B cells. Blood 2013;121(17):3413–9.
134. Genadieva-Stavric S, Cavallo F, Palumbo A. New approaches to management of multiple myeloma. Curr Treat Options Oncol 2014;15(2):157–70.
135. Liebisch P, Dohner H. Cytogenetics and molecular cytogenetics in multiple myeloma. Eur J Cancer 2006;42(11):1520–9.
136. Blade J, Samson D, Reece D, et al. Criteria for evaluating disease response and progression in patients with multiple myeloma treated by high-dose therapy and haemopoietic stem cell transplantation. Myeloma Subcommittee of the EBMT.

European Group for Blood and Marrow Transplant. Br J Haematol 1998;102(5): 1115–23.

137. Harousseau J-L, Moreau P. Autologous hematopoietic stem-cell transplantation for multiple myeloma. N Engl J Med 2009;360(25):2645–54.

138. Rajkumar SV. Treatment of multiple myeloma. Nat Rev Clin Oncol 2011;8(8): 479–91.

139. O'Donnell EK, Raje NS. New monoclonal antibodies on the horizon in multiple myeloma. Ther Adv Hematol 2017;8(2):41–53.

140. Khagi Y, Mark TM. Potential role of daratumumab in the treatment of multiple myeloma. Onco Targets Ther 2014;7:1095–100.

141. Frigyesi I, Adolfsson J, Ali M, et al. Robust isolation of malignant plasma cells in multiple myeloma. Blood 2014;123(9):1336–40.

142. Veillette A, Guo H. CS1, a SLAM family receptor involved in immune regulation, is a therapeutic target in multiple myeloma. Crit Rev Oncol Hematol 2013;88(1): 168–77.

143. Puig N, Sarasquete ME, Balanzategui A, et al. Critical evaluation of ASO RQ-PCR for minimal residual disease evaluation in multiple myeloma. A comparative analysis with flow cytometry. Leukemia 2014;28(2):391–7.

144. Rasmussen T, Poulsen TS, Honore L, et al. Quantitation of minimal residual disease in multiple myeloma using an allele-specific real-time PCR assay. Exp Hematol 2000;28(9):1039–45.

145. Ladetto M, Bruggemann M, Monitillo L, et al. Next-generation sequencing and real-time quantitative PCR for minimal residual disease detection in B-cell disorders. Leukemia 2014;28(6):1299–307.

146. Avet-Loiseau H, Corre J, Lauwers-Cances V, et al. Evaluation of minimal residual disease (MRD) by next generation sequencing (NGS) is highly predictive of progression free survival in the IFM/DFCI 2009 trial. Blood 2015;126(23):191.

147. Martinez-Lopez J, Lahuerta JJ, Pepin F, et al. Prognostic value of deep sequencing method for minimal residual disease detection in multiple myeloma. Blood 2014;123(20):3073–9.

148. Munshi NC, Minvielle S, Tai Y-T, et al. Deep Igh sequencing identifies an ongoing somatic hypermutation process with complex and evolving clonal architecture in myeloma. Blood 2015;126(23):21.

149. Gormley NJ, Turley DM, Dickey JS, et al. Regulatory perspective on minimal residual disease flow cytometry testing in multiple myeloma. Cytometry B Clin Cytom 2016;90(1):73–80.

150. Salem D, Stetler-Stevenson M, Yuan C, et al. Myeloma minimal residual disease testing in the United States: evidence of improved standardization. Am J Hematol 2016;91(12):E502–3.

151. Logan AC, Zhang B, Narasimhan B, et al. Minimal residual disease quantification using consensus primers and high-throughput IGH sequencing predicts post-transplant relapse in chronic lymphocytic leukemia. Leukemia 2013; 27(8):1659–65.

152. Wu D, Sherwood A, Fromm JR, et al. High-throughput sequencing detects minimal residual disease in acute T lymphoblastic leukemia. Sci Transl Med 2012; 4(134):134ra163.

153. van der Velden VH, Hochhaus A, Cazzaniga G, et al. Detection of minimal residual disease in hematologic malignancies by real-time quantitative PCR: principles, approaches, and laboratory aspects. Leukemia 2003;17(6):1013–34.

154. Paiva B, Gutierrez NC, Rosinol L, et al. High-risk cytogenetics and persistent minimal residual disease by multiparameter flow cytometry predict unsustained

complete response after autologous stem cell transplantation in multiple myeloma. Blood 2012;119(3):687–91.

155. Paiva B, Martinez-Lopez J, Vidriales MB, et al. Comparison of immunofixation, serum free light chain, and immunophenotyping for response evaluation and prognostication in multiple myeloma. J Clin Oncol 2011;29(12):1627–33.

156. Rawstron AC, Paiva B, Stetler-Stevenson M. Assessment of minimal residual disease in myeloma and the need for a consensus approach. Cytometry B Clin Cytom 2016;90(1):21–5.

157. Paiva B, van Dongen JJM, Orfao A. New criteria for response assessment: role of minimal residual disease in multiple myeloma. Blood 2015;125(20):3059.

Paroxysmal Nocturnal Hemoglobinuria Assessment by Flow Cytometric Analysis

Mike Keeney, ART, FCSMLS(D)[a],*,
Andrea Illingworth, MS, H(ASCP), SCYM[b], D. Robert Sutherland, MS[c]

KEYWORDS

- PNH • FLAER • Aplastic anemia • MDS • Flow cytometry

KEY POINTS

- Paroxysmal nocturnal hemoglobinuria (PNH) is a serious life-threatening disease that is difficult to recognize clinically.
- PNH clones may be found in other bone marrow failure-related states, for example, aplastic anemia and myelodysplastic syndrome.
- Small PNH clones may develop into clinical PNH disease over time.
- White blood cell clone size (neutrophil or monocyte) reflects actual clone size because of the impact of hemolysis or previous transfusions on red blood cell clone size.
- Flow cytometry is ideally suited to recognize both small and large clones in PNH.

INTRODUCTION

Paroxysmal nocturnal hemoglobinuria (PNH) is a rare acquired hematopoietic stem cell disorder resulting from the somatic mutation of the X-linked phosphatidylinositol-glycan complementation class A (PIG-A) gene.[1] In PNH, a mutation in the PIG-A gene leads to nonmalignant clonal expansion of cells with a partial or absolute loss in glycosylphosphatidylinositol (GPI)-anchored proteins, the consequences of which include intravascular hemolysis (that leads to hemoglobinuria) and thrombosis, with the latter

Disclosure: M. Keeney and the laboratory have received funding from Alexion Pharmaceuticals, Canada; A. Illingworth is a consultant for and has received speaker fees from Alexion Pharmaceuticals; the laboratory has received funding from Alexion Pharmaceuticals; R. Sutherland has received funding from, is a consultant for, and has received speaker fees from Alexion Pharmaceuticals, Canada.
[a] Pathology and Laboratory Medicine, London Health Sciences Centre, 800 Commissioners Road East, ON N6A 5W9, Canada; [b] Dahl Chase Diagnostic Services, Bangor, ME 04401, USA; [c] Laboratory Medicine Program, Toronto General Hospital, University Health Network, Toronto, 200 Elizabeth Street, ON M5G2C4, Canada
* Corresponding author.
E-mail address: Mike.keeney@lhsc.on.ca

Clin Lab Med 37 (2017) 855–867
http://dx.doi.org/10.1016/j.cll.2017.07.007
0272-2712/17/© 2017 Elsevier Inc. All rights reserved.

labmed.theclinics.com

being a major cause of morbidity and mortality.[2] Before the advent of the complement C5 inhibitor eculizumab, 35% of patients with PNH died within 5 years of diagnosis even with the best available treatment.[2] Eculizumab is a humanized monoclonal antibody approved for the treatment of patients with hemolytic PNH. This drug significantly reduces hemolysis, transfusion requirements, and thrombosis and has been shown to improve both quality of life and life expectancy.[3] There is also a well-documented relationship between PNH and other bone marrow failure syndromes, such as aplastic anemia (AA)[2,4] and low-grade MDS. With modern, high-sensitivity assays, up to 60% of patients with AA have PNH clones,[5] 10% to 25% of which may exhibit clonal expansion and progression to clinical PNH. Small populations of GPI-deficient PNH clones have been reported in patients with early stage myelodysplastic syndrome (MDS).[4]

PATIENT GROUPS WHO SHOULD BE SCREENED FOR PAROXYSMAL NOCTURNAL HEMOGLOBINURIA

PNH is a very rare disease with a prevalence of about 16 cases per million and only about 1.3 new cases diagnosed per million per year. As such, PNH testing should not be used as a front-line screening test and more common causes of hemolysis should always be ruled out first. Nevertheless, the life-threatening and progressive nature of PNH warrants testing of appropriate patient populations at risk of PNH with early diagnosis essential for improved patient management and prognosis.[6,7] Such groups include:

1. Unexplained cytopenias with evidence of hemolysis, that is, increased levels of lactate dehydrogenase, low haptoglobin, or elevated reticulocyte count.
2. All patients with AA and those with low-grade refractory-anemia MDS with evidence of hemolysis.
3. Unexplained thrombosis despite anticoagulation; in patients with cytopenia; less than 50 years of age; in unusual sites, for example, cerebral, hepatic portal, dermal vein; with evidence of hemolysis; or with other clinical manifestations of PNH (abdominal pain, chest pain, dyspnea, dysphagia, severe fatigue).
4. All patients with unexplained direct antiglobulin test–negative hemolytic anemia, hemoglobinuria, and/or hematuria.

HISTORY OF PAROXYSMAL NOCTURNAL HEMOGLOBINURIA TESTING

PNH was initially recognized as a hemolytic anemia; therefore, assays to detect the disease focused on red blood cells (RBCs). These tests included the Ham test and the sugar-hemolysis test, both of which demonstrated the increased sensitivity of PNH RBC to complement-mediated hemolysis. These tests were laborious, difficult to standardize, and neither specific nor sensitive. Since the early 1990s, flow cytometric detection of cells lacking expression of GPI-anchored surface molecules has become the method of choice for diagnosing and monitoring PNH. Early methods to detect PNH relied on detecting the loss of CD55 and CD59, 2 GPI-linked complement-regulatory structures expressed on normal RBCs and white blood cells (WBCs).[8]

Although the ability to rapidly detect GPI-deficient cells by flow has led to improved diagnosis, patient management, and prognosis in PNH and related disorders, simple CD55/CD59-based approaches were neither accurate nor sensitive at less than the 1% to 4% clone size, rendering them inadequate to detect small PNH clones present in PNH+ AA and MDS cases.[9]

Because 40% of samples positive for the presence of PNH cells contain GPI-deficient cells at a level of 1% or less (Illingworth A, unpublished observations), the development and validation of sensitive, standardized methodologies is essential to reliably detect small populations of GPI-deficient PNH phenotypes. The International Clinical Cytometry Society (ICCS) published generic guidelines for the diagnosis and monitoring of PNH and related disorders by flow cytometry.[6] However, this document was not prescriptive in that specific assay cocktails were not specified and analytical strategies were not detailed.

ASSAYS FOR PAROXYSMAL NOCTURNAL HEMOGLOBINURIA RED BLOOD CELLS AND WHITE BLOOD CELLS

As in any high-sensitivity assay, scrupulous attention to reagent quality and assay-specific instrument setup (light-scatter, photomultiplier tube [PMT] voltages, and optimal fluorescence compensation) is essential. Once established, the frequencies of PNH phenotypes in all 3 lineages in multiple normal samples must be determined. Additionally, the sensitivities of the assays have to be determined by titrating (spiking) a PNH sample into a normal sample.[10] Furthermore, there is much variability between different antibody clones/conjugates used in the analysis of PNH in RBC and WBC lineages. To successfully develop highly sensitive assays that are also accurate and reproducible, careful selection and titration of antibody clones/conjugates for lineage-specific gating (RBCs, neutrophils, and monocytes) and specific GPI-antigen detection within each cell lineage are required.[10]

ANTIBODY CLONE/CONJUGATE SELECTION FOR HIGH-SENSITIVITY PAROXYSMAL NOCTURNAL HEMOGLOBINURIA RED BLOOD CELL ASSAY

CD235a (glycophorin A) is the only gating reagent available that specifically identifies mature RBCs. Although loss of the GPI-linked CD55 and CD59 structures was traditionally used to detect PNH RBCs,[8] CD55 is inferior to CD59[6] because of its dim expression and inability to delineate type II and type III PNH RBCs. The authors, thus, focused on identifying CD59PE conjugates that offered the best separation of type I, type II, and type III RBCs. Because CD235a (in particular) and CD59 conjugates can cause massive aggregation of RBCs when used at saturation levels, careful selection and extensive titration is required to minimize aggregation while retaining good signal-to-noise characteristics of the assay.[10] Screening of many CD235a clones/conjugates showed that negatively charged FITC conjugates generated significantly less aggregation than their PE-conjugated counterparts. Similar screening and titration of many CD59PE conjugates was used to identify the best-performing CD59 reagents. A summary of recommended CD235a and CD59 clones/conjugates is shown in **Table 1**. To avoid the

Table 1
Recommended red blood cell antibody panels: Beckman Coulter and Becton Dickinson instruments

Target	Antibody Conjugates	Purpose	Clone and Vendor
RBC	CD235a-FITC	Gating on RBC	YTH 89.1 (Cedarlane Laboratories, Burlington, ON, Canada)
			10F7MN (eBioscience/Thermo Fisher Scientific, Waltham, MA, USA [eBio])
			KC16 (BC)
			JC159 (DAKO, Agilent Technologies, CA, USA)
	CD59-PE	GPI-linked for RBC	OV9A2 (eBio)
			MEM-43 (Invitrogen, Carlsbad, CA, USA)
			MEM-43 (ExBio, Prague Czech Republic)

generation of false negatives, it is highly recommended that cocktails of the chosen CD235aFITC and CD59PE reagents be premixed and diluted with clean phosphate-buffered saline (PBS) to aid the accurate addition of reagents for this assay.[10]

INSTRUMENT SETUP RED BLOOD CELL

Using a normal blood sample diluted in PBS, RBCs can be used to establish forward-angle (FS) and side-angle (SS) light-scatter voltages in log:log format such that unstained normal RBCs can be identified toward the middle of the bivariate histogram (**Fig. 1**A, plot 1). The discriminator/threshold should be set to exclude as much debris

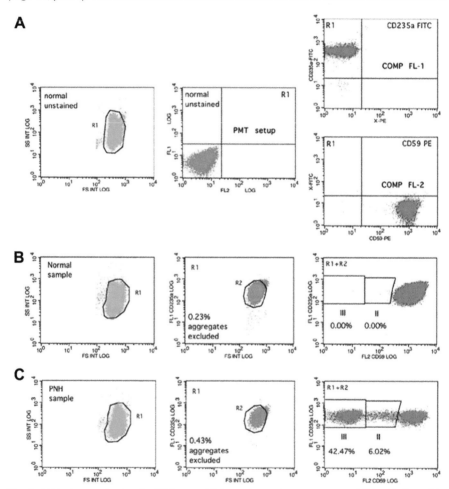

Fig. 1. (*A*) Instrument setup for RBC assay. Light-scatter voltages were established in logarithmic mode such that RBCs from a diluted normal PB sample clustered in the middle of the plot (*left*). Gated RBCs from region R1 with PMT voltages set to have RBCs on-scale (*middle*). Samples were single stained with either CD235aFITC (*top right*) or CD59PE (*bottom right*) and compensation adjusted to reduce spectral overlap. (*B*) Analysis of normal RBCs. (*A*) RBCs gated in R1 (*left*) and displayed on CD235aFITC versus FS plot (*middle*). RBCs were gated in R2 (*doublets excluded*). Cells from R1 and R2 were displayed on CD235aFITC versus CD59PE (*right*). (*C*) Analysis of fresh PNH sample, analyzed as described for the normal sample (*panel B*). The sample contained 42.47% PNH type III cells and 6.02% PNH type II cells.

as possible while not excluding any of the RBC target population. For setting the FL-1 and FL-2 PMT voltages, all compensation is set to zero and the PMT voltages are established without the use of baseline offset or other artifactual displays. Gated RBCs from plot 1 are displayed on an FL-1 versus FL-2 plot and the PMT voltages adjusted so that the cells are on scale and not crushed against the axis (see **Fig. 1**A, plot 2). Two-color compensation adjustments are then performed with samples individually stained with CD235aFITC (see **Fig. 1**A upper-right plot) and CD59PE (see **Fig. 1**A, lower-right plot). Instrument setup can be verified by analyzing a fresh normal sample stained, as outlined later, with the optimized CD235aFITC/CD59PE antibody cocktail (see **Fig. 1**B, plots 1–3).

RED BLOOD CELL SAMPLE PREPARATION METHOD

Anticoagulated (ethylenediaminetetraacetic acid is preferred, but heparin can also be used) peripheral-blood samples should be less than 48 hours old. If possible, these samples should be kept refrigerated, which may extend their stability.

1. Prepare a 1:100 dilution of the sample with clean PBS.
2. Pipette 100 μL of diluted blood sample into the bottom of a test tube using reverse pipetting to avoid aerosol generation, and remove the pipette carefully to avoid leaving blood trails on the inside of the tube.
3. Prepare the CD235aFITC/CD59PE antibody cocktail: Add 15 μL (1.5 μL per test) of CD235aFITC (clone KC16) and 5 μL (0.5 μL per test) of CD59PE (clone MEM43) to 180 μL PBS.

Note that these volumes reflect the authors' currently used reagents and should be validated/titrated by each laboratory to confirm optimal performance.

4. Pipette 20 μL of this diluted cocktail directly into the diluted blood sample and mix by gently swirling the sample using a low-speed vortex.
5. Incubate the sample in the dark for 20 minutes at room temperature (incubation up to 60 minutes has been validated).
6. Wash twice with PBS by centrifugation and resuspend in 0.5 to 1.0 mL of PBS.
7. Rack the sample (drag across a hard plastic or metal test tube rack several times) to disrupt any RBC aggregates generated by the staining/washing procedure immediately before acquisition on the cytometer.
8. Acquire the sample immediately, as delays longer than 15 minutes after the final washing step can show decreased CD235a staining and increased levels of reaggregation.
9. Acquire a minimum of 100,000 RBCs (gated on FS log versus CD235a). If 2 or more events were displayed in the type III PNH RBC region, data acquisition should be continued until 1 million events are acquired.

An example of the assay performed on a known PNH case is shown in **Fig. 1**C. With appropriate sample processing, the level of observed aggregates should be 1.5% or less.

HIGH-SENSITIVITY WHITE BLOOD CELL ASSAYS
Gating Reagents and GPI-Specific Reagents

The ICCS's guidelines[6] stressed the need to use an antibody for gating and 2 GPI-specific markers for each lineage. CD33 has been used successfully to gate on both neutrophils and monocytes[11]; but, as detailed elsewhere, CD15 is superior to CD33 for gating mature neutrophils,[10] whereas CD64 is similarly superior for gating monocytes for high-sensitivity assays.[10,12] Because of the different PMTs and filter sets used by different instrument manufacturers, selection of specific clones/conjugates for gating may be instrument specific, depending on the number of PMTs used. The inclusion of CD45 for debris exclusion and pattern recognition is also recommended in all reagent combinations used for PNH WBC analysis.[10] The recommended gating reagents for neutrophils and monocytes for various 4-, 5- and 6-color reagent sets are shown in **Tables 2–5** for Beckman Coulter (BC; Brea, CA, USA) and Becton Dickinson (BD; Franklin Lakes, NJ, USA) instruments, respectively. Examples of 5-color and 6-color methods are shown in **Figs. 2** and **3**, respectively.

GPI-SPECIFIC REAGENTS

As detailed elsewhere, combinations of fluorescent-labeled proaerolysinc (FLAER) and CD24[10] or FLAER and CD157[13] represent the most tested combinations of reagents to detect GPI-deficient granulocytes/neutrophils, whereas FLAER in combination with either CD14 or CD157 [10,13] represents the most tested combination of reagents to detect GPI-deficient monocytes. After much empirical testing of multiple clones and instrument-specific conjugates, recommended clones/conjugates of GPI-specific reagents for use on instruments equipped with 4, 5, and 6 (or more) PMTs are shown in **Tables 2–5** for Beckman Coulter and BD cytometers, respectively.

PRESENCE OF TYPE II POPULATIONS IN NEUTROPHILS AND MONOCYTES

The presence of RBCs with intermediate expression of CD59 (type II RBCs) has been reported extensively in the literature, describing RBCs with a partial protection from complement-mediated lysis, which have an intermediate life span between normal type I RBCs and type III PNH RBCs (complete absence of CD59). Although type II phenotypes can be frequently detected in granulocytes and monocytes, particularly with more modern techniques that use cocktails of thoroughly validated reagent combinations, the clinical significance, if any, of such populations is unknown at this time. It is, therefore, recommended that only the total (type III plus type II phenotypes when present) be reported for PNH granulocyte and monocyte clone sizes.

ANTIBODY CLONE/CONJUGATE SELECTION FOR 4, 5 AND 6 COLOR HIGH-SENSITIVITY PNH WHITE BLOOD CELL ASSAYS

Other than CD24 and CD14 on neutrophils and monocytes, respectively, the expression of CD157 is another GPI-linked structure expressed on both neutrophils and

Table 2
Recommended white blood cell antibody panels: Beckman Coulter

	FITC	PE	ECD	PC5	eF710	PC7	APC	APC-A700	KrO	eF450
4-C Grans	FLAER	CD24	—	CD15	—	CD45	—	—	—	—
4-C Monos	FLAER	CD14	—	CD64	—	CD45	—	—	—	—
5-C Grans + monos	FLAER	CD157	CD64	CD15	—	CD45	—	—	—	—
6-C Grans + monos	FLAER	CD24	—	CD15	—	CD64	—	CD14	CD45	—
6-C Grans + monos	FLAER	CD157	—	—	CD15	CD64	CD24	—	—	CD45

Abbreviations: Grans, granulocytes; monos, monocytes.

Table 3
Recommended white blood cell antibodies and clones: Beckman Coulter

Target	Antibody Conjugates	Purpose	Clone (Vendor)
WBC	FLAER-Alexa488	GPI-linked (grans and monos)	NA (Cedarlane Laboratories, Burlington, ON, Canada)
	CD24-PE (4C,6C)	GPI-linked (grans)	SN3 (eBioscience/Thermo Fisher Scientific, Waltham, MA, USA [eBio]), ALB9 (BC)
	CD24-APC		SN3 (eBio)
	CD14-PE (4C)	GPI-linked (monos)	61D3 (eBio), RMO52 (BC)
			Tuk4 (Invitrogen, Carlsbad, CA, USA)
	CD14-APC700 (6C)		RMO52 (BC)
	CD157-PE (5C)	GPI-linked (grans + monos)	SY11B5 (eBio)
	CD64-PC5 (4C)	Gating on monos	22 (BC)
	CD64-ECD (5C)		
	CD64-PC7 (6C)		
	CD15-PC5 (4C, 5C)	Gating on grans	80H5 (BC)
	CD15-PerCP-eF710		MMA (eBio)
	CD45-PC7 (4C, 5C)	Debris exclusion and pattern recognition	J33 (BC)
	CD45-KO (6C)		
	CD45-eF450 (6C)		2D1 (eBio)

Abbreviations: grans, granulocytes; monos, monocytes.

monocytes that is useful for the detection of GPI-deficient cells.[14] The availability of a PE-conjugated version of CD157 (clone SY11B5, eBioscience/Thermo Fisher Scientific, Waltham, MA, USA) allowed direct comparison with CD24PE and with CD14PE in the 4-C neutrophil and 4-C monocyte protocols, respectively. The excellent performance of the CD157PE conjugate in these assays subsequently led to the development of a single 5-color combination of FLAER, CD157, CD64, CD15, and CD45 that could be used to simultaneously evaluate GPI-deficient neutrophils and monocytes with a single tube for those with access to cytometers with 5 or more PMTs.[13] Of note, rare non-PNH cases that fail to express (in total or in part) detectable CD157 in both neutrophil and monocyte lineages have been noted. Although the cause of this is currently under investigation, the fact that FLAER is expressed at normal levels in these cases and the RBC assay shows normal expression of CD59 makes it unlikely that such a sample would ever be misdiagnosed as a case of bona fide PNH.[13]

Table 4
Recommended white blood cell antibody panels: Becton Dickinson cytometers

	FITC	PE	PerCP	PCP-eF710	PC7	APC	APC-H7	eF450
4-C Grans	FLAER	CD24	CD45	—	—	CD15	—	—
4-C Monos	FLAER	CD14	CD45	—	—	CD64	—	—
5-C Grans + monos[a]	FLAER	CD157	CD45	—	—	CD64	—	CD15
5-C Grans + monos[b]	FLAER	CD157	—	CD15	—	CD64	CD45	—
6-C Grans + monos[a]	FLAER	CD24	CD45	—	CD64	CD14	—	CD15
6-C Grans + monos[b]	FLAER	CD24	—	CD15	CD64	CD14	CD45	—
6-C Grans + monos[a]	FLAER	CD157	—	CD15	CD64	CD24	—	CD15

Abbreviations: Grans, granulocytes; monos, monocytes.
[a] Three-laser Canto.
[b] Two-laser Canto.

Table 5
Recommended white blood cell antibodies and clones: Becton Dickinson

Target	Antibody Conjugates	Purpose	Clone (Vendor)
WBC	FLAER-Alexa488	GPI-linked (grans and monos)	NA (Cedarlane Laboratories, Burlington, ON, Canada)
	CD24-PE (4C, 6C)	GPI-linked (grans)	SN3 (eBioscience/Thermo Fisher Scientific, Waltham, MA, USA [eBio]), ML5 (BD)
	CD24-APC		SN3 (eBio)
	CD14-PE (4C)	GPI-linked (monos)	61D3 (eBio), MOP9 (BD), TUK4
	CD14-APC (6C)		(Invitrogen, Carlsbad, CA, USA)
	CD157-PE (5C)	GPI-linked (grans + monos)	SY11B5 (eBio)
	CD64-APC (4C, 5C)	Gating on monos	10.1 (BD, eBio)
	CD64-PC7 (6C)		10.1 (BD)
	CD15-APC (4C)	Gating on grans	HI98 (BD)
	CD15-eF450 (5C, 6C)[a]		MMA (eBio)
	CD15-PCP-eF710 (5C, 6C)[a,b]		MMA (eBio)
	CD45-eF450 (6C)[a]	Debris exclusion and pattern recognition	2D1 (eBio)
	CD45-PerCP (4C, 5C)[b]		2D1 (eBio)
	CD45 APC-H7(5C, 6C)[b]		2D1 (BD)

Abbreviations: grans, granulocytes; monos, monocytes.
[a] Three-laser Canto.
[b] Two-laser Canto.

Instrument Setup Considerations for White Blood Cell Assay

The CD157/FLAER-based 5-color assay can be performed on FC500, Navios (Beckman Coulter), and Canto (Becton Dickinson) cytometers, with minor changes in conjugated forms used.[15] Regardless of instrument platform, light-scatter voltage and PMT voltage setup and compensation methodologies for this assay are very similar. In the example shown from a Navios cytometer, 100 µL of a lysed and washed normal-blood sample was used to establish FS and SS light-scatter voltages in linear mode such that all major leukocyte subsets, including lymphocytes, were clearly visible at greater than the FS threshold (see **Fig. 2**, plot 1). PMT voltages were set with all compensation set to zero (baseline offset off at all times). The FL1 PMT was set using a sample stained with a pretitrated volume CD3-Alexa488, ensuring that the unstained B-cell population was properly on scale. A second sample was stained with CD3PE, and the FL2 PMT voltage was adjusted to ensure that B lymphocytes were also comfortably on scale. This procedure was repeated using CD3ECD for FL3 and CD3PC5 for FL4. The FL5 PMT voltage was set using a sample stained with the pretitrated volume of CD45PC7, and the PMT was set so that lymphocytes were positioned at the end of the third decade of fluorescence of the 4-decade log scale. These voltages were used for the compensation process. Compensation adjustments were made using individual VersaComp (Beckman Coulter) beads stained with CD3-Alexa488 (FL1), CD157PE (FL2), CD64ECD (FL3), CD15PC5 (FL4), and CD45PC7 (FL5). The compensation matrix was established using Kaluza software and verified with a fresh PNH sample stained with the same 5 (cocktailed) reagents. The same 5-color assay has been established on the 5-C FC500 cytometer.[13]

For the 8-color FACSCanto II, light-scatter and PMT settings were established in 4.5-decade format (without the biexponential modification) as described earlier for the FL1 PMT. The FL2 (CD157PE), FL3 (CD45PerCPCy5.5), FL4 (CD64APC), and FL7 (CD15eFluor450) PMTs were set to get unstained lymphocytes in the individually

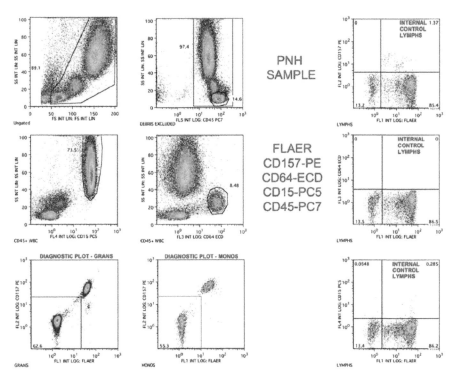

Fig. 2. Five-color, single-tube, CD157-based assay for PNH neutrophils and monocytes. A fresh sample from a patient with long-term PNH was stained with FLAER Alexa488, CD157PE, CD64ECD, CD15PECy5, and CD45PECy7; data were acquired on a 10-C Navios. Debris was removed with light scatter (*top row, left*) and CD45 gating (*top row, middle*). Neutrophils (*middle row, left*) and monocytes (*middle row, middle*) were identified and gated based on CD15 and CD64 expression, respectively. Gated neutrophils (*bottom row, left*) and monocytes (*bottom row, middle*) were displayed on FLAER versus CD157 plots, and PNH neutrophils and monocytes (FLAER negative, CD157 negative) were identified. Gated lymphocytes (internal controls) were identified and sequentially gated based on CD45 and SS (*top row, middle*) and lack of CD64 staining (not shown) and displayed on FLAER versus CD157 (*top row, right*) or FLAER versus CD64 (*middle row, right*) and FLAER versus CD15 (*bottom row, right*). GRANS, granulocytes; MONOS, monocytes.

stained samples comfortably on scale. Compensation was performed with Versa-Comp antibody-capture beads stained with CD3, CD157, CD45, CD64, and CD15 as described earlier and the compensation matrix established in DIVA software (BD Biosciences). The compensation matrix was verified using a PNH sample stained with FLAER, CD157PE, CD45PerCPCy5.5, CD64APC, and CD15eFluor450. This same reagent set can also be used without modifications on Navios instruments.

STAINING PROCEDURE FOR HIGH SENSITIVITY NEUTROPHIL/MONOCYTE ASSAY

All individual antibodies were verified for appropriate reactivity with target cells and titrated to optimize specific staining performance before being cocktailed for use in the single-tube 5-color assay. The ICCS and practical guidelines recommended staining samples within the first 48 hours from sample draw.[6,10]

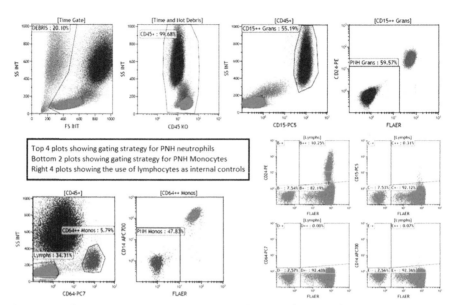

Fig. 3. Six-color, single-tube, FLAER-based assay for identification of PNH neutrophils and PNH monocytes. A 24-hour-old sample from a patient with PNH was stained with FLAER-Alexa488, CD24-PE, CD15-PC5, CD64-PC7, CD14-APC700, and CD45-KrO; data were acquired on a 10-C Navios. Debris was removed with light scatter (*top row, first plot*) and CD45 gating (*top row, second plot*). Neutrophils were identified and gated based on CD15 expression (*top row, third plot*). Gated neutrophils were displayed on FLAER versus CD24 plot (*top row, fourth plot*) identifying PNH neutrophils (FLAER-negative, CD24-negative). Monocytes (*bottom row, first plot*) were identified and gated based on CD64 expression, and gated monocytes were displayed on FLAER versus CD14 plot (*bottom row, second plot*) identifying PNH monocytes (FLAER-negative, CD14-negative). Gated lymphocytes (internal controls) were identified and displayed on FLAER versus CD24, CD14, CD15, and CD64 to verify instrument setup and antibody performance (*4 plots on the right*). Grans, granulocytes; Monos, monocytes.

1. Using reverse-pipetting, pipette 100 μL of fresh peripheral blood carefully into the bottom of a test tube without touching the side of the tube.
2. Add an appropriate volume of premixed and validated cocktail directly to the blood aliquot in the bottom of the tube, and mix very gently but thoroughly as described earlier for the RBC assay.
3. Incubate for 20 minutes at room temperature in the dark.
4. Lyse the RBCs using an appropriate lysing agent. ImmunoPrep (BC), Versalyse (BC), FACSLyse (BD), or ammonium chloride-based lysing agents are all acceptable; those containing fixatives may help retain cellular integrity better than those that do not.
5. After lysing, wash cells once with PBS, resuspend in 1 mL of PBS, and acquire on the cytometer. Note: Samples should be acquired immediately, as delays can cause light-scatter changes, especially when fixative-free lysing agents are used.
6. Acquire a minimum of 50,000 neutrophils and 5000 monocytes in list mode for clinical test samples.
7. If small numbers of GPI-deficient cells are observed, acquisition times should be increased until a statistically reliable number of PNH phenotypes are acquired (20–50 cells).

QUALITY ASSURANCE

Before introducing a high-sensitivity assay to detect GPI-deficient PNH cells in the clinical laboratory, it is important not only to optimize instrument and reagent performance but also to validate accuracy, specificity, sensitivity, imprecision, linearity, carryover, reportable range, stability, and reference range. Validation guidance of an assay such as this can be found in the International Council for Standardization of Hematology/ICCS's guidelines for the validation of flow cytometric laboratory-developed tests.[16]

In addition, ongoing quality control needs to be in place to ensure that established analytical specifications are controlled during patient testing. For the presence of a PNH clone, which essentially is determined by a loss of antigen expression, the presence of internal cell populations that are positive will ensure that the assay is performing appropriately. These internal-control cells verify not only antibody/reagent performance but can also indicate possible issues within the patient sample, which may not be apparent in normal controls. Finally, rigorous monitoring of such internal cellular controls allows the cytometrist to monitor instrument performance, including PMT and compensation settings.

Because very small numbers of PNH phenotypes can be detected in some patients with AA and MDS, it is important to know the sensitivity of the assays deployed in the clinical laboratory. Assay sensitivity is determined by 2 factors: the absolute lower limit of detectability of bona fide PNH phenotypes and the assay background (number of PNH phenotypes) on normal samples. Blood samples from normal individuals have been shown previously to contain very small numbers of neutrophils with PNH phenotypes.[17] Twenty normal samples were screened[10,13,15] with each assay in keeping with recently established international guidelines.[15,18,19] For the RBC protocol, a range of 2 to 6 events falling in the type III RBC region per million RBCs was found[10] (see example shown in **Fig. 1**B). Spiking experiments of PNH cells into whole blood have established that as few as 20 type III PNH RBCs can be detected in a list mode file of 1 million RBCs with the authors' assay.[10] Similar experiments performed with the 4-color neutrophil, 4-color monocyte, and 5 and 6 color combined assays[10,13] showed that as few as 10 PNH phenotypes per 100,000 neutrophils could be detected, with the monocyte assays slightly less sensitive because of the lower frequencies of monocytes in PB samples.

These data establish the RBC assay sensitivity at better than 0.01%. Neutrophil and monocyte assays described here have sensitivities in the 0.05% and 0.1% ranges, respectively.[10,13]

External quality control is also available through the College of American Pathologists in North America and the United Kingdom National External Quality Assessment Service in Europe. Using the initial standardized 4-color neutrophil and monocyte assays described earlier on stabilized PNH whole-blood preparations, results have demonstrated very good interlaboratory performance characteristics among expert laboratories.[20] Using fresh samples and the same standardized 4-color assays, another recent study demonstrated good intralaboratory and interlaboratory performance characteristics for both precision and reproducibility analyses and excellent correlation and agreement between centers for all target PNH clone sizes, even in laboratories with little prior experience performing PNH testing.[21]

REFERENCES

1. Rosse WF, Ware RE. The molecular basis of paroxysmal nocturnal hemoglobinuria. Blood 1995;86(9):3277–86.

2. Hillmen P, Lewis SM, Bessler M, et al. Natural history of paroxysmal nocturnal hemoglobinuria. N Engl J Med 1995;333(19):1253–8.

3. Varela JC, Brodsky RA. Paroxysmal nocturnal hemoglobinuria and the age of therapeutic complement inhibition. Expert Rev Clin Immunol 2013;9(11):1113–24.

4. Parker CJ. Bone marrow failure syndromes: paroxysmal nocturnal hemoglobinuria. Hematol Oncol Clin North Am 2009;23(2):333–46.

5. Scheinberg P, Marte M, Nunez O, et al. Paroxysmal nocturnal hemoglobinuria clones in severe aplastic anemia patients treated with horse anti-thymocyte globulin plus cyclosporine. Haematologica 2010;95(7):1075–80.

6. Borowitz MJ, Craig FE, Digiuseppe JA, et al. Guidelines for the diagnosis and monitoring of paroxysmal nocturnal hemoglobinuria and related disorders by flow cytometry. Cytometry B Clin Cytom 2010;78(4):211–30.

7. Parker C, Omine M, Richards S, et al. Diagnosis and management of paroxysmal nocturnal hemoglobinuria. Blood 2005;106(12):3699–709.

8. van der Schoot CE, Huizinga TW, van 't Veer-Korthof ET, et al. Deficiency of glycosyl-phosphatidylinositol-linked membrane glycoproteins of leukocytes in paroxysmal nocturnal hemoglobinuria, description of a new diagnostic cytofluorometric assay. Blood 1990;76(9):1853–9.

9. Sutherland DR, Kuek N, Davidson J, et al. Diagnosing PNH with FLAER and multiparameter flow cytometry. Cytometry B Clin Cytom 2007;72(3):167–77.

10. Sutherland DR, Keeney M, Illingworth A. Practical guidelines for the high-sensitivity detection and monitoring of paroxysmal nocturnal hemoglobinuria clones by flow cytometry. Cytometry B Clin Cytom 2012;82(4):195–208.

11. Sutherland DR, Kuek N, Azcona-Olivera J, et al. Use of a FLAER-based WBC assay in the primary screening of PNH clones. Am J Clin Pathol 2009;132(4):564–72.

12. Dalal BI, Khare NS. Flow cytometric testing for paroxysmal nocturnal hemoglobinuria: CD64 is better for gating monocytes than CD33. Cytometry B Clin Cytom 2013;84(1):33–6.

13. Sutherland DR, Acton E, Keeney M, et al. Use of CD157 in FLAER-based assays for high-sensitivity PNH granulocyte and PNH monocyte detection. Cytometry B Clin Cytom 2014;86(1):44–55.

14. Hernandez-Campo PM, Almeida J, Acevedo MJ, et al. Detailed immunophenotypic characterization of different major and minor subsets of peripheral blood cells in patients with paroxysmal nocturnal hemoglobinuria. Transfusion 2008;48(7):1403–14.

15. Sutherland DR, Illingworth A, Keeney M, et al. High-sensitivity detection of PNH red blood cells, red cell precursors, and white blood cells. Curr Protoc Cytom 2015;72. 6.37.1-30.

16. ICSH/ICCS Workgroup. Validation of cell-based fluorescence assays: practice guidelines from the International Council for Standardization of Haematology and International Clinical Cytometry Society. Cytometry B Clin Cytom 2013;84(5):281.

17. Hu R, Mukhina GL, Piantadosi S, et al. PIG-A mutations in normal hematopoiesis. Blood 2005;105(10):3848–54.

18. Davis BH, McLaren CE, Carcio AJ, et al. Determination of optimal replicate number for validation of imprecision using fluorescence cell-based assays: proposed practical method. Cytometry B Clin Cytom 2013;84(5):329–37.

19. Davis BH, Keeney M, Brown R, et al. 2nd edition. H52–A2 red blood cell diagnostic testing using flow cytometry; approved guideline, vol. 34. Wayne (PA): Clinical and Laboratory Standards Institute; 2014.

20. Fletcher M, Sutherland DR, Whitby L, et al. Standardizing leucocyte PNH clone detection: an international study. Cytometry B Clin Cytom 2014;86(5):311–8.
21. Marinov I, Kohoutova M, Tkacova V, et al. Intra- and interlaboratory variability of paroxysmal nocturnal hemoglobinuria testing by flow cytometry following the 2012 practical guidelines for high-sensitivity paroxysmal nocturnal hemoglobinuria testing. Cytometry B Clin Cytom 2013;84(4):229–36.

Mast Cell Disease Assessment by Flow Cytometric Analysis

Jacqueline M. Cortazar, MD, David M. Dorfman, MD, PhD*

KEYWORDS

- Flow cytometry • Mast cell disease • Mastocytosis
- Immunophenotype of mast cells

KEY POINTS

- Mast cells are present at low frequency in the bone marrow and require highly sensitive and standardized techniques for adequate acquisition of cells by flow cytometry.
- Mast cells can be identified by flow cytometric immunophenotypic analysis based on bright CD117 expression and variable side scatter, and neoplastic mast cells can be identified based on aberrant expression of CD25 and/or CD2, but not in all cases.
- Mast cells in systemic mastocytosis typically demonstrate event clustering within the flow cytometric CD117 x SSC gate, which can be assessed using statistical and/or clustering algorithms.
- CD30 may be helpful as an additional marker to identify neoplastic mast cells in systemic mastocytosis, including cases of well-differentiated systemic mastocytosis.

INTRODUCTION: MAST CELLS AND MAST CELL DISORDERS

Mast cells play an essential role in the innate immune system and allergic reactions.[1,2] Upon cross-linking of the surface high-affinity immunoglobulin E (IgE) receptor (FcεRI), multiple signaling pathways are initiated that lead to degranulation of cytoplasmic contents including histamine, heparin, and proteases, de novo synthesis of arachidonic acid metabolites, and production of various cytokines and chemokines.[1,3] Release of these mediators leads to clinical symptoms such as flushing, pruritus, urticaria, angioedema, bronchoconstriction, increased vascular permeability, and anaphylaxis.[1] Patients who present with this constellation of symptoms may be evaluated for an underlying mast cell disorder.

Disclosure Statement: The authors have nothing to disclose.
Department of Pathology, Brigham and Women's Hospital, Harvard Medical School, 75 Francis Street, Boston, MA 02115, USA
* Corresponding author.
E-mail address: ddorfman@bwh.harvard.edu

Clin Lab Med 37 (2017) 869–878
http://dx.doi.org/10.1016/j.cll.2017.07.008
0272-2712/17/© 2017 Elsevier Inc. All rights reserved.

labmed.theclinics.com

Mast cell disorders include both primary and secondary disorders. Primary mast cell disorders, which fall under the category of mastocytosis, are a heterogenous group, all characterized by an accumulation of abnormal populations of mast cells that express aberrant cell markers and genetic mutations, in at least 1 organ. These disorders range in severity from benign entities involving skin to malignant rapidly progressive malignant neoplasms, such as mast cell sarcoma (**Box 1**).

Mastocytosis is defined in the 2016 revision to the World Health Organization classification of myeloid neoplasms and acute leukemia[4] as 3 distinct entities: cutaneous mastocytosis, systemic mastocytosis (SM), and mast cell sarcoma (MCS). SM is subcategorized into 5 separate entities: indolent systemic mastocytosis (ISM), smoldering systemic mastocytosis (SSM), systemic mastocytosis with an associated hematological neoplasm (SM-AHN), aggressive systemic mastocytosis (ASM), and mast cell leukemia (MCL, **Box 1**). The 2008 World Health Organization (WHO) classification of tumors of haematopoietic and lymphoid tissues established well-defined criteria for the diagnosis of SM that include 1 major criterion (multifocal clusters of >15 mast cells in extracutaneous organs) and 4 minor criteria (atypical mast cell morphology, aberrant CD2 and/or CD25 expression on mast cells, presence of D816V KIT mutation, or persistently elevated serum tryptase levels of >20 ng/mL, **Box 2**).[5] The diagnosis of SM can be made when the major criterion and 1 minor criterion or at least 3 minor criteria are present. In addition to the established variants of SM, a potential new variant of SM has recently been described, termed well-differentiated systemic mastocytosis (WDSM), in which the mast cells harbor the D816V KIT mutation but are of normal morphology and do not express aberrant CD2 or CD25.[6–9]

Secondary mast cell disorders include several entities under the broad category of mast cell activation syndromes. In these disorders, mast cells are present in normal numbers but are hyper-responsive and fulfill 1 or more of the minor diagnostic criteria for systemic mastocytosis.[1,10,11] Monoclonal mast cell activation syndrome requires the presence of 1 or 2 minor criteria for mastocytosis.[1] Additionally, patients with idiopathic anaphylaxis have been demonstrated to harbor the D816V KIT mutation and aberrantly express CD25 on their mast cells.[10] Other mast cell-driven processes such as allergic disorders, physical urticarias, chronic autoimmune urticaria, and

---

Box 1
Word Health Organization (WHO) classification of mastocytosis (2016 revision to the 2008 WHO classification)

1. Cutaneous mastocytosis (CM)

2. Systemic mastocytosis
   a. Indolent systemic mastocytosis (ISM)
   b. Smoldering systemic mastocytosis (SSM)
   c. Systemic mastocytosis with an associated hematological neoplasm (SM-AHN)[a]
   d. Aggressive systemic mastocytosis (ASM)
   e. Mast cell leukemia (MCL)

3. Mast cell sarcoma

[a] Equivalent to the previously described category "systemic mastocytosis with an associated clonal hematological non-mast cell lineage disease (SMAHNMD)"

From Swerdlow SH, Campo E, Harris NL, et al. WHO Classification of Tumours of Haematopoietic and Lymphoid Tissues. 4th Ed. 2008; with permission.

Box 2
World Health Organization criteria for cutaneous and systemic mastocytosis

Cutaneous mastocytosis (CM)

Skin lesions demonstrating the typical clinical findings of urticaria pigmentosa (UP)/ maculopapular cutaneous mastocytosis (MPCM), diffuse cutaneous mastocytosis, or solitary mastocytoma, and typical histologic infiltrates of mast cells in a multifocal or diffuse pattern in an adequate skin biopsy; in addition, a diagnostic prerequisite for the diagnosis of CM is the absence of features/criteria sufficient to establish the diagnosis of SM

Systemic mastocytosis

The diagnosis of SM can be made when the major criterion and 1 minor criterion or at least 3 minor criteria are present

Major criterion:
  Multifocal, dense infiltrates of mast cells ($\geq$15 mast cells in aggregates) detected in sections of bone marrow and/or other extracutaneous organ(s)

Minor criteria:
1. In biopsy sections of bone marrow or other extracutaneous organs, greater than 25% of the mast cells in the infiltrate are spindle-shaped or have atypical morphology, or, of all mast cells in bone marrow aspirate smears, greater than 25% are immature or atypical mast cells
2. Detection of an activating point mutation at codon 816 of *KIT* in bone marrow, blood, or another extracutaneous organ
3. Mast cells in bone marrow, blood, or other extracutaneous organs express CD2 and/or CD25 in addition to normal mast cell markers
4. Serum total tryptase persistently exceeds 20 ng/mL (unless there is an associated clonal myeloid disorder, in which case this parameter is not valid)

From Swerdlow SH, Campo E, Harris NL, et al. WHO classification of tumours of haematopoietic and lymphoid tissues, vol. 2. 4th edition. 2. print. Lyon: International Agency for Research on Cancer; 2008; with permission.

---

idiopathic angioedema are among other entities that result from hyper-responsive mast cells.[1]

IMMUNOPHENOTYPE OF MAST CELLS

Mast cells are derived from CD34 positive hematopoietic progenitor cells, which, in response to stimulation with stem cell factor/kit ligand, develop into mature mast cells.[3] The immunophenotypic analysis of mast cells has been limited by the low frequency of mast cell precursors and mature mast cells, with mast cell precursors demonstrated to be less than 0.001% to 0.02% of the CD34-positive cells.[12] Because of this, the mast cell immunophenotype has primarily been elucidated through in vitro models.[6,13–17] Based on these studies, mast cell precursors have been demonstrated to express CD34, CD117(c-kit), CD33, CD13, CD38, interleukin (IL)-3R alpha (CD123), GMCSF receptor, and rarely HLA-DR, and are negative for FcεRI, CD14, and CD17.[3,6] As the cells mature, they express proteins associated with mast cell function including FcεRI, mast cell chymase and tryptase, and histamine, and lose expression of markers of immaturity.[6,18] Immature and mature mast cells have been demonstrated to express CD117, CD58, CD63, CD147, CD151, CD203c, and CD172a (**Fig. 1**).[6,18] In comparison to normal or reactive mast cells, MCs in mastocytosis aberrantly express low-affinity IL-2R alpha (CD25) and CD2.[6,12,19,20] Additionally, quantitative differences in antigen expression can be seen, including increased expression of complement-associated molecules CD35

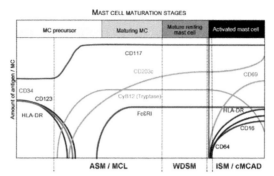

Fig. 1. Immunophenotypic findings at various stages of mast cell development and correlation with immunophenotypic findings in patients with different subtypes of systemic mastocytosis. Abbreviations: MC, mast cell; ASM/MCL, aggressive systemic mastocytosis/mast cell leukemia; WDSM, well-differentiated systemic mastocytosis; ISM/cMCAD, indolent systemic mastocytosis/clonal mast cell activation disorder. (*From* Sánchez-Muñoz L, Teodosio C, Morgado JMT, et al. Flow cytometry in mastocytosis: utility as a diagnostic and prognostic tool. Immunol Allergy Clin North Am 2014;34(2):297–313; with permission.)

and CD11c, activation markers CD69 and CD63, and the complement regulatory protein CD59.[6,18,21] In cases of suspected mastocytosis, flow cytometric analysis can be effective to identify mast cell populations and identify aberrant surface marker expression.

FLOW CYTOMETRIC ANALYSIS FOR THE DIAGNOSIS OF SYSTEMIC MASTOCYTOSIS

Flow cytometry is a valuable tool to evaluate surface and cytoplasmic protein expression on single cells. Because of the low frequency of mast cells in bone marrow biopsies, which typically represent less than 1% of nucleated cells, this technique is well suited to assess their immunophenotype, if sufficient numbers of mast cells are evaluated.[19] In order to detect this population, sensitive and specific methodological approaches are required to ensure the acquisition of a sufficient number of mast cells for evaluation.[6,21]

The original demonstration of the utility of multiparametric flow cytometry for mast cell diseases demonstrated that mast cells can be identified by their light-scatter properties and high level of CD117 expression.[19] The current techniques for acquiring mast cells utilize this finding, and gate on CD117 bright cells with variable side scatter, and allow for adequate acquisition of large numbers of cells within that gate (**Fig. 2**). At the Brigham and Women's Hospital, cases of suspected mast cell disorders are evaluated by collecting at least 200,000 total events (up to 1,000,000 total events) whenever possible. Immunophenotypic analysis of mast cells is performed within a uniform mast cell gate defined by variable SSC and a high level of CD117 expression.[22]

The current panel of makers used for the diagnosis of mastocytosis includes CD45, CD117, CD25, and CD2. This combination of markers allows for the identification of both normal mast cells by CD117 expression, and CD25 and CD2 to detect aberrant protein expression on neoplastic mast cells; assessment of CD2 and CD25 expression is made in comparison with isotype controls. The detection of a CD117-positive mast cell population that expresses CD25 and/or CD2 is consistent with a

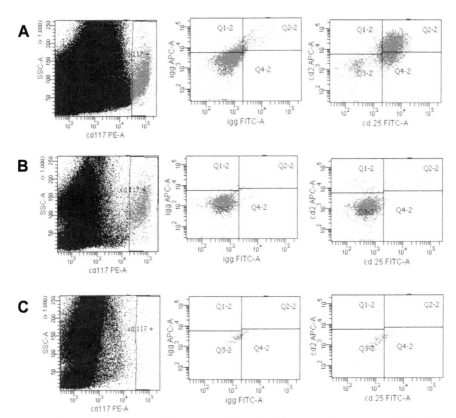

Fig. 2. (*A*) Example of positive flow cytometric analysis for systemic mastocytosis based on the presence of a discrete population of CD117 bright cells with variable side scatter that show coexpression of CD2 and CD25 based on a comparison of staining for CD2 and isotype control and CD25 and isotype control. (*B*) Example of positive flow cytometric analysis for systemic mastocytosis based on the presence of a discrete population of CD117 bright cells with variable side scatter with absence of coexpression of CD2 and CD25. (*C*) Example of negative flow cytometric analysis for systemic mastocytosis based on the lack of a discrete population of CD117 bright cells and the lack of cells showing coexpression of CD2 and CD25 within the mast cell gate.

neoplastic mast cell population and fulfills 1 of the minor criteria for the diagnosis of mastocytosis (see **Fig. 2**).[4,21,23,24]

Flow cytometric analysis has been found to have greater sensitivity for the detection of CD2 expression by mast cells than immunohistochemical staining (14 of 23 cases [61%] versus 9 of 23 cases [39%]), and flow cytometric analysis and immunohistochemical staining have been found to have comparable high sensitivity for the detection of CD25 expression by mast cells.[24] Not all cases of SM exhibit aberrant CD2 expression, and studies have identified patients who fulfill the diagnostic criteria for systemic mastocytosis in which neoplastic mast cells are negative for CD2, CD25, or both by flow cytometric analysis.[22,25,26] WDSM accounts for at least some of these cases.[6–9] Of note, a recent study found that aberrant expression of CD2 and/or CD25 may be seen in patients who do not fulfill the diagnostic criteria for systemic mastocytosis, particularly after chemotherapy for another hematopoietic neoplasm. However, in that study, at least 60% of mast cells were found to express CD25 in cases of systemic mastocytosis, with minimal false positivity using this cut-off for CD25 expression.[26] The identification of cases of systemic mastocytosis that lack CD2 or CD2 and CD25 expression may be challenging, and requires the fulfillment of other criteria for the diagnosis of SM. As a result, several studies have investigated the utility of other markers and characteristics of mast cells to aid in the detection of neoplastic mast cell populations by flow cytometric analysis.

NEW FLOW CYTOMETRIC MARKERS AND APPROACHES FOR THE DIAGNOSIS OF SYSTEMIC MASTOCYTOSIS

One recent set of flow cytometric studies examined the presence of discrete and expanded CD117-positive mast cell populations in cases of SM, and demonstrated that these populations may be present in cases of SM lacking CD2 and CD25 (see **Fig. 2**) but not in bone marrow specimens negative for SM.[22] In the first study, the majority of SM cases had a discrete and expanded population of mast cells within the CD117-positive mast cell gate (24 of 39 cases [62%]), including 7 cases (29%) that did not demonstrate aberrant expression of CD2 and or CD25, and were originally interpreted as negative for the presence of a mast cell neoplasm by flow cytometric analysis. Bone marrow biopsy specimens that were negative for SM did not display discrete and expanded CD117-positive mast cell populations. When the presence of a discrete and expanded CD117-positive mast cell population was considered a criterion for the presence of a neoplastic mast cell neoplasm, the sensitivity of flow cytometric analysis for the detection of SM increased from 77% to 95%.[22] The presence of discrete clusters of CD117-positive mast cells in SM is presumably a result of the clonal expansion of neoplastic mast cells that have similar CD117 staining intensity and side scatter characteristics.

A follow-up study, to quantitate the presence of discrete and expanded mast cell populations in SM by flow cytometric analysis in 75 patients with systemic mastocytosis and 124 patients negative for systemic mastocytosis, demonstrated that the populations of mast cells in cases of systemic mastocytosis showed significantly lower coefficients of variation for side scatter and CD117 compared with the populations of mast cells in cases negative for systemic mastocytosis (46.1% vs 61.0%, $P<.0001$, and 64.5% vs 80.5%, $P<.0001$, respectively, **Fig. 3**). These discrete and expanded mast cell populations with lower coefficients of variation for side scatter and CD117 were also noted in SM cases that were negative for CD25 and/or CD2.[27] In addition, the presence of discrete clusters of mast cells was independent of the number of events within the mast cell gate. Based on these findings, cases of SM and bone marrow specimens negative for SM were analyzed using FLOCK (FLOw Clustering without K) cluster analysis, a computational approach to identify cell subsets in multidimensional flow cytometry data in an unbiased, automated fashion. FLOCK analysis identified discrete mast cell populations in most cases of SM but only a minority of non-SM cases (**Fig. 4**).[28] The FLOCK-identified mast cell populations accounted for a statistically significantly increased percentage of total cells on average in SM cases compared with non-SM cases (2.46% vs 0.9%, $P<.0001$) and were diagnostic of SM with a sensitivity of 75%, a specificity of 86%, a positive predictive value of 76%, and a negative predictive value of 85%.[28] ROC analysis of FLOCK data found that relatively large-sized FLOCK-identified mast cell populations were highly specific for SM; populations of at least 0.07% of the total population were 90% specific for SM and populations of at least 0.15% of the total population were 98% specific for SM.[28] In addition, preliminary analysis found that the

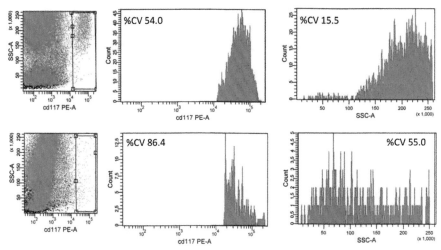

Fig. 3. Gating strategy and identification of coefficient of variation (CV) of CD117 and side scatter. A broad, uniform mast cell gate included all CD117-bright events (*X* axis between 10^4 and 10^5 on the logarithmic scale) and all events on the *Y* axis (SSC-A, linear axis) and followed 2 distribution patterns: discrete cluster formation (*top row*) and scattered events (*bottom row*) within the mast cell gate. The CV of CD117 and side scatter was calculated based on means and standard deviations of histograms generated from events within the mast cell gate.[27] Populations of mast cells in cases of systemic mastocytosis showed significantly lower coefficients of variation for CD117 and side scatter compared with the populations of mast cells in cases negative for systemic mastocytosis (64.5% vs 80.5%, *P*<.0001, and 46.1% vs 61.0%, *P*<.0001, respectively).

relative density of FLOCK-identified mast cell populations was significantly greater in SM cases compared with non-SM cases.[28]

The intensity of expression of CD45 on neoplastic mast cells, as assessed by flow cytometric immunophenotypic analysis, has been demonstrated to detect neoplastic mast cells in combination with CD25.[29] Thirty-one cases of mastocytosis and 71 specimens not involved by mastocytosis were compared, and it was found that bright CD45 expression, defined as greater than 20% of CD117-positive mast cells showing brighter CD45 expression than the average CD45 expression on lymphocytes, was found to have a positive predictive value for systemic mastocytosis of 90%.[29]

CD30 expression by flow cytometric immunophenotypic analysis has also been shown to be a diagnostically useful marker in the assessment of patients with possible mastocytosis. In a cohort of 142 patients with the diagnosis of SM and 21 patients negative for SM, CD30 expression was present in most cases of SM (114 of 132 cases, 80%) and detected in only 1 case that was negative for SM (1 of 21 cases, 4.8%).[7] The WDSM cohort, which was negative for CD2 and CD25, was positive for CD30 in 8 of 9 patients (89%). The levels of CD30 expression were similar in all subgroups of SM, except mast cell leukemia, which was negative for CD30. Additionally, the level of expression of CD30 by bone marrow mast cells was significantly higher in cases of SM than in normal/reactive bone marrow mast cells.[7] These results suggest that CD30 may a useful diagnostic marker to identify neoplastic mast cells, particularly in CD2- and CD25-negative SM cases.[29]

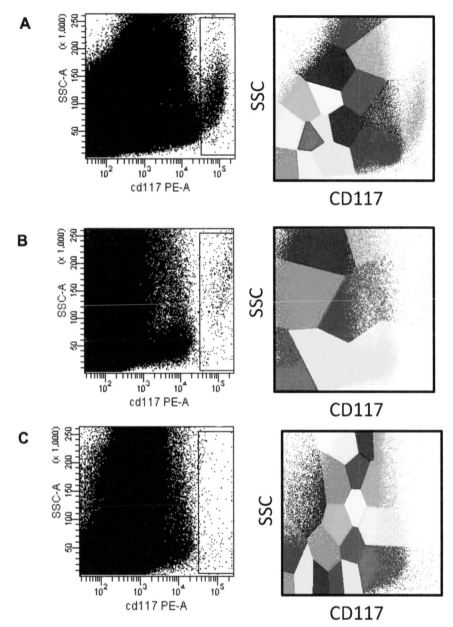

Fig. 4. Representative flow cytometry findings and FLOCK analysis findings in SM and non-SM cases. (*A*) An SM case showing a significant population of cells with event clustering within the broadly defined CD117/SSC mast cell gate by flow cytometric analysis (*left panel*) and with a discrete mast cell population identified by FLOCK analysis (*right panel*). (*B*) An SM case showing a small population of cells with event clustering within the broadly defined CD117/SSC mast cell gate by flow cytometric analysis (*left panel*) and with a discrete mast cell population identified by FLOCK analysis (*right panel*). (*C*) A bone marrow specimen negative for SM showing absence of event clustering within the broadly defined CD117/SSC mast cell gate by flow cytometric analysis (*left panel*) and without a discrete mast cell population identified by FLOCK analysis (*right panel*). *From* Dorfman DM, LaPlante CD, Pozdnyakova O, et al. FLOCK cluster analysis of mast cell event clustering by high-sensitivity flow cytometry predicts systemic mastocytosis. Am J Clin Pathol 2015;144(5):764–70; with permission.)

REFERENCES

1. Akin C. Mast cell activation syndrome: proposed diagnostic criteria. J Allergy Clin Immunol 2010;126(6):1104.e4. Available at: http://www.sciencedirect.com/science/article/pii/S0091674910013333.
2. Metcalfe DD. Mast cells and mastocytosis. Blood 2008;112(4):946–56.
3. Okayama Y, Kawakami T. Development, migration, and survival of mast cells. Immunol Res 2006;34(2):97–115.
4. Arber DA, Orazi A, Hasserjian R, et al. The 2016 revision to the World Health Organization classification of myeloid neoplasms and acute leukemia. Blood 2016; 127(20):2391–405.
5. Swerdlow SH, Campo E, Harris NL, et al. 4th edition. WHO classification of tumours of haematopoietic and lymphoid tissues, vol. 2. Lyon (France): Internat. Agency for Research on Cancer; 2008. 2. print.
6. Sánchez-Muñoz L, Teodosio C, Morgado JMT, et al. Flow cytometry in mastocytosis: utility as a diagnostic and prognostic tool. Immunol Allergy Clin North Am 2014;34(2):297–313.
7. Morgado JM, Perbellini O, Johnson RC, et al. CD30 expression by bone marrow mast cells from different diagnostic variants of systemic mastocytosis. Histopathology 2013;63(6):780–7. Available at: http://onlinelibrary.wiley.com/doi/10.1111/his.12221/abstract. Accessed August 29, 2017.
8. Álvarez-Twose I, Jara-Acevedo M, Morgado JM, et al. Clinical, immunophenotypic, and molecular characteristics of well-differentiated systemic mastocytosis. J Allergy Clin Immunol 2016;137(1):178.e1.
9. Akin C, Escribano L, Nuñez R, et al. Well-differentiated systemic mastocytosis: a new disease variant with mature mast cell phenotype and lack of codon 816 c-kit mutations. J Allergy Clin Immunol 2004;113(2):S327.
10. Akin C, Scott LM, Kocabas CN, et al. Demonstration of an aberrant mast-cell population with clonal markers in a subset of patients with "idiopathic" anaphylaxis. Blood 2007;110(7):2331–3.
11. Iwaki S, Spicka J, Tkaczyk C, et al. Kit- and fc epsilonRI-induced differential phosphorylation of the transmembrane adaptor molecule NTAL/LAB/LAT2 allows flexibility in its scaffolding function in mast cells. Cell Signal 2008;20(1):195–205.
12. Matarraz S, López A, Barrena S, et al. The immunophenotype of different immature, myeloid and B-cell lineage-committed CD34+ hematopoietic cells allows discrimination between normal/reactive and myelodysplastic syndrome precursors. Leukemia 2008;22(6):1175–83.
13. Schernthaner GH, Hauswirth AW, Baghestanian M, et al. Detection of differentiation- and activation-linked cell surface antigens on cultured mast cell progenitors. Allergy 2005;60(10):1248–55.
14. Shimizu Y, Suga T, Maeno T, et al. Detection of tryptase-, chymase+ cells in human CD34 bone marrow progenitors. Clin Exp Allergy 2004;34(11):1719–24.
15. Tedla N, Lee C, Borges L, et al. Differential expression of leukocyte immunoglobulin-like receptors on cord-blood-derived human mast cell progenitors and mature mast cells. J Leukoc Biol 2008;83(2):334–43.
16. Dahl C, Hoffmann HJ, Saito H, et al. Human mast cells express receptors for IL-3, IL-5 and GM-CSF; a partial map of receptors on human mast cells cultured in vitro. Allergy 2004;59(10):1087–96.
17. Yokoi H, Myers A, Matsumoto K, et al. Alteration and acquisition of siglecs during in vitro maturation of CD34+ progenitors into human mast cells. Allergy 2006; 61(6):769–76.

18. Teodosio C, García-Montero AC, Jara-Acevedo M, et al. Mast cells from different molecular and prognostic subtypes of systemic mastocytosis display distinct immunophenotypes. J Allergy Clin Immunol 2010;125(3):726.e4.
19. Orfao A, Escribano L, Villarrubia J, et al. Flow cytometric analysis of mast cells from normal and pathological human bone marrow samples: identification and enumeration. Am J Pathol 1996;149(5):1493–9.
20. Escribano L, Diaz-Agustin B, López A, et al. Immunophenotypic analysis of mast cells in mastocytosis: when and how to do it. proposals of the Spanish network on mastocytosis (REMA). Cytometry B Clin Cytom 2004;58(1):1–8.
21. Escribano L, Diaz-Agustin B, Bellas C, et al. Utility of flow cytometric analysis of mast cells in the diagnosis and classification of adult mastocytosis. Leuk Res 2001;25(7):563–70.
22. Pozdnyakova O, Kondtratiev S, Li B, et al. High-sensitivity flow cytometric analysis for the evaluation of systemic mastocytosis including the identification of a new flow cytometric criterion for bone marrow involvement. Am J Clin Pathol 2012;138(3):416–24.
23. Pardanani A, Kimlinger T, Reeder T, et al. Bone marrow mast cell immunophenotyping in adults with mast cell disease: a prospective study of 33 patients. Leuk Res 2004;28(8):777–83.
24. Jabbar KJ, Medeiros LJ, Wang SA, et al. Flow cytometric immunophenotypic analysis of systemic mastocytosis involving bone marrow. Arch Pathol Lab Med 2014;138(9):1210–4.
25. Morgado JMT, Sanchez-Munoz L, Teodosio CG, et al. Immunophenotyping in systemic mastocytosis diagnosis: 'CD25 positive' alone is more informative than the 'CD25 and/or CD2' WHO criterion. Mod Pathol 2012;25(4):516–21.
26. Cherian S, McCullouch V, Miller V, et al. Expression of CD2 and CD25 on mast cell populations can be seen outside the setting of systemic mastocytosis. Cytometry B Clin Cytom 2016;90B:387–92.
27. Pozdnyakova O, Laplante CD, Li B, et al. High-sensitivity flow cytometric analysis of mast cell clustering in systemic mastocytosis: a quantitative and statistical analysis. Leuk Lymphoma 2015;56(6):1735–41.
28. Dorfman DM, LaPlante CD, Pozdnyakova O, et al. FLOCK cluster analysis of mast cell event clustering by high-sensitivity flow cytometry predicts systemic mastocytosis. Am J Clin Pathol 2015;144(5):764–70.
29. Chisholm KM, Merker JD, Gotlib JR, et al. Mast cells in systemic mastocytosis have distinctly brighter CD45 expression by flow cytometry. Am J Clin Pathol 2015;143(4):527–34.

Flow Cytometry in Pediatric Hematopoietic Malignancies

Jie Li, MD[a,b], Gerald Wertheim, MD, PhD[a,b], Michele Paessler, DO[a],
Vinodh Pillai, MD, PhD[a,b],*

KEYWORDS

- Pediatric flow cytometry • Hematogones • Lymphoblasts • Leukemia • Lymphoma

KEY POINTS

- There are several differences between pediatric and adult hematologic samples that inform the approach and differential diagnosis of hematopoietic neoplasms.
- Hematogones can cause diagnostic difficulty with leukemic blasts on bone marrow aspirate smears or biopsy morphology but can be resolved by flow cytometric evaluation.
- Increasing the use of novel therapies, such as chimeric antigen receptor therapy and newer monoclonal antibodies, raises special issues for the identification of residual and relapsed leukemia.
- Myeloid neoplasms, such as transient myeloproliferative disorder of Down syndrome and juvenile myelomonocytic leukemia, are unique to this age group and need incorporation of clinical, laboratory, and cytogenetic findings in addition to flow cytometry.

INTRODUCTION

There is significant overlap between pediatric and adult hematopoietic malignancies, but there are several differences that are relevant while approaching pediatric cases. B lymphoblastic leukemia, Burkitt lymphoma, primary mediastinal large B-cell lymphoma, and diffuse large B-cell lymphoma (DLBCL) constitute most cases. Acute myeloid leukemia (AML) and myelodysplastic syndrome are less frequent compared with the adult population. Minimal residual disease (MRD) analysis is widely used in the risk stratification and follow-up of both lymphoblastic and myeloid leukemias. Among the myeloid malignancies, juvenile myelomonocytic leukemia (JMML) and

The authors have nothing to disclose.
[a] Department of Pathology and Laboratory Medicine, Division of Hematopathology, Children's Hospital of Philadelphia, Philadelphia, PA, USA; [b] Department of Pathology and Laboratory Medicine, Hospital of University of Pennsylvania, Perelman School of Medicine, University of Pennsylvania, Philadelphia, PA, USA
* Corresponding author. Department of Pathology and Laboratory Medicine, 34th and Civic Center Boulevard, Philadelphia, PA 19104.
E-mail address: pillaiv1@email.chop.edu

transient myeloproliferative disorder of Down syndrome (TMD) are only encountered in the pediatric age group. Small B-cell lymphomas are typically high in the differential in adult hematopathology but are markedly decreased in the pediatric age group. Marginal zone lymphoma and pediatric-type follicular lymphoma are the only small, mature B-cell lymphomas that are encountered in any frequency. Chronic lymphocytic leukemia, mantle cell lymphoma, and plasma cell neoplasms are essentially nonexistent, though there are rare case reports. There are also differences in samples between pediatric and adult hematopoietic neoplasms. Counterintuitively, pediatric bone marrow and lymph node biopsy samples are generous compared with adult samples because of the use of general anesthesia in the pediatric age group and limited use of interventional radiology-guided biopsies. Bilateral bone marrow biopsies for solid tumors, staging bone marrow biopsies for all neoplasms, and lumbar puncture for cerebrospinal fluid involvement are frequently performed compared with the adult population. There are several non-neoplastic conditions, such as hemophagocytic lymphohistiocytosis, aplastic anemia, and bone marrow failure syndrome, that are frequently encountered in the pediatric age group. However, flow cytometry has a limited role in these disorders and is primarily used to exclude malignancies that are frequently in the differential diagnosis. Flow cytometry is also extensively used in the evaluation of immunodeficiency syndromes and is reviewed separately in this issue.

NORMAL LYMPHOID MATURATION AND ABERRANT B LYMPHOBLASTS

A recurring issue in pediatric flow cytometry is the distinction between normal hematogones and B lymphoblasts. Hematogones refer to normal physiologic lymphoid progenitors in the bone marrow and is a term primarily used by hematopathologists. The term *hematogones* (blood-maker) was first used to describe these cells of uncertain significance in pediatric sternal aspirates.[1] Hematogones correspond to the pro–B cell, pre–B cell, and immature B-cell stages that are more commonly used by immunologists.[2] The number of hematogones is usually 5% of the total bone marrow cells in adult bone marrow specimens.[3] However, many hematogones can be observed in infants and young children, sometimes even constituting 50% of the total cellularity.[1] *Hematogones* as a term refers to the earliest, intermediate, and late stage of maturing B cells referred to as stage I, stage II, and stage III hematogones, respectively (**Fig. 1**A). Stage I hematogones are large cells with dispersed chromatin, nucleoli, scant cytoplasm, and a high nuclear/cytoplasmic (N:C) ratio and resemble lymphoblasts. Stage III hematogones resemble small mature lymphocytes but with a higher N:C ratio and immature chromatin and can be seen in the circulation in very young children. Stage II hematogones have an appearance that is intermediate between the two. Hematogones resemble mature lymphocytes in bone marrow biopsies and may sometimes be confused morphologically with immature erythroid cells on hematoxylin-eosin–stained sections and may be better appreciated with a periodic acid–Schiff stain. The various stages of maturation cannot be reliably discerned on biopsies.

The high percentage of hematogones that can occur in normal pediatric marrows and the fact that leukemic B lymphoblasts may be difficult to distinguish from hematogones by morphology can complicate the microscopic diagnosis of acute lymphoblastic leukemia. Fortunately, hematogones have distinct flow cytometric characteristics that greatly aid in this distinction.[3,4] The best initial parameters for evaluating all the hematogones is CD45 versus side scatter (SSC) gate (see **Fig. 1**B). All 3 of the hematogone populations have a low side scatter but progressively increasing CD45 expression, and cell numbers typically increase as maturation progresses.

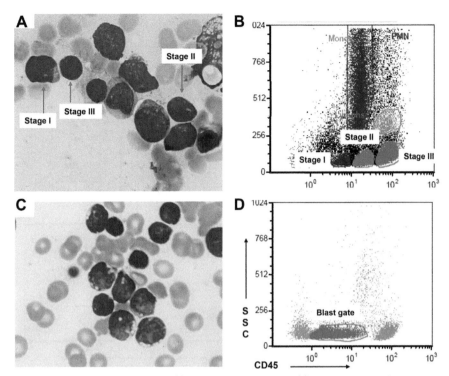

Fig. 1. Characteristic appearance of hematogones on stained bone marrow aspirate smears (Wright Giemsa, original magnification ×500) and flow cytometric dot plots compared with B lymphoblasts (Giemsa). (*A*) Morphologic appearance of various stages of hematogones. (*B*) CD45 versus SSC dot plot shows position of stage I, II, and III hematogones. (*C*) Variably sized B lymphoblasts with cytoplasmic vacuoles. (*D*) Typical CD45 versus SSC dot plot shows a large population of CD45 dim variable B lymphoblasts.

These properties impart a "ducks-in-a-row" pattern. By contrast, leukemic B lympho-blasts (see **Fig. 1**C) typically show lower CD45 expression (see **Fig. 1**D) and occasion-ally increased side scatter (particularly if blasts have vacuoles). Additional flow cytometric markers can aid in hematogone evaluation. Stage I hematogones (**Fig. 2**A) express CD34, dim CD19, bright CD38, and bright CD10, with a low level of CD22 expression and lack of CD20 expression. Stage II hematogones (see **Fig. 2**B) usually show decreased level of CD10 with slightly increased level of CD20 and CD22, and lack CD34 compared to stage II hematogones. Stage III hematogones (see **Fig. 2**C) lose CD10 expression variably and have bright CD20 and CD22 expres-sion. CD38 and CD58 are uniformly expressed by all stages (with minor variations) and are very useful in identifying all stages of hematogones. Mature B cells are negative for CD10. A CD10 versus CD20 plot of all the stages of hematogones shows the "inverted S" pattern, with CD10-postive CD20-early hematogones, CD20-positive CD10-mature B cells, and cells undergoing this phenotypic maturation with variable expres-sion of both. Surface expression of kappa and lambda light chains is negative in stage I and II but is positive in stage III hematogones. Stage III hematogones can show CD5 expression, which may be associated with atopic conditions and does not necessarily indicate a CD5-positive hematologic neoplasm.

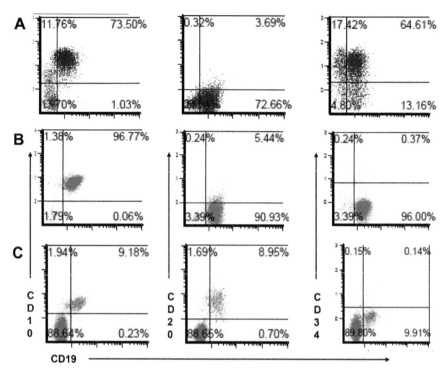

Fig. 2. Expression of CD19, CD10, CD20, and CD34 in normal hematogones. (*A*) The earliest stage I hematogones (*blue*) are CD10 bright, CD19 positive, CD34 positive, and CD20 negative. (*B, C*) As they mature (stage II *colored teal* and stage III *colored green*), they start losing CD10 (dimmer) and CD34 and gaining CD20. Mature B cells lose CD10 and are not prominent here.

Leukemic B lymphoblasts show aberrant phenotypic expression if carefully compared with the baseline expression of normal hematogones. Aberrant expression (underexpression or overexpression) of CD45, CD10, and CD38 is frequently noted in leukemic B lymphoblasts (**Fig. 3**). Discordant expression of antigens may also be seen. For example, expression of CD20 (along with CD34) is never physiologically seen with CD45 levels equivalent to stage I hematogones and would strongly suggest malignancy. Aberrant myeloid antigen expression, such as CD13, CD15, or CD33 on lymphoblasts, can be observed in up to 80% of B-cell acute lymphoblastic leukemia (B-ALL) cases[3] and occasionally suggests specific genetic alterations (see later discussion). Other useful features include lack of normal maturation as the CD45 expression increases. Because the fluorescence intensity associated with various antigens can vary depending on the fluorochrome used, one must be familiar with normal patterns in specific flow panels. Comparison of potential leukemic cases with flow cytometry studies recently performed on cases with normal hematogones helps resolve many difficult cases. Usually the immunophenotype does not change in the short time span after diagnosis when residual disease is measured. Although the immunophenotype can change slightly in later relapses, it would still be extremely unusual for multiple antigens to be significantly different. These concepts also form the basis of MRD detection in lymphoblastic leukemia.[5] In addition, MRD flow cytometric studies collect 500,000 to 1 million total events compared with 20,000 to 50,000 total events

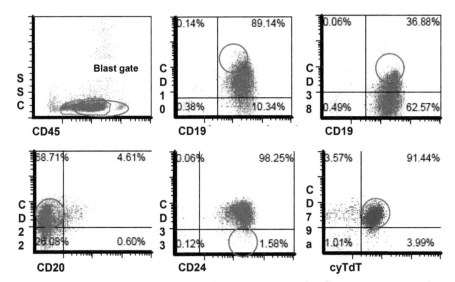

Fig. 3. Distinction of B lymphoblasts from hematogones. Further flow cytometric data from the B-lymphoblastic leukemia shown in **Fig. 1**B. A large CD45dim population with multiple aberrancies compared with normal hematogones, such as dim CD10 and dim CD38 and CD33 expression. The red circles indicate the position of normal stage I hematogones for comparison. cyTDT, cytoplasmic TDT.

collected in routine flow cytometric studies. MRD detection in B-lymphoblastic leukemia is discussed separately in this issue (see Andreas Boldt and colleagues article, "Flow Cytometric Evaluation of Primary Immunodeficiencies").

Other frequently used antigens in flow panels, such as CD9, CD24, and HLA-D related (HLA-DR), are not critical for the distinction from hematogones but correlate with common cytogenetic abnormalities in lymphoblastic leukemia (**Fig. 4**). CD10 and CD24 are frequently lost in MLL-rearranged lymphoblastic leukemia.[6,7] CD9 loss (subset or whole), bright CD10 expression, and aberrant myeloid antigen expression are associated with ETV6-RUNX1 rearrangements.[6] B-ALL with t(1:19) frequently shows a more mature phenotype with loss of CD34 and dim or subset expression of CD20.[8] Aberrant expression of myeloid antigens is frequently seen in association with BCR-ABL1 and, as mentioned, ETV6-RUNX1–rearranged lymphoblastic leukemias. Antigenic aberrancies in the provisional category of Ph-like lymphoblastic leukemias have not been well studied but show CD10 loss in the authors' experience. However, a subset of Ph-like B-ALL cases harbors translocations that lead to overexpression of the cell surface protein CRLF2; flow cytometry can be used to identify these cases.

CIRCULATING AND TISSUE HEMATOGONES

Although all stages of hematogones are predominantly found in the bone marrow, stage III hematogones are frequently seen in the peripheral blood of infants, especially premature infants. These cells could raise the possibility of leukemia, especially in the setting of cytopenias that frequently occur in premature infants for various non-neoplastic reasons, such as infections and prematurity. Many of these circulating cells in infants have an immature appearance with distinct nucleoli, larger size, and slightly immature chromatin (often referred to as baby lymphs). Flow cytometry of these normal circulating cells (**Fig. 5**) reveals that they have polytypic immunoglobulin light

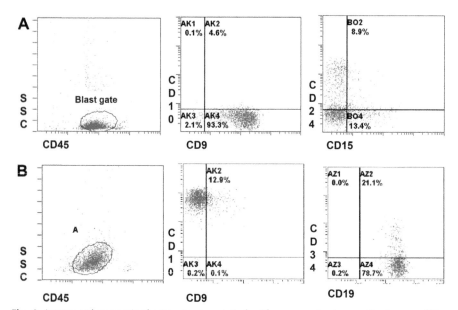

Fig. 4. Immunophenotypic aberrancies associated with recurrent cytogenetic abnormalities. (*A*) KMT2A/MLL-rearranged B-lymphoblastic leukemia with loss of CD10 and CD24. (*B*) B-lymphoblastic leukemia with ETV6-RUNX1 translocation showing loss of CD9.

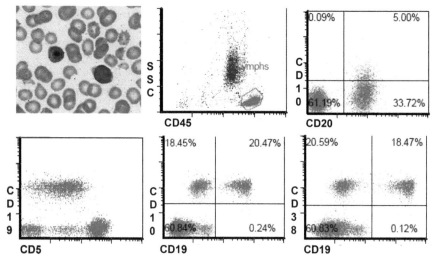

Fig. 5. Circulating stage III hematogones in premature infant with multi-lineage cytopenias. Peripheral smear (Wright Giemsa, original magnification ×500) shows immature lymphoid cell (and nucleated erythroid). Peripheral flow cytometry shows mature CD45 bright lymphocytes that are polytypic for kappa and lambda immunoglobulin light chains and show dim CD5 expression and dim subset expression of CD10. No aberrant blast population was noted in the CD45dim region, and follow-up was uneventful.

chain expression with variable expression of CD10 and CD5 may be dimly present. Dim CD5 expression is seen in normal circulating stage III hematogones and some mature B cells but not seen in earlier stages of hematogones.[9] Terminal deoxy transferase (TdT)-positive cells are also frequently found in tissue pediatric lymph node and tonsil specimens.[10] Double immunohistochemical stains have showed that these are positive for CD79a and CD10 as well, consistent with hematogones. Clusters and loose aggregates can be noted that are not larger than 2 to 5 cells. Large aggregates or sheets of cells should raise the suspicion of leukemia.

HEMATOGONE HYPERPLASIA

Hematogone hyperplasia is defined arbitrarily as greater than 5% of the cellularity for adult marrows.[1] There is no such number for pediatric marrows, because hematogones can comprise most cellular elements in infants and young children. Many hematogones have been associated with chemotherapy or stem cell transplant, viral infections, and autoimmune disorders.[11] The authors frequently detect increased hematogones in the setting of chimeric antigen therapy after the loss of chimeric cells targeting CD19. Hematogones are usually scattered and in loose aggregates on bone marrow biopsies when evaluated by immunostains. Immunostains will reveal that CD19 stains the highest numbers of these cells followed by TdT and much less by CD34. It is important to note that hematogone hyperplasia involves stage II or stage III hematogones and never stage I hematogones. Hence, clusters or focal increase in CD34-positive cells (which are only expressed in stage I hematogones) are not seen in hematogone hyperplasia. Clusters containing more than 5 CD34-positive cells without intervening negative cells have been associated with impending relapse of lymphoblastic leukemia.[12] It is not unusual to see increased TdT positivity or loose clustering in hematogone hyperplasia because of its expression in stage II hematogones and should not be relied on for suspicion of lymphoma.

ANTIGEN LOSS WITH NOVEL TARGETED THERAPIES

Second- and third-generation monoclonal antibodies and chimeric antigen receptor T (CART) cells are increasingly being used in the treatment of relapsed/refractory B-lymphoblastic leukemia.[13,14] However, they raise special issues for identifying both normal hematogones and recurrent B lymphoblasts.[15] Among the chimeric antigen therapies, CD19 is the most common target. Blinatumomab, a bispecific T-cell engager antibody against CD19/CD3, is the most frequently used monoclonal antibody. CD19 is expressed by virtually all B-lymphoblastic leukemias, though there are rare cases of de-novo CD19-negative B-ALL that are associated with lytic lesions, hypercalcemia, and an aleukemic presentation.[16] There are de novo leukemias that are dim for CD19 expression. However, it is not clear whether levels of CD19 expression strictly correlate with response to CD19-targeted therapy. Presence of a substantial population of CD19-negative cells due to prior CD19 therapy is an indication that patients may be more susceptible to a CD19-negative relapse. CD19 is best assessed by bright fluorochromes so that weak CD19 expression can be distinguished from true negatives. Chimeric T cells targeting CD19 are derived from patients' T cells. They are usually infused once or twice at the beginning of therapy. A preinfusion chemotherapy regimen of cyclophosphamide and fludarabine minimizes leukemia (and consequently cytokine storm) while maximizing T-cell engraftment.[17] Chimeric antigen therapy rapidly kills CD19-expressing B lymphoblasts and induces B-cell aplasia. B-cell aplasia is followed by flow cytometric quantification of circulating CD19-positive B cells in peripheral blood. B-cell aplasia persists for 3 to 6 months before normal

CD19-positive B cells return. Patients are typically followed every few months for a year. In the early stages after chimeric antigen therapy, an unusual CD19-negative hematogone population is noted by flow cytometry and immunostains that can some-times be interpreted as CD19-negative B-lymphoblastic leukemia, especially in MRD studies. These CD19-negative cells that are positive for CD79a, PAX-5, and CD34 by immunohistochemistry are not prominent normally and seem to be expanded under CART-19 treatment pressure. By flow, there seems to be 2 CD19-negative progenitor populations that are present even in individuals who have not been treated with tar-geted therapy.[15] One population shows low CD22, bright CD34, and decreased CD38 and is negative for CD10, whereas the other expressed brighter CD22, CD38, and CD34 and dim CD10. There is no maturation of normal B cells beyond these early stages if there are persisting CART-19 cells. CD19-positive normal hematogones re-turn 6 months after CART-19 infusion if there is loss of CART-19 cells and there no further infusions. Although early relapses (<1 month) after CART-19 therapy is due to ineffective expansion or function of CART-19 cells, later relapses in the presence of CART-19 expansion is due to abnormalities of CD19 expression. Abnormalities in CD19 are attributed to various mechanisms and include mutations in the CD19 gene that prevent optimal surface expression or expression of alternate isoforms.[18–20] These B lymphoblasts are usually identical to patients' pre-CART lymphoblasts except for diminished surface CD19 expression (**Fig. 6**). Hence, comparison with prior flow immunophenotype is very useful in identifying relapsed disease. A CD22- and CD24-based approach is useful for detecting MRD level disease.[15] CD66 is helpful in excluding myeloid cells that are positive for CD24. MRD assessment can detect relapsed CD19-negative cells earlier than routine flow cytometry and is recommended for monitoring relapse. Immunostains on bone marrow biopsies can be misleading because they stain for cytoplasmic and membranous CD19. Hence, it is important to look for surface CD19 expression specifically by flow cytometry, which is more pre-dictive of a lack of response to CART-19 therapy. CART-19 treatment pressure can induce a phenotypic switch in some B-lymphoblastic leukemias. MLL-rearranged leu-kemias can relapse as a CD19-negative myeloperoxidase (MPO)-expressing acute

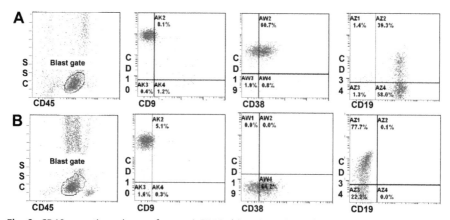

Fig. 6. CD19-negative relapse after anti-CD19 chimeric antigen therapy. Panel (*A*) shows the immunophenotype before therapy. B lymphoblasts (blast gate) are aberrantly CD10 bright, CD9 negative, CD38dim, and CD34 (subset) positive. Panel (*B*) shows the immunophenotype after therapy. The immunophenotype is essentially similar with the same aberrancies except for loss of surface CD19.

myelomonocytic leukemia after chimeric antigen or blinatumomab therapy and are treated as AML.[21,22] It can occur as early as 1 month after therapy. It is, therefore, important to perform a complete flow cytometric evaluation with MPO and multiple myeloid markers in patients who relapse after CD19-directed therapy.

CD22 is a leading target for both chimeric antigen receptor cells and for monoclonal antibodies, such as inotuzumab ozogamicin and moxetumomab pasudotox, because it is expressed by a high proportion of B-lymphoblastic leukemias.[23] Lymphoblastic leukemias with MLL rearrangements have a lower site density of CD22 compared with other leukemias. Interestingly, CD22 levels do not seem to strictly correlate with response to therapy. Also, loss of CD22 was not seen in patients treated with anti-CD22 therapy, though some relapses show dim CD22 expression on B lymphoblasts.

MYELOID NEOPLASMS

The myeloid neoplasms unique to the pediatric age group includes TMD, myeloid leukemia of Down syndrome, and juvenile myelomonocytic leukemia. TMD or transient abnormal myelopoiesis usually resembles megakaryocytic leukemia. TMD affects 5% to 10% of infants with Down syndrome and usually presents in the first few days of life. TMD resolves spontaneously, but 20% to 30% of patients develop AML in 1 to 3 years.[24] Chemotherapy is recommended when hepatomegaly and life-threatening symptoms occur. Peripheral blood smears show a high white blood cell count with numerous large cells with dispersed chromatin, nucleoli, and basophilic cytoplasm with blebs, consistent with megakaryoblasts (**Fig. 7**). Flow cytometry

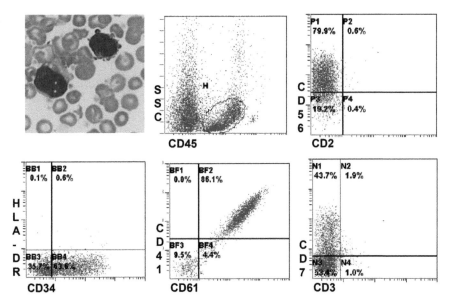

Fig. 7. TMD. A 1 day old with trisomy 21 presented with coagulopathy, multiorgan failure with white blood cell count of 915,000/μL, hemoglobin 10.8 gm/dL, and platelet count of 1,191,000/μL. Peripheral blood smear shows large atypical cells with dispersed chromatin and basophilic cytoplasm with blebbing. Flow cytometry reveals an aberrant population of CD45dim blasts (gated events) that are positive for CD56, CD7, CD34 (*subset*), megakaryocytic markers CD41, CD61, and negative for MPO; HLA-DR consistent with megakaryoblasts.

reveals that the cells are CD45 (negative to dim to moderate) cells that are typically positive for CD7, CD56, CD41, CD61, CD42b, CD33, CD36, and CD38, variably positive for CD34 and HLA-DR, and negative for MPO.[25,26] TMD is indistinguishable from acute megakaryoblastic leukemia (AMKL) by morphology, flow, or routine molecular studies. However, AMKL was found more likely to express CD13 and CD11b compared with TMD.[25] GATA1 mutations are noted in 100% of both TMD and AMKL.[27] Down syndrome AMKL blasts were found more likely to express CD7 and CD11b compared with adult AMKL and pediatric non-Down syndrome AMKL.[28] Down syndrome AMKL was also found more likely to express CD13, CD33, and CD36 compared with pediatric non-Down syndrome AMKL.

JMML is a myeloproliferative/myelodysplastic neoplasm occurring in 1- to 3-year-old children. Patients typically present with monocytosis, anemia, and hepatosplenomegaly. Peripheral smear examination reveals atypical monocytes and sometimes dysplastic granulocytes. Flow cytometric analysis reveals an increased mature monocytic population that may show aberrant expression of myelomonocytic antigens (**Fig. 8**). There are limited immunophenotypic studies of monocytic populations in JMML and chronic myelomonocytic leukemia (CMML) in the literature. Abnormalities of myelomonocytic maturation and aberrancies of CD14, CD13, CD33, CD15, CD64, CD56, and CD7 have been noted, though none are specific for the entities and are shared by AML and myelodysplastic syndrome.[29,30] Although CD56 can be aberrantly expressed in some reactive monocytes, myelomonocytic neoplasms had 2 or more immunophenotypic abnormalities.[31] Viral infections and autoimmune diseases can cause monocytosis that can be difficult to distinguish from neoplastic monocytosis.

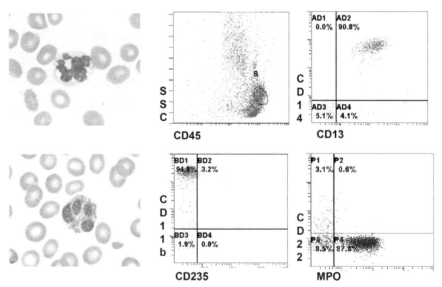

Fig. 8. Juvenile myelomonocytic syndrome. A 13 month old presented with malaise, difficulty walking, and vomiting. Complete blood count reveals a white blood cell count of 34,500/μL with 34% monocytes, hemoglobin 2.6 g/dL, and platelet 126,000/μL. Clinical examination revealed hepatosplenomegaly. Bone marrow aspirate showed atypical monocytes and granulocytes that were also noted in the peripheral blood (Wright Giemsa, original magnification ×1000). Flow cytometric analysis performed on the bone marrow aspirate did not reveal an increased CD45dim blast population but showed an atypical CD14 bright positive monocytic population (gated) that aberrantly expressed bright CD11b and MPO.

Quantification of the CD14-positive CD16-classic monocyte subset distinguished CMML (>94% of total monocytes) from reactive monocytosis and other hematologic malignancies, which had a lower fraction of this subset.[32] It remains to be seen whether a similar assay can be used in the diagnosis of JMML as well. Mutations in NRAS, KRAS, PTPN11, CBL, NF1, and monosomy 7 are present in most patients with JMML; hence, incorporation of cytogenetic and molecular findings is frequently necessary for the diagnosis. Mutations in genes involved in chromatin modification, RAS pathway, DNA methylation can occur in JMML, CMML and MDS. However, mutations in spliceosome genes are rare in JMML compared to CMML and MDS.[33,34]

AML is in the differential diagnosis of atypical monocytosis. Assessment of blasts, monoblasts, and promonocytes is primarily defined by morphology on aspirate; flow cytometry has a limited role in that distinction. It is especially important to rule out AML with inv(16)(p13.1q22) or t(16;16)(p13.1;q22);CBFB-MYH11, which can present with atypical monocytes in the peripheral blood and abnormally granulated eosinophils in the bone marrow.

AML is uncommon compared with acute lymphoblastic leukemia in the pediatric age group and is certainly less common in children compared with adults. Interestingly, the frequency of specific genetically defined subtypes of AML show a distinct distribution in different age groups. Infants with AML have a high frequency of KMT2A translocations, whereas AML in young children shows a higher frequency of RUNX1-RUNX1T1 or MYH11-CBFB fusions relative to adults.

As with B-ALL, antigen expression frequently correlates with chromosomal alterations and can be used to guide further genetic studies. For instance, KMT2A-translocated inv16, t(16:16) and t(8:16) AML typically shows monocytic marker expression; a monoblastic flow cytometric pattern should prompt fluorescence in situ hybridization analysis for those genes. Other genotypic-immunophenotypic correlations include AML with RUNX1-RUNX1T1 fusions associating with expression of B-lymphoid antigens and acute promyelocytic leukemia with PML exon 3 fusions displaying CD2 expression.

An important use of flow cytometry in patients with pediatric AML involves detection of MRD during therapy. Studies have shown that MRD measured by multiparameter flow cytometry is an independent poor prognostic factor in children with AML.[35] The main difficulty with MRD flow involves distinguishing leukemic blasts from regenerating myeloid blasts in normal hematopoiesis. Several groups have identified common leukemia-associated immunophenotypes that may aid in this distinction. These immunophenotypes are not typically seen physiologically and include lineage infidelity (eg, expression of lymphoid markers, such as CD19 or CD7 on myeloid blasts), aberrant antigen levels (eg, bright or dim CD13 or CD33), or antigen dyssynchrony (eg, coexpression of CD34 and CD15). Determination of normal and abnormal antigen expression patterns requires extensive testing of control samples, reproducible determination of antigen levels, and interpretive expertise. MRD analysis in AML is discussed separately in this issue (see Jie Xu and colleagues article, "How Do We Use Multicolor Flow Cytometry to Detect Minimal Residual Disease in Acute Myeloid Leukemia?").

MATURE B-CELL NEOPLASMS IN PEDIATRIC PATIENTS

Reactive lymph nodes and tonsils are frequently excised in the pediatric age group for various reasons. A touch preparation and/or frozen section triage help in limiting flow cytometric evaluation to cases whereby leukemia or lymphoma is suspected. Reactive lymph nodes and tonsils usually show polytypic immunoglobulin light chain expression, but light chain bias can be noted in some cases of exuberant reactive hyperplasia. Hodgkin lymphoma can show an increased CD4:CD8 ratio. Flow cytometry is more useful in detecting clonal populations in DLBCL and Burkitt lymphoma but can sometimes be negative in DLBCL. Routine flow cytometry usually does not detect clonal populations in primary mediastinal large B-cell lymphoma, nodular lymphocyte-predominant Hodgkin lymphoma, and classic Hodgkin lymphoma. Pediatric-type follicular lymphoma shows light chain restricted populations, but these may be difficult to discern when neoplastic cells are present in a reactive background. Hence, additional studies to rule out clonality (ie, immunoglobulin light chain gene rearrangement molecular studies) may be required when flow cytometry is negative, yet morphologic suspicion is high. Post-transplant lymphoproliferative disorders are noted in setting of solid organ transplants for congenital abnormalities. The criteria for evaluation of those disorders are similar to those used in adults.

T-LYMPHOBLASTIC LEUKEMIA/LYMPHOMA VERSUS THYMOCYTES

Lymphoblastic leukemia, Hodgkin lymphoma, primary mediastinal large B-cell lymphoma, and thymic lesions can all present with a mediastinal mass. T-lymphoblastic leukemia/lymphoma can present as a rapidly enlarging mediastinal mass with pressure symptoms. Such patients are not candidates for general anesthesia (because of the inability to intubate), and only a limited biopsy may be obtained. Flow cytometric analysis is key in these situations for a rapid definitive diagnosis.[4] T lymphoblasts show low side scatter and dim to negative CD45 and are positive for TdT, CD7, and cytoplasmic CD3. Surface CD3 is usually negative but can be positive. Blasts are frequently CD4 and CD8 double positive or double negative. However, single CD4 or CD8 positivity can be seen in occasional cases. Approximately one-third of cases show CD10 positivity. Other T-cell markers, such as CD2 or CD5, can be lost in the neoplastic cells. In addition to TdT, the other markers that are helpful for the diagnosis include CD99, CD1a, and CD34. The coexpression of myeloid markers, such as CD13 or CD33, or other B-cell markers, such as CD79a, can be seen in subset of cases but should not be called mixed phenotype leukemia unless other criteria for lineage assessment are met.[36] T/myeloid mixed phenotype leukemias are a lot more common that B/T mixed lineage leukemia. Early T-cell precursor (ETP) phenotype acute lymphoblastic leukemia in adolescents and adults has been associated with poorer prognosis in some studies.[37] They are negative for CD1a, CD8, and CD5 (or dim) and have CD34 or other myeloid antigens. CD4 is usually negative and CD7 is positive.[38] Distinction between lymphoblastic lymphoma (B and T) and leukemia is based on bone marrow involvement. Greater than 25% involvement is regarded as leukemia by convention.

T lymphoblasts must be distinguished from thymocytes in thymocyte-rich thymoma or thymic hyperplasia.[39] Thymocytes share immunophenotypic similarities with T-lymphoblastic leukemia/lymphoma cells, such as double CD4 and CD8 positivity and TdT. However, thymocytes show variable surface CD3 expression that is not characteristic of T lymphoblasts. CD4 and CD8 double positive cells may account for most maturing thymocytes; however, cells with heterogeneous expression of CD4 or CD8 are always present. Double-positive thymocytes also lack expression of CD10, CD34, and HLA-DR. Morphologic examination is very helpful if flow is not definitive. Thymic hyperplasia (thymic rebound after chemotherapy) shows normal thymic architecture. Thymoma shows effaced architecture with increased epithelial cells. Type B1 thymomas can be problematic because of the predominance of small lymphocytes; but a P40 or P63 stain highlights the interspersed epithelial elements, and a AE1/AE3 or CK5/6 immunostain highlights the meshwork characteristic of those neoplasms. It is important to note that ectopic thymic tissue can form a cervical mass and could be mistaken for a neoplasm.[40]

REFERENCES

1. Sevilla DW, Colovai AI, Emmons FN, et al. Hematogones: a review and update. Leuk Lymphoma 2010;51:10–9.
2. LeBien TW, Tedder TF. B lymphocytes: how they develop and function. Blood 2008;112:1570–80.
3. McKenna RW, Washington LT, Aquino DB, et al. Immunophenotypic analysis of hematogones (B-lymphocyte precursors) in 662 consecutive bone marrow specimens by 4-color flow cytometry. Blood 2001;98:2498–507.
4. Kroft SH. Role of flow cytometry in pediatric hematopathology. Am J Clin Pathol 2004;122(Suppl):S19–32.
5. Wood BL. Principles of minimal residual disease detection for hematopoietic neoplasms by flow cytometry. Cytometry B Clin Cytom 2016;90:47–53.
6. Gandemer V, Aubry M, Roussel M, et al. CD9 expression can be used to predict childhood TEL/AML1-positive acute lymphoblastic leukemia: proposal for an accelerated diagnostic flowchart. Leuk Res 2010;34:430–7.
7. Schwartz S, Rieder H, Schläger B, et al. Expression of the human homologue of rat NG2 in adult acute lymphoblastic leukemia: close association with MLL rearrangement and a CD10(-)/CD24(-)/CD65s(+)/CD15(+) B-cell phenotype. Leukemia 2003;17:1589–95.
8. Borowitz MJ, Hunger SP, Carroll AJ, et al. Predictability of the t(1;19)(q23;p13) from surface antigen phenotype: implications for screening cases of childhood acute lymphoblastic leukemia for molecular analysis: a Pediatric Oncology Group study. Blood 1993;82:1086–91.
9. Fuda FS, Karandikar NJ, Chen W. Significant CD5 expression on normal stage 3 hematogones and mature B lymphocytes in bone marrow. Am J Clin Pathol 2009; 132:733–7.
10. Onciu M, Lorsbach RB, Henry EC, et al. Terminal deoxynucleotidyl transferase-positive lymphoid cells in reactive lymph nodes from children with malignant tumors: incidence, distribution pattern, and immunophenotype in 26 patients. Am J Clin Pathol 2002;118:248–54.
11. Chantepie SP, Cornet E, Salaun V, et al. Hematogones: an overview. Leuk Res 2013;37:1404–11.
12. Rimsza LM, Viswanatha DS, Winter SS, et al. The presence of CD34+ cell clusters predicts impending relapse in children with acute lymphoblastic leukemia receiving maintenance chemotherapy. Am J Clin Pathol 1998;110:313–20.
13. Jabbour E, O'Brien S, Ravandi F, et al. Monoclonal antibodies in acute lymphoblastic leukemia. Blood 2015;125:4010–6.
14. Maude SL, Frey N, Shaw PA, et al. Chimeric antigen receptor T cells for sustained remissions in leukemia. N Engl J Med 2014;371:1507–17.
15. Cherian S, Miller V, McCullouch V, et al. A novel flow cytometric assay for detection of residual disease in patients with B-lymphoblastic leukemia/lymphoma post anti-CD19 therapy. Cytometry B Clin Cytom 2016. http://dx.doi.org/10.1002/cyto.b.21482.
16. Hussein S, Pinkney K, Jobanputra V, et al. CD19-negative B-lymphoblastic leukemia associated with hypercalcemia, lytic bone lesions and aleukemic presentation. Leuk Lymphoma 2015;56:1533–7.
17. Turtle CJ, Hanafi LA, Berger C, et al. CD19 CAR-T cells of defined CD4+:CD8+ composition in adult B cell ALL patients. J Clin Invest 2016;126:2123–38.

18. Sotillo E, Barrett DM, Black KL, et al. Convergence of acquired mutations and alternative splicing of CD19 enables resistance to CART-19 immunotherapy. Cancer Discov 2015;5:1282–95.

19. PIllai V, Sotillo E, Harrington C, et al. Changes in CD19 localization after CD19-directed chimeric antigen receptor T cell therapy for primary mediastinal large B cell lymphoma. British Journal of Haematology 2015;171(S1):176.

20. Evans AG, Rothberg PG, Burack WR, et al. Evolution to plasmablastic lymphoma evades CD19-directed chimeric antigen receptor T cells. Br J Haematol 2015. http://dx.doi.org/10.1111/bjh.13562.

21. Gardner R, Wu D, Cherian S, et al. Acquisition of a CD19-negative myeloid phenotype allows immune escape of MLL-rearranged B-ALL from CD19 CAR-T-cell therapy. Blood 2016;127:2406–10.

22. Rayes A, McMasters RL, O'Brien MM. Lineage switch in MLL-rearranged infant leukemia following CD19-directed therapy. Pediatr Blood Cancer 2016;63: 1113–5.

23. Shah NN, Stevenson MS, Yuan CM, et al. Characterization of CD22 expression in acute lymphoblastic leukemia. Pediatr Blood Cancer 2015;62:964–9.

24. Gamis AS, Alonzo TA, Gerbing RB, et al. Natural history of transient myeloproliferative disorder clinically diagnosed in Down syndrome neonates: a report from the Children's Oncology Group Study A2971. Blood 2011;118:6752–9 [quiz: 6996].

25. Karandikar NJ, Aquino DB, McKenna RW, et al. Transient myeloproliferative disorder and acute myeloid leukemia in Down syndrome. An immunophenotypic analysis. Am J Clin Pathol 2001;116:204–10.

26. Langebrake C, Creutzig U, Reinhardt D. Immunophenotype of Down syndrome acute myeloid leukemia and transient myeloproliferative disease differs significantly from other diseases with morphologically identical or similar blasts. Klin Padiatr 2005;217:126–34.

27. Hitzler JK, Cheung J, Li Y, et al. GATA1 mutations in transient leukemia and acute megakaryoblastic leukemia of Down syndrome. Blood 2003;101:4301–4.

28. Wang L, Peters JM, Fuda F, et al. Acute megakaryoblastic leukemia associated with trisomy 21 demonstrates a distinct immunophenotype. Cytometry B Clin Cytom 2015;88:244–52.

29. Harrington AM, Schelling LA, Ordobazari A, et al. Immunophenotypes of chronic myelomonocytic leukemia (CMML) subtypes by flow cytometry: a comparison of CMML-1 vs CMML-2, myeloproliferative vs dysplastic, De Novo vs therapy-related, and CMML-specific cytogenetic risk subtypes. Am J Clin Pathol 2016; 146:170–81.

30. Oliveira AF, Tansini A, Vidal DO, et al. Characteristics of the phenotypic abnormalities of bone marrow cells in childhood myelodysplastic syndromes and juvenile myelomonocytic leukemia. Pediatr Blood Cancer 2017;64. http://dx.doi.org/10.1002/pbc.26285.

31. Xu Y, McKenna RW, Karandikar NJ, et al. Flow cytometric analysis of monocytes as a tool for distinguishing chronic myelomonocytic leukemia from reactive monocytosis. Am J Clin Pathol 2005;124:799–806.

32. Selimoglu-Buet D, Wagner-Ballon O, Saada V, et al. Characteristic repartition of monocyte subsets as a diagnostic signature of chronic myelomonocytic leukemia. Blood 2015;125:3618–26.

33. Hirabayashi S, Flotho C, Moetter J, et al. Spliceosomal gene aberrations are rare, coexist with oncogenic mutations, and are unlikely to exert a driver effect in childhood MDS and JMML. Blood 2012;119:e96–9.

34. Stieglitz E, Taylor-Weiner AN, Chang TY, et al. The genomic landscape of juvenile myelomonocytic leukemia. Nat Genet 2015;47:1326–33.
35. Loken MR, Alonzo TA, Pardo L, et al. Residual disease detected by multidimensional flow cytometry signifies high relapse risk in patients with de novo acute myeloid leukemia: a report from Children's Oncology Group. Blood 2012;120: 1581–8.
36. Swerdlow SH, Campo E, Harris NL, et al. WHO classification of tumours of haematopoietic and lymphoid tissues. 4th edition. Lyons (France): IARC; 2008.
37. Jain N, Lamb AV, O'Brien S, et al. Early T-cell precursor acute lymphoblastic leukemia/lymphoma (ETP-ALL/LBL) in adolescents and adults: a high-risk subtype. Blood 2016;127:1863–9.
38. Allen A, Sireci A, Colovai A, et al. Early T-cell precursor leukemia/lymphoma in adults and children. Leuk Res 2013;37:1027–34.
39. Li S, Juco J, Mann KP, et al. Flow cytometry in the differential diagnosis of lymphocyte-rich thymoma from precursor T-cell acute lymphoblastic leukemia/lymphoblastic lymphoma. Am J Clin Pathol 2004;121:268–74.
40. Scott KJ, Schroeder AA, Greinwald JH Jr. Ectopic cervical thymus: an uncommon diagnosis in the evaluation of pediatric neck masses. Arch Otolaryngol Head Neck Surg 2002;128:714–7.

Flow Cytometric Evaluation of Primary Immunodeficiencies

Andreas Boldt, PhD*,1, Michael Bitar, MSc1, Ulrich Sack, MD

KEYWORDS

- Immunodeficiency • Flow cytometry • T-cell defect • B-cell defect
- Immunophenotyping

KEY POINTS

- Flow cytometric procedures allow the detection of abnormalities in peripheral blood of primary immunodeficiency patients.
- In the first step, immunophenotyping of B-, NK-, CD4+, and CD8+ cells, and HLA-DR/CD38 analysis is recommended to differentiate between normal activation and abnormalities in lymphocyte subsets.
- In a second step, a further differentiation of T, B, and/or NK cell subsets is necessary, for example, in common variable immunodeficiency or DiGeorge syndrome.
- As a third step, functional tests are indispensable in many immunodeficiencies, for example, chronic granulomatous disease or hyper immunoglobulin M syndrome.

FLOW CYTOMETRY AND IMMUNODEFICIENCIES

The term immunodeficiency describes the insufficient immune response to potentially harmful antigens. In general, immunodeficiencies can be divided into primary immunodeficiency diseases (PID) and secondary immunodeficiency diseases.

Primary Immunodeficiency Diseases

PIDs are genetic disorders that mostly cause susceptibility to infections and are sometimes associated with autoimmune and malignant diseases.[1] Mutations can affect cells and molecules of the innate (chronic granulomatous disease [CGD]; complement deficiencies; leukocyte adhesion defects) as well as the adaptive immune system (T and/or B cells). Further, PIDs are part of complex inherited

Disclosure Statement: The authors have nothing to disclose.
Medical Faculty, Department of Diagnostics, Institute of Clinical Immunology, University of Leipzig, Johannisallee 30, Leipzig D-04103, Germany
1 Both authors contributed equally.
* Corresponding author.
E-mail address: Andreas.boldt@medizin.uni-leipzig.de

Clin Lab Med 37 (2017) 895–913
http://dx.doi.org/10.1016/j.cll.2017.07.013
0272-2712/17/© 2017 Elsevier Inc. All rights reserved.

labmed.theclinics.com

syndromes. In the Online Mendelian Inheritance in Man (OMIM) database,[2] hundreds of mutations causing immunodeficiencies or diseases associated with immune dysfunctions have been described. In the United States, the incidence of PID is estimated to be around 1:1200.[3] The first signs of an immune dysfunction can be found in children, often in the early childhood, but also in adults; this depends on the underlying defect.[4] In general, the clinical representation can be dominated by infections, tumors, chronic inflammation,[5] or even signs of autoimmunity[6] or allergy,[7] but there are also patients without any symptoms. This difference is caused by immune dysfunctions inducing simultaneously deficient and autoreactive actions.[8,9] Despite clinical diversity, severe and recurrent infections remain the cardinal signs of immunodeficiencies.[10]

According to the International Union of Immunological Societies Primary Immunodeficiency Diseases Classification Committee of the World Health Organization, PID can be classified into the following groups[11]:

1. Immunodeficiencies affecting cellular and humoral immunity;
2. Combined immunodeficiency disease with associated syndromic features;
3. Predominant antibody deficiencies (recurrent bacterial infections);
4. Diseases of immune dysregulation;
5. Congenital defects of phagocyte number, function; or both;
6. Defects in intrinsic and innate immunity;
7. Autoinflammatory disorders;
8. Complement deficiencies; and
9. Phenocopies of PID.

First, a patient suspicious for a primary immunodeficiency should be evaluated by a thorough clinical and family history as along with a physical examination. Owing to the heterogeneity of clinical symptoms caused by immunodeficiencies, clinical awareness remains crucial.[10,12] Specific therapeutic options remain limited to immunoglobulin replacement therapy and stem cell transfer. First approaches with gene therapy and reports about targeted therapies with biologicals are rare. In most cases, treatment is limited to symptomatic therapy as well as the prevention of complications. The first pass laboratory tests include complete blood cell count followed by the testing of more specific immune parameters, including quantitative serum immunoglobulin levels and specific antibody determination.[13,14]

The most appropriate and encompassing screening of the cellular immune system is accomplished by flow cytometry (FCM) for specific subset markers or indicators for functional abnormalities.[15] Today, FCM allows parallel detection of multiple parameters in many individual cells.[16,17] Immunophenotyping of PID provides diagnostic clues for classifying patients and predicting clinical outcome. In addition, the evaluation of intracellular proteins associated with selected PIDs has been proven as a useful diagnostic method.

As a first step, a general cellular overview with simple immunophenotyping of B cells, natural killer (NK), CD4+, CD8+, and double-negative T cells and analysis of HLA-DR/CD38 is recommended to differentiate between normal activation and severe deficiencies of lymphocyte subsets. For example, the general cellular overview is useful to detect the loss of B cells in Brutons disease; CD4+ and CD8+ deficiencies in DiGeorge syndrome (DGS); T, B, and/or NK cell deficiencies in SCID; or greater numbers of double-negative T cells in autoimmune lymphoproliferative syndrome (ALPS). Alternatively, for severe combined immunodeficiencies with absence of T and/or B cells, newborn screening assays are promising[18]; however, these tests commonly miss immunodeficiencies without profound cytopenia.

In most cases, a further differentiation of T, B, and NK subsets is necessary. This is the case in common variable immunodeficiency (CVID), the most common form of PID in adults.[19] CVID is characterized by reduced to absent immunoglobulin levels in peripheral blood.[3] The underlying B-cell defects are still under investigation; nevertheless, only few percent of known cases could be characterized at a molecular level.[20]

Defects of T cells are often severe and less common. Deficiencies of innate immunity such as complement deficiencies are often not considered and are, therefore, not diagnosed.[21]

Besides immunophenotyping, functional tests are indicative for many immunodeficiencies. Intracellular protein phosphorylation is a critical step in cellular activation induced by the binding of different ligands to cell surface receptors. This process is initiated by activation of specific protein-tyrosine kinases that are associated with intracellular domains of the respective ligand receptor.[22] One important pathway in this cell activation process involves Janus kinases (JAK) family linked to signal transducer and activator of transcription (STAT) proteins.[23] The JAK-STAT pathway is a membrane to nucleus mechanism for rapid induction of gene expression. Independent of the particular cell functions affected in immunodeficiencies, the JAK-STAT pathway remains a central player in all of the key cells, ranging from CD4 helper cell subsets to alternatively activated macrophages.[24]

Herein, we describe exemplary laboratory findings in patients with secondary immunodeficiencies (**Figs. 1** and **2**) and PID patients suffering from Bruton's disease (X-linked agammaglobulinemia [XLA]; **Fig. 3**), CVID (**Fig. 4**), hyper-IgM syndrome (**Fig. 5**), ALPS (**Fig. 6**), DGS (**Fig. 7**), CGD (**Fig. 8**), CINCA syndrome (**Fig. 9**), MECP2-duplication syndrome (**Fig. 10**), ataxia teleangiectasia,[25] immune dysregulation, polyendocrinopathy, enteropathy, X-linked inheritance (IPEX) syndrome,[26] and STAT1/STAT3 mutations.[27]

Secondary Immunodeficiency Diseases

In contrast with PIDs with genetic disorders resulting in infections, secondary immunodeficiencies are caused by infections, tumors, irradiation, compounds interacting with pathways relevant for immune functions, and even by lifestyle, mental diseases, nutrition, aging, and others.[28] With the increasing use of biologicals and novel immunotherapeutics, the frequency of immunodeficiencies induced by therapeutic intervention increases again. Thus, iatrogenic immunosuppression is a relevant indication for cellular phenotyping and to check the immune function today. A well-known example is the analysis of antigen-specific memory T cells after previous infection by *Mycobacterium tuberculosis* that can be suppressed under

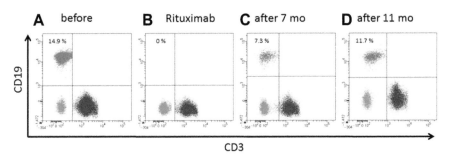

Fig. 1. Exemplary flow cytometric monitoring of B-cell numbers before (*A*) and after (*B*) Rituximab treatment (male, 13 years old) and the process of normalization (*C*, *D*).

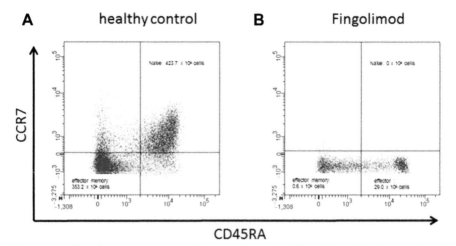

Fig. 2. Exemplary flow cytometric monitoring of naïve T-cell numbers after (*B*) Fingolimod treatment (female, 44 years old) compared with a healthy control (*A*). Staining with CD45RA and CCR7 was used to separate naive (CD45RA$^+$ CCR7$^+$) from effector memory cells (CD45RA$^-$CCR7$^-$) and effector cells (CD45$^+$ CCR7$^-$).

anti-tumor necrosis factor therapies, causing reactivation of tuberculosis.[29] Antibody therapies, which are targeted at cellular components, cause complete or partial deficiencies of specific lymphocyte subsets. For example, the treatment of an anti-CD20 antibody (rituximab) induces the loss of all peripheral B cells (see **Fig. 1**), while a sphingosin-1-phosphat-analogon (fingolimod) dramatically reduces naïve T and B cells in the periphery, by inhibiting lymphocyte traffic outside the lymph nodes (**Fig. 2**). In both cases, a flow cytometric monitoring of the target cells before and after drug treatment is necessary to monitor immune function under therapy.

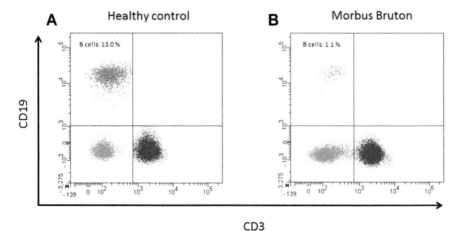

Fig. 3. Exemplary flow cytometric B-cell analysis (*red population*) of a Morbus Bruton patient (*B*) (male, 74 years old) compared with healthy control (*A*). Staining with CD19 and CD3 were used to separate B cells (CD19$^+$) from T cells (CD3$^+$) and others (CD3$^-$CD19$^-$).

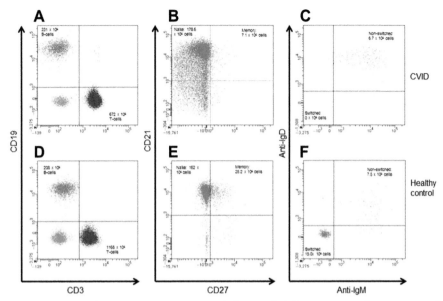

Fig. 4. Exemplary flow cytometric analysis of the B-cell differentiation of a patient with common variable immunodeficiency (CVID; *A–C*; female, 25 years old) compared with a healthy control (*D–F*). The B cells were separated by CD19/CD3 staining (*A, D*). Naïve cells and memory cells were identified by CD21/CD27 staining (*B, E*) and class-switched B cells were double negative for IgM/IgD marker staining (*C, F*). In the present case, the CVID patient has normal B-cell numbers (*A*), but lower memory cells (*B*) and completely deficient class-switched B cells (*C*).

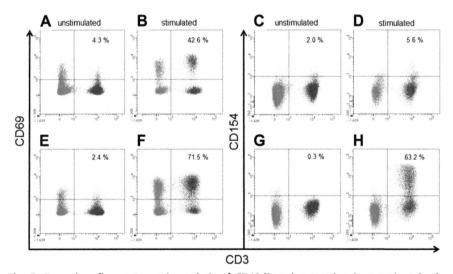

Fig. 5. Exemplary flow cytometric analysis of CD40-ligand expression in a patient (male, 17 years old) with hyper immunoglobulin (IgM) syndrome (*A–D*) compared with a healthy control (*E–H*). Whole blood was stimulated with phorbol myristate acetate (PMA)/ionomycin for 2 hours and stained with CD69 (stimulation control) and CD154. The expression of CD154 was strongly restricted (5.6% of T cells) compared with the healthy control (63.2% of T cells). All data were calculated in relation to the total number of T cells.

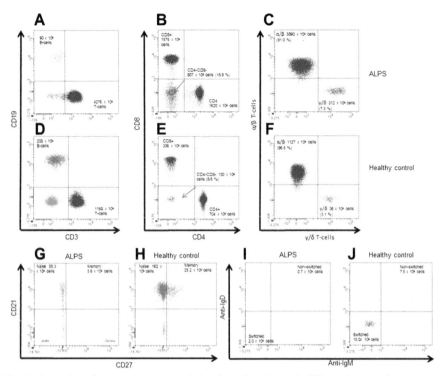

Fig. 6. Exemplary flow cytometric analysis of T-cell and B-cell differentiation of an patient with autoimmune lymphoproliferative syndrome (ALPS; *A–C, G, I*; male, 3 years old) was compared with a healthy control (*D–F, H, J*). In ALPS, there was a normal number of T cells, but the differentiation shows a high amount of CD4⁻CD8⁻ double negative T cells (*B*), which did not correlate with the numbers of γ/δ T cells (*C*). Moreover, B cells (*A*) and the B-cell subgroups naïve/memory cells (*G*) as well as class switched B cells (*I*) were deficient in ALPS.

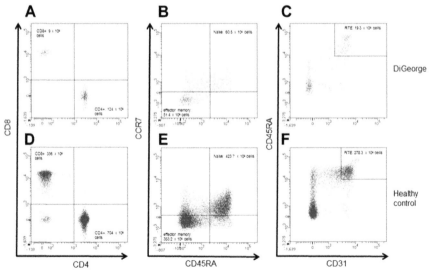

Fig. 7. Exemplary flow cytometric analysis of the T-cell differentiation of a patient (*A–C*; male, 2 years old) with DiGeorge syndrome (*A–C*) compared with a healthy control (*D–F*). The analysis revealed strongly decreased CD4⁺ and CD8⁺ cells (*A*) owing to deficient recent thymic emigrants (*C*), naïve cells, and memory cells (*B*). Memory T cells were defined as CD45RA⁻CCR7⁻, naïve cells were CD45RA⁺ CCR7⁺, and for separating recent thymic emigrants the combination of CD45RA⁺ and CD31⁺ was used.

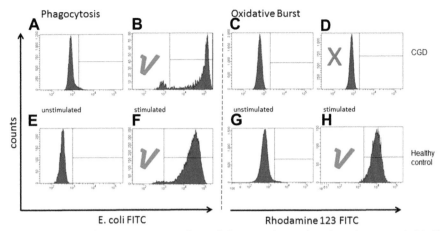

Fig. 8. Exemplary flow cytometric analysis of the granulocyte function phagocytosis (*A, B*) and oxidative burst (*C, D*) in a patient (male, 2 years old) with chronic granulomatous disease (CGD) compared with a healthy control (*E–H*). For analyzing phagocytosis, granulocytes were stimulated with fluorescent *Escherichia coli*. The bacteria will be phagocytosed by the granulocytes resulting in an increase of mean fluorescent intensity (*B, F*). Unstimulated granulocytes were used as negative controls (*A, E*). For analyzing the oxidative burst activity, Di-Rhodamine labeled *E coli* were phagocytosed and intracellularly degraded. In that process, Di-Rhodamine changed to fluorescent Rhodamine 123, resulting in an increase of mean fluorescent intensity of the granulocytes (*H*). Unstimulated granulocytes were used as negative controls (*C, G*). However, in the CGD an increase of mean fluorescent intensity in granulocytes could not be observed typically (*D*), in contrast with normal phagocytosis activity (*B*). FITC, fluorescein isothiocyanate.

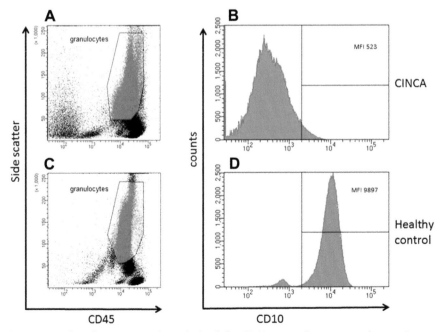

Fig. 9. Exemplary flow cytometric analysis of the CD10 expression on granulocytes in a patient (female, 2 years old) with chronic infantile neurologic cutaneous and articular (CINCA) syndrome (*A, B*) compared with a healthy control (*C, D*).

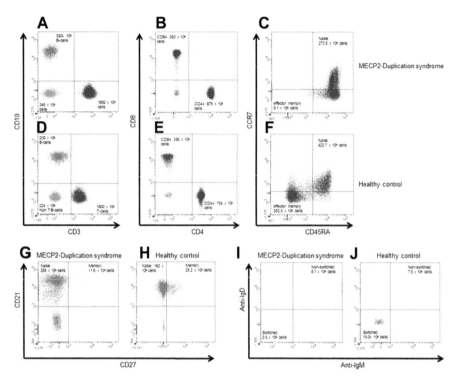

Fig. 10. Exemplary flow cytometric analysis of T-cell and B-cell differentiation of a patient (*A–C, G, I;* male, 2 years old) with MECP2-duplication syndrome compared with a healthy control (*D–F, H, J*). The patient has normal B cells, T cells, and CD4⁺ and CD8⁺ cells (*A, B*), but the differentiation showed strong deficient effector memory T cells (*C*), and memory (*G*) and class switched B cells (*I*).

Defects in B Cells

Agammaglobulinemia: X-linked and autosomal recessive

XLA is based on a defect in the Bruton's tyrosine kinase (Btk) gene, which is responsible for normal development and maturation of B cells. There is also an additional form with an autosomal recessive inheritance.[30] Most patients suffer from symptoms caused by seriously reduced or absent levels of the immunoglobulins (IgG, IgM, and/ or IgA). Despite agammaglobulinemia and a normal number of B lymphocyte precursors, there are very few mature B lymphocytes. By using typical B-cell markers CD19 or CD20, a simple flow cytometric B-cell enumeration is indicative. In **Fig. 3**, a typical example of an XLA patient with extremely low B-cell counts is shown in comparison with a healthy control (**Table 1**). Moreover, the laboratory screening can be refined by evaluating intracellular expression of the Btk protein (Btkp) in monocytes by using FCM. The absence of Btkp is strongly suspicious on XLA. Furthermore, analyzing intracellular Btkp can be useful for investigating X-linked maternal carriers. Along this line, it is common that carriers present 2 populations of monocytes, the first of which expresses normal Btk levels, whereas the second one displays absent Btk expression depending on the random inactivation of either normal or the defective X chromosome.[31] Thus, percentage calculation of Btk⁺ monocytes can be used to detect carriers. Determining the definitive genetic cause needs further genetic testing.[31,32]

Table 1
Immunophenotyping of several primary immunodeficiencies and associated genetic defects

Disease	Genetic Defect	Immunophenotyping
XLA	Mutations in Btk gene	CD19$^+$↓↓↓
HIGM	Mutations in CD40 L (CD154)	CD3$^+$ CD154$^-$↓↓↓
ALPS	Mutations in CD95	CD4$^-$ CD8$^-$↑↑↑ γ/δ CD3$^+$↑↑ CD21$^+$ CD27$^-$↓ CD21$^+$ CD27$^+$ IgM$^-$ IgD$^-$↓
CVID	Unknown	CD19$^+$ CD27$^+$ IgM$^-$IgD$^-$↓↓↓
DiGeorge syndrome	22q11.2 deletion	CD4$^+$ CD45RA$^+$ CCR7$^+$↓↓ CD4$^+$ CD45RA$^-$ CCR7$^-$↓↓ CD4$^+$ CD45RA$^+$ CD31$^+$↓↓↓
IPEX	Mutations in FOXP3	CD3$^+$ CD4$^+$ CD25$^+$ FOXP3$^+$↓↓
CINCA	Mutations in CIAS1	CD45$^+$ CD10$^+$↓↓↓
MECP2 duplication syndrome	Mutations in *MECP2*	CD3$^+$ CD45RA$^-$ CCR7$^-$↓↓ CD19$^+$ CD21$^+$ CD27$^+$↓↓ CD19$^+$ CD21$^+$ CD27$^+$ IgD$^-$ IgM$^-$↓↓

Abbreviations: ALPS, autoimmune lymphoproliferative syndrome; Btk, Bruton's tyrosine kinase; CINCA, chronic infantile neurologic cutaneous and articular; CVID, common variable immunodeficiency; HIGM, hyper-IgM syndrome; IPEX, immune dysregulation, polyendocrinopathy, enteropathy, X-linked inheritance syndrome; XLA, X-linked agammaglobulinemia.

Common variable immunodeficiency

CVID is a group of PID, particularly in the second and third decades of life. CVID is characterized by low levels of 2 immunoglobulin classes and lacking antibody responses to vaccination.[11]

In the present literature, various panels for phenotyping of B cells for classification of CVID are proposed.[33–35] The immunophenotypic classification schemes Freiburg (2002),[33] Paris (2003),[34] and EUROclass (2008)[35] are based on the analysis of B cells: memory cells, class-switched B cells as well as transitional cells and CD21 low cells. These panels have been published with different reference ranges, probably caused by the use of different antibodies, gating strategies, or other differences between the laboratories. For further differentiation, additional specific markers should be analyzed. For example, increased CD21^{low} B cells were proven as signs for splenomegaly (rare in healthy donors), whereas an expanded population of transitional B cells (CD38^{++} IgM^{++}) has been linked to lymphadenopathy.[33–35]

However, in all schemes the B-cell subset counts, which are the basis for classification, were specified in percentage of total B cells or parts of them. Because of strong variability of B cells and its subgroups, age, medical treatment, or secondary diseases can lead to false-positive or false-negative results. Therefore, for analysis of individuals with CVID, we modified these panels[17] and recommend the additional report of absolute cell numbers. In an example shown here (see **Fig. 4, Table 1**), we found normal B-cell (CD19$^+$) and T-cell (CD3$^+$) counts in both patients and controls, but the switched memory B cells (CD19$^+$ CD27$^+$IgM$^-$IgD$^-$) in CVID patients were absolutely absent (0 × 10^6 cells/µL), as compared with healthy controls (15 × 10^6 cells/µL). Furthermore, FCM can also be used to investigate 3 of the 4 genetic conditions related to CVID, including:

a. Deficiency of the inducible costimulator, which can be detected by a lack of inducible costimulator upregulation on stimulated T cells, associated with absence of memory switched B cells and a reduction of CXCR5+ CD4+ T cells[35–37];

b. CD19 deficiency, characterized by absence of CD19 with presence of other B cell markers including CD20, CD21 and surface IgM[38,39]; and

c. TACI deficiency in CD27+ B cells.[40,41]

Defects in T Cells

Defects in total T-cell numbers

Distinctly reduced numbers of T cells including naïve ones, with or without decreased B-cell and/or NK cell counts, are common in severe combined immunodeficiency (SCID). Based on the underlying mutations and the absence of cell types, SCID can be classified into several forms. Isolated absence of T cells with the presence of B cells and NK cells (T−B+NK+) can be caused by genetic defects in the IL-7 receptor α chain; the T−B+NK− phenotype is frequently caused by defects in the IL-2-R-γ chain or JAK3 mutations (**Tables 1** and **2**). Because of strong cellular abnormalities in SCID, a suitable flow cytometric approach is to analyze T, B, and NK cells by their commonly used lineage markers. For early detection of SCID before clinical symptoms, newborn screening has been established.[42]

Hyper IgM syndrome

Hyper IgM syndrome (HIGM) is characterized by recurrent bacterial infections and decreased levels of IgG, IgE, and IgA, but normal or elevated IgM. The most frequent type of HIGM is the X-linked HIGM generated by mutations in the CD40 ligand (CD40 L, also CD154) gene.[43] CD40 L is expressed at the surface of activated

---

Table 2
Immunophenotyping characteristics in severe combined immunodeficiency

Phenotype	Gene Defect	OMIM
T-B + NK+	IL-7 R-α- chain	146661
	Protein-tyrosine phosphatase CD45	151460
	CD3 chains	615607, 610163, 186740
	B-cell chronic lymphocytic	15640687
	Leukemia/lymphoma	617237
T-B + NK-	IL-2R-γ (X-linked SCID)	300400
	JAK-3	600802
T-B-NK+	RAG1, RAG2	601457
	Artemis	602450
	DNA-PKcs	600899
T-B-NK-	ADA	267500
	Reticulardysgenesis	—
	MTHFD1	—
CD4-CD8+B + NK+	MHC class II	153390
	p56lck	—
CD4+CD8-B + NK+	CD8-α-chain	608957
	ZAP-70 kinase	176947
	MHC class I expression	604571

Abbreviations: ADA, adenosine deaminase; DNA-PKcs, DANN protein kinase catalytic subunit; IL-2R- γ, interlukin-2 receptor gamma chain; IL-7Rα-chain, interlukin-7 receptor alpha chain; JAK-3, janus kinase 3; MHC, major histocompatibility complex; p56lck, lymphocyte-specific protein-tyrosine kinase; RAG1/2, recombinase-activating genes 1 and 2; ZAP-70kinaseZeta chain associated protein kinase, 70kD.

CD4$^+$ T cells and interacts with CD40 on B cells. Failure of this interaction results in absent activation of B cells, including proliferation, immunoglobulin class switch, and affinity maturation. Surface expression of CD40 L can be measured following ex vivo activation by FCM.

We analyzed CD154 expression on activated T cells in a patient with suspicion of HIGM. We found a strongly reduced CD154 expression on activated T cells compared with a healthy control. Our results correspond with those of Lee and colleagues[44] from 2005 (see **Fig. 5, Table 1**).

Autoimmune lymphoproliferative syndrome

ALPS is a rare PID characterized by the accumulation of lymphocytes and hepatosplenomegaly.[43,45] ALPS is caused by mutations in the protein implicated in the FAS-mediated apoptotic cascade (CD95), only a small group of patients has other mutations, including defects in genes encoding FAS ligand, caspase 10, and caspase 8.[46]

FCM plays an important role in the diagnosis of ALPS, because ALPS patients have a unique phenotypic finding required as a diagnostic criterion. Namely, ALPS patients are characterized by increased double-negative T-cell counts (CD3$^+$CD4$^-$CD8$^-$). Commonly, double-negative T cells found in healthy blood express γ/δ T-cell receptors; in ALPS patients, these double-negative T cells express the α/β T-cell receptor. Therefore, the combination of double-negative T cells with coexpression of α/β but not γ/δ T-cell receptor is an important diagnostic tool to confirm or exclude ALPS.

The analysis of other markers could show further typical cellular changes in ALPS, such as elevated CD8$^+$CD57$^+$ T cells, decreased CD3$^+$CD25$^+$ T cells, decreased memory B cells (CD20$^+$CD27$^+$), and an atypical expression of CD45 and B220 on CD4$^-$CD8$^-$ T cells. Hanlon and colleagues[46] reported functional defects in the apoptotic process despite normal expression of CD95 on T cells.

We analyzed and evaluated the immunophenotype of a patient with ALPS by FCM. We could show that double-negative T cells were strongly increased in ALPS, but not the counts of γ/δ T cells. Therefore, we confirmed that these high double negative T-cell counts were a sign of ALPS but not of an infection. Furthermore, B cells (CD19$^+$) were extremely rare. A detailed investigation of the subsets revealed deficient naïve (CD21$^+$CD27$^-$) and memory B cells (CD21$^+$CD27$^+$) in addition to a decreased number of switched B cells (IgM$^-$IgD$^-$; see **Fig. 6, Table 1**). Our results were corresponding with published data (as discussed elsewhere in this article).

Other Well-Defined Syndromes with Immunodeficiency

Wiskott-Aldrich syndrome

Wiskott-Aldrich syndrome (WAS) is an X-linked, recessive immunodeficiency caused by a genetic defect in WAS protein (WASp) gene resulting in reduced or absent expression of the WASp. Clinically, it is characterized by thrombocytopenia, eczema, recurrent infections, and a high risk of lymphoid malignancy and autoimmune disorders.[43,47,48]

FCM analysis of WASp expression in lymphocytes has been reported as a suitable supporting test for the diagnostics of WAS. The authors noted that intracellular WASp was expressed as a distinctly "bright" phenotype on normal lymphocytes and "dim" phenotype on lymphocytes from WAS patients.[49] Moreover, in peripheral blood of WAS-patients phenotypic abnormalities were observed such as decreased CD8$^+$ cells and B cells, reduced frequency of CD21/CD35-expressing B cells, and CD27$^+$ memory B cells, in contrast with increased NK cells.[50]

Additionally, Yamada and colleagues[51] showed that the flow cytometric analysis of monocytes could also discriminate WAS carriers. The authors found that FCM evaluation was simpler and more rapid than molecular methods, but it may be less sensitive to detect carriers with reduced percentage of WASp^{dim} monocytes.

Ataxia telangiectasia

The syndrome of ataxia telangiectasia (AT) is a rare autosomal recessive disorder, which results from a mutation in chromosome 11q22-23 (OMIM 208900). Immunologic findings include variable immune defects of both humoral and cellular immunity. Common laboratory findings are reduced levels of IgE, IgA, and IgG2 subclass, deficient B-cell receptor, impaired ability to form cytotoxic T lymphocytes, and significantly reduced counts of naïve CD4$^+$ and CD8$^+$ T cells.[52] De Stefano and colleagues[25] (2016) investigated a patient with AT and combined immunophenotyping of T and B cells with functional flow cytometric assays. In a patient with AT they could detect very low class-switched memory B cells and increased total numbers of T cells, caused by an extraordinarily high amount of γ/δ T cells (CD3$^+$CD4$^-$CD8$^-$; >75% of T cells). A detailed subset analysis revealed that naïve T cells and recent thymic emigrants (RTEs) were strongly deficient resulting in decreased CD4$^+$/CD8$^+$ T cells. Flow cytometric measurement of proliferation activity revealed an impaired proliferation activity in T cells, in contrast with normal B-cell proliferation after mitogenic stimulation.

For diagnostics of AT, Porcedda and colleagues[53] (2008) developed a flow cytometric method to analyze the phosphorylation of histone H2AX in peripheral blood mononuclear cells after irradiation with 2 Gy. They could show a significantly lower mean fluorescence intensity of phosphorylated histone H2AX in the AT group, compared with normal phosphorylation of histone H2AX in the healthy control group.[53]

Nijmegen breakage syndrome

Nijmegen breakage syndrome (NBS) is a rare autosomal recessive chromosomal instability syndrome caused by mutations in the NBN gene (OMIM 251260). Immunologically, NBS is characterized by recurrent infections, essentially with respiratory tract involvement as a result of defective cellular as well as humoral immune responses.[54]

Most patients with NBS have low total serum gamma globulin levels, especially IgG and IgA, which have been attributed to general lymphopenia, low B-cell counts, and poor T-B cooperation owing to low T helper lymphocyte counts. Detection of NBS by FCM includes immunophenotyping of B-cell populations, which are characterized by a decreased number of CD19$^+$ cells. Furthermore, low relative and absolute counts of memory (IgD$^-$ CD27$^+$) and naïve (IgD$^+$ CD27$^-$) B cells are related to a significant increase in the natural effector (IgD$^+$ CD27$^+$) B cells.[55]

Piatosa and colleagues[55] studied a group of NBS patients and reported a high proportion of IgM-only memory and a low proportion of IgM-negative cells within CD27$^+$ IgD$^-$ memory B cells. They proposed a class switch recombination defect in these subsets of cells in NBS patients, resulting in insufficient production of immunoglobulins. Because of the low T-cell counts, the T-cell–dependent antigen response is severely defective, connected with a lower frequency of memory B cells. The T-cell–independent B-cell differentiation pathway seems less affected.

DiGeorge syndrome

DGS, also known as chromosome 22q11.2 deletion (del22q11.2) syndrome, is the most common deletion syndrome. Clinically, DGS is characterized by typical facial features, congenital heart defects, diabetic embryopathy, hypocalcemia, immune deficits, and growth and/or developmental retardation.[56,57]

Most cases of DGS patients were classified as partial DGS, which is characterized by a mild to moderate decrease in the T-cell count caused by deficient thymic migration, but with clinical manifestations as described.[56,57] Less than 1% of DGS patients were classified as a complete DGS, without thymic activity and mimicking SCID phenotype.[56,57] Ravkov and colleagues[58] demonstrated that one of the ways to investigate DGS is the detection of RTE cells, namely CD4$^+$ T cells. RTE cells are T cells that have been lately generated in the thymus and exported into circulation. They have reduced proliferation, cytokine production, and transcription factor expression.[58]

The expression of T-cell receptor excision circles (TRECs) is another tool to investigate RTEs.[58] TRECs are created during the T-cell receptor rearrangement within the thymus. Activation and proliferation of cells after migration to secondary lymphoid organs result in diluting TREC copies over time. Naïve T cells that have lately emigrated from the thymus will express moderate to high TREC levels compared with those of aged, stimulated T cells.

Recently, it has been reported that CD31 can be used as a cell surface marker to differentiate CD4$^+$ RTEs (CD4$^+$ CD45RA$^+$ CD31$^+$) with high TRECs content from activated, peripheral, naïve T cells (CD4$^+$).[58] Thus, TREC evaluation (also CD4$^+$CD45RA$^+$ CD31$^+$ T cells by FCM) can be used as a diagnostic confirmation of low thymic output, which would be found in DGS, or to monitor immune reconstitution after bone marrow transplantation.[58] Lima and colleagues[59] studied another marker to identify low thymic output in the 22q11.2 deletion syndrome, measured by CCR9$^+$CD45RA$^+$ T cell counts.

Herein we have presented an exemplary flow cytometric gating strategy to detect T-cell subsets in a DGS patient and in a healthy control. Naïve CD4 T cells (CD45RA$^+$ CCR7$^+$), effector memory cells (CD45RA$^-$ CCR7$^-$), and (CD45RA$^+$ CD31$^+$) RTEs were significantly diminished in DGS compared with healthy controls (see **Fig. 7**, **Table 1**).

Diseases with Immune Dysregulation

Immune dysregulation, polyendocrinopathy, enteropathy, X-linked inheritance syndrome

IPEX syndrome is a rare genetic disease caused by mutations in the forkhead transcription factor FOXP3 (OMIM 300292, 304790). FOXP3 plays an important role in the development and effector function of T-regulatory cells (Treg), which control and suppress immune responses.[43,60]

The patients present with diminished Treg activity and low numbers of circulating Tregs. In flow cytometric analysis, Tregs were typically detected by surface staining of CD4, CD25^{high} (the high-affinity binding subunit of the IL-2 receptor), CD127^{low} (a subunit of the IL-7 receptor), and intracellular staining of FOXP3. However, the presence of FOXP3-positive cells does not exclude IPEX, because a number of mutations have an effect on FOXP3 function, but not on protein stability (see **Table 1**).[43,60]

The importance and complexity of the disease and the benefit of early diagnosis require a simple and rapid screening method, such as the analysis of intracellular FOXP3 expression by FCM. The time between blood collection and measurement should not exceed 36 hours, because of a significant time-dependent spontaneous depletion of FOXP3$^+$ Treg cells. Importantly, the percentage of CD3$^+$ CD4$^+$ CD25$^+$ T cells in the blood of IPEX patients is not decreased making this truncated marker combination inappropriate for IPEX evaluation.[43,60]

X-Linked lymphoproliferative syndrome

X-linked lymphoproliferative (XLP) syndrome is a rare inherited immunodeficiency presenting hypogammaglobulinemia and Epstein-Barr virus–associated lymphomas.[43,61] XLP is a life-threatening primary immunodeficiency. Therefore, a rapid and definitive diagnosis as well as a suitable treatment are very significant for life-saving and improved prognosis for XLP patients. The genetic defect is located on *SH2D1A* gene (XLP1), which encodes the signaling lymphocyte activation molecule–associated protein (SAP). Recently, Rigaud and colleagues[62] described a second causative gene for XLP, the *BIRC4* gene, which encodes the X-linked inhibitor of apoptosis protein (XIAP). Along this line, it seems reasonable to consider that XLP is now divided into 2 different diseases, XLP1 and XLP2.

Deficient expression of SAP and XIAP can be analyzed by intracellular FCM and has been reported as a sensitive screening method for the identification of mutation-positive patients. Furthermore, Marsh and colleagues[63] have described a protocol for intracellular FCM. In brief, upon fixation, lymphocytes were permeabilized and marked with monoclonal anti-SAP or anti-XIAP, and stained for suitable surface markers (CD3$^+$ CD4$^+$, CD8$^+$, CD19$^+$, and CD56$^+$ cells). SAP can be detected in T cells and NK cells, especially after stimulation, compared with clearly decreased or absent SAP expression in XLP1 patients.[64,65]

Moreover, Oliveira and colleagues[43] reported that FCM suitably identifies all patients with mutations in SAP and XIAP. Additionally, very low numbers of invariant NK T cells (CD3$^+$ CD16$^+$56$^+$ VA24$^+$VB11$^+$) were observed in either XLP1 or XLP2 patients, serving as a clue in the diagnostics cascade. Also, Zhao and colleagues[66] reported the use of FCM in the diagnostic cascade in 6 patients with SAP deficiency. They described the clinical value of flow cytometric evaluation of lymphoid SAP expression for the detection of patients with XLP1.

Congenital Defects of Phagocytes

Chronic granulomatous disease

CGD is a rare PID characterized by deficient intracellular killing of pathogens by phagocytes resulting in recurrent life-threatening infections.[67] Laboratory diagnostics of CGD is achieved with FCM, by measurement of phagocytosis and oxidative burst by using fluorescein–labeled *Escherichia coli* and dihydrorhodamine 123 (DHR) as a substrate, respectively. Bacteria are ingested and processed by phagocytes inducing fluorescence signals, measured by FCM.[68] Fluorescence intensity increases strongly when neutrophils are activated. In contrast, patients with CGD present clearly decreased or absent DHR-dependent fluorescence. Furthermore, FCM test can be used to identify maternal carriers of X-linked CGD, which will present a bimodal peak because of random X-inactivation.[43,67,69]

We investigated the phagocytic activity and leukocyte oxidative burst (as mentioned elsewhere in this article) in neutrophil populations in both patients with CGD and control. Upon activation, we observed an absence of fluorescence of DHR 123 in neutrophils from a CGD patient compared with a healthy control. In contrast, phagocytosis was normal in patient and control (see **Fig. 8**).

Autoinflammatory Disorders

Chronic infantile neurologic cutaneous and articular syndrome

Chronic infantile neurologic cutaneous and articular (CINCA) syndrome or neonatal/infantile onset multisystem inflammatory disease is a rare, neonatally onset, severe chronic inflammatory disorder, characterized by central nervous system affection, arthropathy and cutaneous symptoms (OMIM 607115). CINCA syndrome is caused by a failure of a gene encoding the NLPR3 (CIAS1 or cryopyrin) protein, which is essential in the activation of the inflammatory response.[70]

We investigated the CD10 expression on the surface of neutrophils in a CINCA patient and in healthy control by FCM. Unlike Leone and colleagues,[71] who have reported increased ($P<.0005$) surface expression of CD10 in patients with CINCA, we found that it decreased compared with a healthy control (see **Fig. 9**, **Table 1**). We gated the neutrophil population based on side scatter and CD45 (high side scatter CD45$^+$) and evaluated the mean fluorescence intensity of CD10 expression on neutrophils. However, further studies are required to understand the relation between CD10 expression and CINCA syndrome.

MECP2 duplication syndrome

Mutation of the X-linked methyl-CpG-binding protein 2 gene (MECP2; OMIM: 300005) is correlated with infantile hypotonia, serious mental retardation, autistic features, reduced speech development, and recurrent infections particularly of the respiratory tract (often requiring hospitalization and intravenous antibiotics therapy).[72] Children with MECP2 duplication syndrome also display variable immunologic abnormalities. That includes decreased memory T and B cells and NK cells as well as hampered immunoglobulin responses.[73] We investigated peripheral blood of a patient with MECP2 duplication syndrome by FCM. Compared with a heathy control, the immunophenotyping showed a normal enumeration of B cells (CD19$^+$), T helper (CD4$^+$), as well as cytotoxic cells (CD8$^+$). Interestingly, a strong decrease of memory T cells (CD3$^+$CD45RA$^-$CCR7$^-$), memory B cells (CD19$^+$CD21$^+$CD27$^+$) and class-switched B cells (CD19$^+$CD21$^+$CD27$^+$IgD$^-$IgM$^-$) could be found (see **Fig. 10**, **Table 1**). Our results corresponded with Yang and colleagues.[73] Moreover, the same study[73] pointed out, that a duplication of the MECP2 gene causes immunodeficiency partly by restriction of interferon-γ production by CD4$^+$ T cells. FCM analysis of peripheral blood mononuclear cells of children with MECP2 duplication syndrome revealed that MECP2 overexpressed in human T helper cells selectively reduces interferon-γ production, impairs T helper type 1 cell differentiation and deregulates proliferation by acting as a transcriptional repressor and regulator of *ifng* locus accessibility.[73]

SUMMARY

Flow cytometric immunophenotyping is a well-standardized and flexible method for precise identification and characterization of cells and their function. FCM identifies cellular compositions in the peripheral blood as well as defects in the immune function and should be considered as an important tool in the diagnostic cascade. Today, 8- to 10-color staining analyses represent the state of the art in routine laboratories.

REFERENCES

1. Chapel H. Classification of primary immunodeficiency diseases by the International Union of Immunological Societies (IUIS) Expert Committee on Primary Immunodeficiency 2011. Clin Exp Immunol 2012;168:58–9.

2. Online Mendelian Inheritance in Man (OMIM). An online catalog of human genes and genetic disorders. In: Online Mendelian Inheritance in Man. Available at: http://omim.org/. Accessed April 12, 2017.

3. Boyle JM, Buckley RH. Population prevalence of diagnosed primary immunodeficiency diseases in the United States. J Clin Immunol 2007;27:497–502.

4. Notarangelo LD. Primary immunodeficiencies. J Allergy Clin Immunol 2010;125: S182–94.

5. Chinen J, Notarangelo LD, Shearer WT. Advances in clinical immunology in 2015. J Allergy Clin Immunol 2016;138:1531–40.

6. Bacchetta R, Notarangelo LD. Immunodeficiency with autoimmunity: beyond the paradox. Front Immunol 2013;4:77.

7. Navabi B, Upton JE. Primary immunodeficiencies associated with eosinophilia. Allergy Asthma Clin Immunol 2016;12:27.

8. Warnatz K, Voll RE. Pathogenesis of autoimmunity in common variable immuno-deficiency. Front Immunol 2012;3:210.

9. McGonagle D, McDermott MF. A proposed classification of the immunological diseases. PLoS Med 2006;3:e297.

10. O'Sullivan MD, Cant AJ. The 10 warning signs: a time for a change? Curr Opin Allergy Clin Immunol 2012;12:588–94.

11. Bousfiha A, Jeddane L, Al-Herz W, et al. The 2015 IUIS phenotypic classification for primary immunodeficiencies. J Clin Immunol 2015;35:727–38.

12. Wood P, UK Primary Immunodeficiency Network. Primary antibody deficiencies: recognition, clinical diagnosis and referral of patients. Clin Med (Lond) 2009;9: 595–9.

13. Reust C. Evaluation of primary immunodeficiency disease in children. Am Fam Physician 2013;87:773–8.

14. Sack U, Boldt A, Borte M, et al. Novel diagnostic options for immunodeficiencies. Clin Biochem 2014;47:724–5.

15. Abraham RS, Aubert G. Flow cytometry, a versatile tool for diagnosis and moni-toring of primary immunodeficiencies. Clin Vaccine Immunol 2016;23:254–71.

16. Oliveira JB, Notarangelo LD, Fleisher TA. Applications of flow cytometry for the study of primary immune deficiencies. Curr Opin Allergy Clin Immunol 2008;8: 499–509.

17. Boldt A, Borte S, Fricke S, et al. Eight color immunophenotyping of T-, B- and NK cell subpopulations for characterization of chronic immunodeficiencies. Cytome-try B Clin Cytom 2014;86:191–206.

18. Barbaro M, Ohlsson A, Borte S, et al. Newborn screening for severe primary im-munodeficiency diseases in Sweden-a 2-Year Pilot TREC and KREC screening study. J Clin Immunol 2017;37:51–60.

19. Gathmann B, Mahlaoui N, CEREDIH, et al, European Society for Immunodefi-ciencies Registry Working Party. Clinical picture and treatment of 2212 patients with common variable immunodeficiency. J Allergy Clin Immunol 2014;134: 116–26.

20. Pieper K, Grimbacher B, Eibel H. B cell biology and development. J Allergy Clin Immunol 2013;131:959–71.

21. Frazer-Abel A, Sepiashvili L, Mbughuni MM, et al. Overview of laboratory testing and clinical presentations of complement deficiencies and dysregulation. Adv Clin Chem 2016;77:1–75.

22. Fleisher TA, Dorman SE, Anderson JA, et al. Detection of intracellular phosphor-ylated STAT-1 by flow cytometry. Clin Immunol 1999;90:425–30.

23. Uzel G, Frucht DM, Fleisher TA, et al. Detection of intracellular phosphorylated STAT-4 by flow cytometry. Clin Immunol 2001;100:270–6.

24. O'Shea JJ, Plenge R. JAKs and STATs in immunoregulation and immune medi-ated disease. Immunity 2012;36:542–50.

25. De Stefano A, Boldt A, Schmiedel L, et al. Flow cytometry as an important tool in the diagnosis of immunodeficiencies demonstrated in a patient with ataxia-telangiectasia. Laboratoriumsmedizin 2016;40:255–61.

26. Boldt A, Kentouche K, Fricke S, et al. Differences in FOXP3 and CD127 expression in Treg-like cells in patients with IPEX syndrome. Clin Immunol 2014;153: 109–11.

27. Bitar M, Boldt A, Binder S, et al. Flow cytometric measurement of STAT1 and STAT3 phosphorylation in CD4+ and CD8+ T cells - clinical applications in primary immunodeficiency diagnostics. J Allergy Clin Immunol 2017;S0091-6749(17):30915–6.

28. Cantoni N, Recher M. Primary and secondary immunodeficiencies. Ther Umsch 2014;71:31–43.

29. Xie X, Li F, Chen JW, et al. Risk of tuberculosis infection in anti-TNF-α biological therapy: from bench to bedside. J Microbiol Immunol Infect 2014;47:268–74.

30. Ferrari S, Lougaris V, Caraffi S, et al. Mutations of the Igbeta gene cause agammaglobulinemia in man. J Exp Med 2007;204:2047–51.

31. Kanegane H, Futatani T, Wang Y, et al. Clinical and mutational characteristics of X-linked agammaglobulinemia and its carrier identified by flow cytometric assessment combined with genetic analysis. J Allergy Clin Immunol 2001;108: 1012–20.

32. Futatani T, Miyawaki T, Tsukada S, et al. Deficient expression of Bruton's tyrosine kinase in monocytes from X-linked agammaglobulinemia as evaluated by a flow cytometric analysis and its clinical application to carrier detection. Blood 1998; 91:595–602.

33. Warnatz K, Denz A, Drager R, et al. Severe deficiency of switched memory B cells (CD27(+)IgM(-) IgD(-)) in subgroups of patients with common variable immunodeficiency: a new approach to classify a heterogeneous disease. Blood 2002;99: 1544–51.

34. Piqueras B, Lavenu-Bombled C, Galicier L, et al. Common variable immunodeficiency patient classification based on impaired B cell memory differentiation correlates with clinical aspects. J Clin Immunol 2003;23:385–400.

35. Wehr C, Kivioja T, Schmitt C, et al. The EUROclass trial: defining subgroups in common variable immunodeficiency. Blood 2008;111:77–85.

36. Berrón-Ruiz L, López-Herrera G, Vargas-Hernández A, et al. Impaired selective cytokine production by CD4(+) T cells in Common Variable Immunodeficiency associated with the absence of memory B cells. Clin Immunol 2016;166–167: 19–26.

37. Bossaller L, Burger J, Draeger R, et al. ICOS deficiency is associated with a severe reduction of CXCR51CD4 germinal center Th cells. J Immunol 2006;177: 4927–32.

38. van Zelm MC, Reisli I, van der BM, et al. An antibody-deficiency syndrome due to mutations in the CD19 gene. N Engl J Med 2006;354:1901–12.

39. Kanegane H, Agematsu K, Futatani T, et al. Novel mutations in a Japanese patient with CD19 deficiency. Genes Immun 2007;8:663–70.

40. Salzer U, Chapel HM, Webster AD, et al. Mutations in TNFRSF13B encoding TACI are associated with common variable immunodeficiency in humans. Nat Genet 2005;37:820–8.

41. Pan-Hammarstrom Q, Salzer U, Du L, et al. Reexamining the role of TACI coding variants in common variable immunodeficiency and selective IgA deficiency. Nat Genet 2007;39:429–30.

42. Borte S, von Döbeln U, Fasth A, et al. Neonatal screening for severe primary immunodeficiency diseases using high-throughput triplex real-time PCR. Blood 2012;15(119):2552–5.
43. Oliveira JB, Fleisher TA. Laboratory evaluation of primary immunodeficiencies. J Allergy Clin Immunol 2010;125:S297–305.
44. Lee W-I, Torgerson TR, Schumacher MJ, et al. Molecular analysis of a large cohort of patients with the hyper immunoglobulin M (IgM) syndrome. Blood 2005;105:1881–90.
45. Fleisher TA. The autoimmune lymphoproliferative syndrome: an experiment of nature involving lymphocyte apoptosis. Immunol Res 2008;40:87–92.
46. Hanlon MG, Gacis ML, Kakakios AM, et al. Investigation of suspected deficient Fas-mediated apoptosis in a father and son. Cytometry 2001;43:195–8.
47. Simon KL, Anderson SM, Garabedian EK, et al. Molecular and phenotypic abnormalities of B lymphocytes in patients with Wiskott-Aldrich syndrome. J Allergy Clin Immunol 2014;133:896–9.
48. Castiello MC, Bosticardo M, Pala F, et al. Wiskott-Aldrich Syndrome protein deficiency perturbs the homeostasis of B cell compartment in humans. J Autoimmun 2014;50:42–50.
49. Yamada M, Ohtsu M, Kobayashi I, et al. Flow cytometric analysis of Wiskott-Aldrich syndrome (WAS) protein in lymphocytes from WAS patients and their familial carriers. Blood 1999;93:756–7.
50. Park JY, Shcherbina A, Rosen FS, et al. Phenotypic perturbation of B cells in the Wiskott-Aldrich syndrome. Clin Exp Immunol 2005;139:297–305.
51. Yamada M, Ariga T, Kawamura N, et al. Determination of carrier status for the Wiskott-Aldrich syndrome by flow cytometric analysis of Wiskott-Aldrich syndrome protein expression in peripheral blood mononuclear cells. J Immunol 2000;165:1119–22.
52. Schubert R, Reichenbach J, Zielen S. Deficiencies in CD4+ and CD8+ T cell subsets in ataxia telangiectasia. Clin Exp Immunol 2002;129:125–32.
53. Porcedda P, Turinetto V, Brusco A, et al. A rapid flow cytometry test based on histone H2AX phosphorylation for the sensitive and specific diagnosis of ataxia telangiectasia. Cytometry A 2008;73:508–16.
54. Chrzanowska KH, Gregorek H, Dembowska-Bagińska B, et al. Nijmegen breakage syndrome (NBS). Orphanet J Rare Dis 2012;28;7:13.
55. Piatosa B, van der Burg M, Siewiera K, et al. The defect in humoral immunity in patients with Nijmegen breakage syndrome is explained by defects in peripheral B lymphocyte maturation. Cytometry A 2012;81:835–42.
56. van Vu Q, Wada T, Toma T, et al. Clinical and immunophenotypic features of atypical complete DiGeorge syndrome. Pediatr Int 2013;55:2–6.
57. Dar N, Gothelf D, Korn D, et al. Thymic and bone marrow output in individuals with 22q11.2 deletion syndrome. Pediatr Res 2015;77:579–85.
58. Ravkov E, Slev P, Heikal N. Thymic output: assessment of CD4+ recent thymic emigrants and T cell receptor excision circles in infants. Cytometry B Clin Cytom 2017;92(4):249–57.
59. Lima K, Abrahamsen TG, Foelling I, et al. Low thymic output in the 22q11.2 deletion syndrome measured by CCR9+CD45RA+ T cell counts and T cell receptor rearrangement excision circles. Clin Exp Immunol 2010;161:98–107.
60. Torgerson TR, Ochs HD. Immune dysregulation, polyendocrinopathy, enteropathy, X-linked: forkhead box protein 3 mutations and lack of regulatory T cells. J Allergy Clin Immunol 2007;120:744–50.

61. Nichols KE, Ma CS, Cannons JL, et al. Molecular and cellular pathogenesis of X-linked lymphoproliferative disease. Immunol Rev 2005;203:180–99.
62. Rigaud S, Fondaneche M-C, Lambert N, et al. XIAP deficiency in humans causes an X-linked lymphoproliferative syndrome. Nature 2006;444:110–4.
63. Marsh RA, Bleesing JJ, Filipovich AH. Using flow cytometry to screen patients for X-linked lymphoproliferative disease due to SAP deficiency and XIAP deficiency. J Immunol Methods 2010;362:1–9.
64. Shinozaki K, Kanegane H, Matsukura H, et al. Activation-dependent T cell expression of the X-linked lymphoproliferative disease gene product SLAM-associated protein and its assessment for patient detection. Int Immunol 2002;14:1215–23.
65. Tabata Y, Villanueva J, Lee SM, et al. Rapid detection of intracellular SH2D1A protein in cytotoxic lymphocytes from patients with X-linked lymphoproliferative disease and their family members. Blood 2005;105:3066–71.
66. Zhao M, Kanegane H, Kobayashi C, et al. Early and rapid detection of X-linked lymphoproliferative syndrome with SH2D1A mutations by flow cytometry. Cytometry B Clin Cytom 2011;80:8–13.
67. Rosenzweig SD, Holland SM. Phagocyte immunodeficiencies and their infections. J Allergy Clin Immunol 2004;113:620–6.
68. Filias A, Theodorou GL, Mouzopoulou S, et al. Phagocytic ability of neutrophils and monocytes in neonates. BMC Pediatr 2011;11:29.
69. Elloumi HZ, Holland SM. Diagnostic assays for chronic granulomatous disease and other neutrophil disorders. Methods Mol Biol 2014;1124:517–35.
70. Finetti M, Omenetti A, Federici S. Chronic infantile neurological cutaneous and articular (CINCA) syndrome: a review. Orphanet J Rare Dis 2016;11:167.
71. Leone V, Presani G, Perticarari S, et al. Chronic infantile neurological cutaneous articular syndrome: CD10 over-expression in neutrophils is a possible key to the pathogenesis of the disease. Eur J Pediatr 2003;162:669–73.
72. van Esch H. MECP2 duplication syndrome. Mol Syndromol 2012;2:128–36.
73. Yang T, Ramocki MB, Neul JL, et al. Overexpression of methyl-CpG binding protein 2 impairs T(H)1 responses. Sci Transl Med 2012;4:163ra158.

Cost-Effective Flow Cytometry Testing Strategies

Catherine P. Leith, MB BChir

KEYWORDS

- Flow cytometry • Laboratory test utilization • Laboratory test algorithms
- Evidence-based laboratory medicine • Physician education

KEY POINTS

- Use clinical and pathology data to decide if FC is the method of choice for making a diagnosis; hold FC testing until further clinical/pathology data are available if its role in diagnosis is unclear.
- Do not compromise morphology and possible immunohistochemistry studies by sending excessive tissue sample for FC. This is particularly problematic with needle core biopsies; setting criteria in pathology for which samples are sent for FC, and which cases require pathologist morphology review before FC testing is performed, can limit unnecessary testing, and ensure adequate tissue is available for morphology/immunohistochemistry.
- Develop standard FC panels based on commonly seen diseases, with additional add-on markers available for uncommon entities; not every case needs every marker.
- Develop limited triage panels to use where likelihood of disease is low, and where FC will rule out disease, with follow-up FC assays for positive cases.
- Establish rules for the flow laboratory to identify cases for triage based on easily obtainable numeric parameters (eg, patient age, complete blood cell count data). Successful triage requires training flow laboratory technical staff to interpret initial data, and add on additional markers in positive cases.

INTRODUCTION

This article looks at strategies to make flow cytometry (FC) testing more cost effective and efficient in the clinical laboratory, particularly for initial diagnosis of disease. There is no one size fits all system for FC testing; an on-site hospital laboratory with access to the electronic medical record (EMR) will likely develop systems quite different from a reference laboratory to which samples are sent where access to clinical data is limited.

Disclosures: The author has nothing to disclose.
Department of Pathology and Laboratory Medicine, University of Wisconsin School of Medicine and Public Health, K4/434, 600 Highland Avenue, Madison, WI 53792, USA
E-mail address: cpleith@wisc.edu

Clin Lab Med 37 (2017) 915–929
http://dx.doi.org/10.1016/j.cll.2017.07.012   labmed.theclinics.com
0272-2712/17/© 2017 Elsevier Inc. All rights reserved.

The 2006 Bethesda International Consensus group listed a wide range of medical indications for performing FC, summarized in **Table 1**, and also developed guidelines on panel selection based primarily on specimen type, with information on medical indication, patient history, and morphology taken into account if available.[1,2]

When developing strategies to develop cost-effective FC assays, it is important to consider the direct costs associated with the flow test, but also how testing may affect costs elsewhere in the health care system. For example, if a patient with mild lymphocytosis is referred for hematology oncology consultation, an FC study performed up front could rule out a lymphoproliferative disorder (LPD), saving the patient a clinic visit, and therefore patient, physician, and clinic time and costs. Thus the costs of the FC assay are more than recouped through other savings. Alternatively, if the FC assay demonstrates an LPD, the hematologist is able to plan the clinic visit more precisely knowing the diagnosis/differential diagnosis.

Setting up cost-effective FC assays requires taking into consideration factors related to individual patient samples and to the overall system in which FC takes place, and then applying this information to develop cost-effective FC testing strategies, using general guiding principles for test utilization (**Table 2**).[3]

THE INDIVIDUAL PATIENT AND THEIR SPECIMEN
What is Suspected Clinical Diagnosis and How Useful Will Flow Cytometry Be?

Deciding the role FC will play in diagnosis assists in determining if FC studies are done "up front" before morphology review (useful for cases where flow is critical) or should wait for morphology.

Is flow cytometry critical to make the suspected diagnosis?
FC is fundamental for the diagnosis and categorization of LPD and acute leukemia, and plays an important role in diagnosis of B-cell lymphoma, plasma cells disorders, and myelodysplasia. FC plays a more limited role in diagnoses where tissue architecture is important, and plays a very limited role in diagnosis of Hodgkin lymphoma where morphology and immunohistochemistry studies are key with a limited FC role.[4,5] FC for suspected T-cell lymphoma is also much more challenging than for B-cell lymphoma, and may not be the best approach.[6] FC is not useful in diagnosis of myeloproliferative neoplasms. Thus FC performed "up front" without morphologic correlate makes sense for diseases with a critical FC role.

| Table 1 | | |
| Indications for FC of hematolymphoid neoplasms | | |
Specimen	Abnormality	
Blood	Cytopenias other than isolated anemia	
	Leukocytosis	Lymphocytosis
		Monocytosis
		Eosinophilia
Blood, marrow, fluids	Atypical cells/blasts	
Bone marrow	Monoclonal gammopathy	
Tissues	Suspected tissue based hematopoietic disease	

Adapted from Davis BH, Holden JT, Bene MC, et al. 2006 Bethesda International Consensus recommendations on the flow cytometric immunophenotypic analysis of hematolymphoid neoplasia: Medical indications. Cytometry B Clin. Cytom 2007;72(Suppl 1):S5–13; with permission.

Table 2	
Factors to consider in development and implementation of cost-effective FC tests	

Factors related to the individual specimen	What is suspected clinical diagnosis and will FC be useful?
	 What is the specimen and what is its longevity?
	 What other data are available?
	    Complete blood cell count and clinical laboratory data
	    Clinical history
	    Imaging data
	 What is the likely disease based on the disease prevalence and
	    patient data?

Factors related to the laboratory and the health care system	Is the FC laboratory a reference or in-house laboratory? What is the work flow and experience level in the FC laboratory? Who is ordering FC, a diverse or uniform medical group? How do FC data impact other areas of health care system?

Is flow cytometry critical to "rule out" the suspected diagnosis?

FC is often ordered to rule out hematolymphoid disease but is obviously only useful in this regard if the disease being ruled out is easily diagnosed by FC. Thus FC is excellent to distinguish reactive from neoplastic lymphocytosis but is not useful to distinguish reactive from neoplastic neutrophilia. The "rule out" cases are excellent targets to develop more limited FC assays.

Will flow cytometry answer the clinical question?

Sometimes FC is the wrong modality to use to answer a specific question. Transformation of chronic lymphocytic leukemia (CLL) or follicular lymphoma to diffuse large B-cell lymphoma are examples where morphology is critical, and FC adds little information. In other cases FC studies may be irrelevant. For example, FC on a fine-needle aspirate of a lymph node in a patient with suspected head and neck cancer and with known CLL does not answer the critical clinical question of whether there is a solid tumor present.

Setting criteria for the laboratory to determine on specimen arrival if FC testing should proceed based on likely diagnosis, or wait for morphology review, is essential for smooth laboratory operations.

Table 3 outlines some examples showing the likelihood of a positive flow result in different clinical scenarios, and the role of FC in such cases. Cases where FC is being used to "rule out" disease are particularly good targets for limited flow studies.

What is the Specimen and What is Its Longevity

The specimen type and longevity influence the FC strategy, whether testing should be performed up front, and who needs to decide which test to perform.

Liquid samples with abundant cells (blood, bone marrow)

If FC is critical to make the suspected diagnosis, upfront FC testing and subsequent integration with morphology and other data makes sense; holding these specimens pending hematopathology morphology review is inefficient and impracticable. The specific FC panel to perform depends on the likely diagnosis and index of suspicion of disease and can be decided according to preset laboratory criteria. Because these specimens have high cell counts, further flow testing can always be performed if the initial choice of panel was incorrect or did not answer the clinical question (**Fig. 1** is an example). In some cases, particularly marrow samples where the differential is

Table 3
Examples to show how the likelihood of a positive flow study based on known clinical/pathology data is used to direct FC studies

Likelihood that FC Will Aid in Diagnosis	Clinical/Pathology Scenario	Example	Role of FC
High	Morphology shows hematolymphoid neoplasm	Acute leukemia marrow in 30 y old	FC diagnostic study
		Blood lymphocytosis >10 K/μL in elderly patient	FC diagnostic study
		Lymph node morphology effaced by likely lymphoma	FC diagnostic study
Intermediate	Suspected malignancy with limited/time sensitive sample	CSF for suspected brain lymphoma	"Rule in" study
		FNA from patient with adenopathy	"Rule in" study
Low	Suspected malignancy; FC sample low yield but helpful if positive	Blood on 50 y old with unexplained splenomegaly	"Rule out" study
	Malignancy unlikely; flow to rule out disease	Blood on 50 y old with borderline lymphocytosis	"Rule out" study
Very low	FC unlikely to be helpful in diagnosis	Lymph node biopsy shows Hodgkin lymphoma	Potential to cancel FC
		Lymph node biopsy for potential Richter transformation	Recommend tissue submission for morphology
		Blood on 50 y old man with leukocytosis, morphology suggests CML	Potential to cancel FC
		CSF on patient with neurologic symptoms; morphology/imaging not worrisome for LPD	Potential to cancel FC

Cases highly likely to be malignant have complete diagnostic FC. FC is useful in cases with intermediate/low likelihood of positive result, but a limited panel often suffices.

Abbreviations: CML, chronic myelogenous leukemia; CSF, cerebrospinal fluid; FNA, fine-needle aspiration.

broader, FC studies may still be better held pending morphology review, and with a focused approach dependent on morphology findings.[7]

Liquid samples with limited cells (fine-needle aspiration, cerebrospinal fluid specimens)

Specimens with low cellularity, such as fine-needle aspirates or cerebrospinal fluid (CSF) specimens, need to have a decision regarding FC made quickly to ensure there are enough cells for analysis. These samples, despite low cellularity, can be diagnostic (**Fig. 2**). However, unlike blood specimens where abundant material allows additional FC testing as needed, it is essential to choose the correct FC test up front. Therefore close communication with hematopathology and morphology review are generally needed before processing. **Fig. 3** is an example of CSF sent to rule out lymphoma. Review of the EMR showed a history of plasmablastic lymphoma, and FC was thus directed toward plasma cell antigens. The routine B-cell lymphoma FC tube would not have been useful in this case.

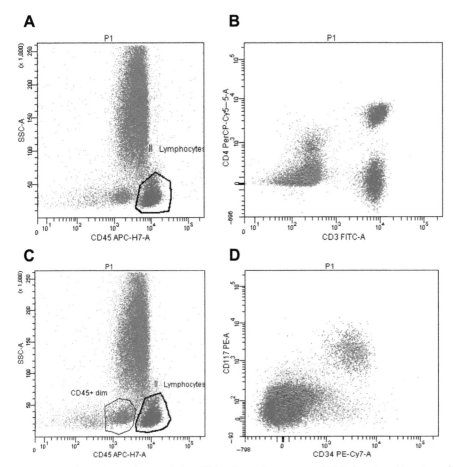

Fig. 1. FC study performed on peripheral blood sent for suspected LPD showing detection of unexpected blast population. (*A*) CD45 versus side scatter dot plot showing lymphocytes identified in *green*. (*B*) CD3 versus CD4. The lymphocytes are mostly CD4$^+$ and CD4$^-$ T cells. (*C*) CD45 versus side scatter dot plot, now also identifying distinct CD45 dim population (*red*). (*D*) CD34 versus CD117. The *red* blast population expresses CD34 and CD117.

Tissue samples

Up front FC assays before morphology review are often less useful in evaluation of tissue specimens. This is partly because architecture plays such a critical role in these tissue samples, and partly because the differential is often wider, including such entities as Hodgkin lymphoma, where FC has a more limited role. Thus it is better to hold FC testing pending morphology review, or if not practicable, as in the reference laboratory setting, to perform an initial limited panel. Core needles are replacing excisional biopsies of lymph nodes in many institutions. It is crucial not to compromise morphology by sending too much tissue for FC; a positive flow result without concomitant morphology is of limited value. With the expanding armamentarium of antibodies available for immunohistochemistry, most diagnoses are made by morphology and immunohistochemistry. In our institution, we process the entire core sample for histology with rare exceptions. Each institution needs to come up with its own guidelines for how to handle these small tissue specimens.

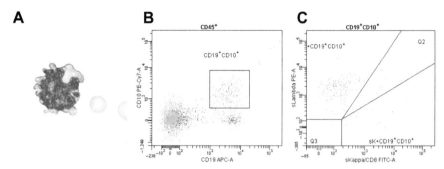

Fig. 2. FC can identify malignancy even if cell numbers are low. CSF study performed on CSF for suspected lymphoma. Single FC tube with CD45/CD19/CD20/kappa/lambda/CD3/CD4/CD8/CD10. (*A*) Wright Giemsa–stained cytospin of CSF shows scattered large atypical cells. (*B*) CD19 versus CD10 on CD45+ gated cells. A small population of CD19+/CD10+ cells is identified (*colored red in box*). (*C*) Kappa versus lambda on gated CD19+/CD10+ cells. The population shows monoclonal lambda expression.

What Other Data Are Available?

Access to other clinical and laboratory data is key to deciding what flow panel to run, or if flow is needed at all. Data that are immediately available and readily evaluable by the FC technologists is the most useful for setting up focused flow panels; patient age and complete blood cell count data for blood or cell count data for body fluids meet these criteria. The EMR can obviously provide far more data including detailed clinical history, imaging data, and other laboratory results. However, EMR review is time consuming, and for practical purposes should be used to understand the clinical situation where the flow study order is unclear or makes little sense. **Table 4** lists some examples of specimen data and how it can be used to decide which flow studies to perform.

What is the Most Likely Diagnosis Based on Available Data?

Some diseases are much more common than others, so performing flow assays that focus on the most likely diseases makes sense. Importantly such focused panels must

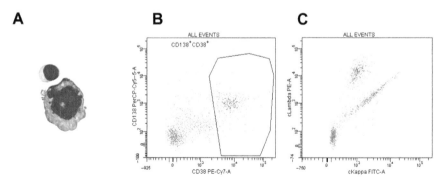

Fig. 3. FC study performed on CSF in a patient with history of plasmablastic lymphoma. Single FC tube with CD45/CD38/CD138/ckappa/clambda. (*A*) Wright Giemsa–stained cytospin of CSF shows large abnormal cells next to a small lymphocyte. (*B*) CD38 versus CD138 expression. A distinct CD38+/CD138+ population is identified, consistent with plasma cells. (*C*) cKappa versus cLambda. The *purple* CD38+/CD138+ population is monoclonal for lambda.

Table 4
Patient factors that are used to direct the FC panel using peripheral blood as an example

Factor	Easy to Find and Interpret?	Suspected Diagnosis Example	Background	Examples of Use in Deciding FC Panel
Age	Yes; numeric data interpretation	LPD	LPD more common in older patients and rare in young patients	Limit work-up in patients <55 y — Full work-up in patients >55 y
		Acute leukemia	AML more likely in patients >40 y ALL more common in children T-ALL mainly in teenagers	Panel with full range B-cell markers in patients <40 y — AML-centric panel in patients >40 y
Cell counts	Yes Numeric data	LPD	LPD more likely with higher ALC	Limit work-up if ALC <5000/μL — Full work-up if ALC >5000/μL
Historical CBC data	Medical record dependent but not immediately available; numeric data	LPD	LPD more likely with sustained lymphocytosis	Limit work-up if single elevated ALC Cancel work-up if ALC elevation transient — Perform full work-up if ALC persistently elevated
Radiology data	Medical record dependent; not easily interpretable	LPD	Splenomegaly/ adenopathy seen in lymphoma	Easier for laboratory to perform flow according to ALC rules than access imaging data

Factors that are easily available and interpretable by FC laboratory staff (eg, numeric data) are most useful for panel determination.
Abbreviations: ALC, absolute lymphocyte count; ALL, acute lymphoblastic leukemia; AML, acute myeloid leukemia; CBC, complete blood cell count; T-ALL, T-acute lymphoblastic leukemia.

still be capable of identifying rare diseases so these entities are not missed. The most obvious example where a panel focused on a single disease makes sense is in the work-up of blood LPDs. CLL and monoclonal B-cell lymphocytosis are much more common than such diseases as peripheralizing marginal zone, mantle cell, or follicular lymphoma. Similar examples are found in other disease groups; acute leukemia in a patient older than 50 years is much more likely to be acute myeloid leukemia than B-lymphoblastic leukemia, whereas T-lymphoblastic leukemia is rare in this age group. Conversely, in children, B-lymphoblastic leukemia is more common than acute myeloid leukemia. Thus a panel focused on acute myeloid leukemia makes sense for older patients but not for children.

SYSTEMIC FACTORS
Is the Flow Laboratory a Reference or In-House Laboratory?

The overall approach to FC and types of panels used depends in part on whether the FC laboratory is a reference or in-house laboratory. Reference laboratories often have more limited access to the clinical history and other laboratory and radiologic data, and may not receive morphology slides to help guide which flow tests to perform. In addition, specimens are older on receipt because of transport time. As a result a broader FC approach is needed, to rule out a wider variety of possible diseases (because of lack of morphology/clinical correlates) and because an algorithmic approach is less feasible due to specimen age. In contrast, targeted and algorithmic flow approaches are easier in local laboratories, where specimens are collected on site and where clinical data are readily available.

The flow strategy used also depends on the individual laboratory operation and work flow. Some approaches, such as that used in the Euroflow panels, use a single screening tube in the initial work-up, with the further work-up dependent on these initial results.[8] This method requires a fast reliable evaluation of the initial data, so that the relevant reflex panel can be set up, and a laboratory work schedule that allows for an overall longer time for complete case analysis, both factors that may be difficult to reproduce consistently in every laboratory. When considering setting up a reflex test model, it is important to consider the experience level of the laboratory staff. A successful model is one that is reliably executed by even the least experienced laboratory member.

Who is Ordering Flow Cytometry: A Diverse or Uniform Medical Group?

Some strategies to limit FC testing may not be noticeable to referring physicians because they still receive an FC report with a diagnosis. However, cancellation of unnecessary FC tests requires close communication with ordering physicians to explain the rationale and to educate them about testing indications.[9] Case-by-case communication is time consuming, so long-term strategies to decrease unnecessary FC testing require systematic physician education, and use of tools, such as changes in electronic orders, something much easier to implement with a single physician group than in a referral laboratory setting.

How Do Flow Cytometry Data Impact Other Areas of the Health Care System?

FC studies that seem inappropriate may sometimes be useful if they positively affect the patient and other parts of the health care system. For example, if a patient with mild lymphocytosis is referred for hematology-oncology consultation, an FC study performed up front before a clinic visit could rule out an LPD, saving the patient a clinic visit, and the ensuing patient, physician, and clinic time and costs. Thus the costs of the FC assay are more than recouped through other savings. A well-structured panel is effective in the previously mentioned scenario at reasonable cost.

STRATEGIES TO SET UP AND PERFORM COST-EFFECTIVE FLOW CYTOMETRY PANELS

Cost-effective testing in the FC laboratory means performing only the testing required to reach a diagnosis and/or answer the clinical question, and doing so in the most time-efficient manner. This requires effective overall panel design, identification of cases with low likelihood of disease amenable to more limited flow testing, and development of algorithms to add additional markers if needed based on initial flow results. The algorithm concept has the potential to contain the total number of antigens tested in each case, and thus cost. The disadvantage of this approach is the increased technical time and expertise needed to follow the algorithm correctly, and the risk, especially in reference laboratories, that the lengthier test time may affect specimen viability. In addition, if a high proportion of cases undergo reflex testing, the increased labor cost of the two-step system increases the total panel cost compared with an upfront full panel without concomitant increase in revenue. Thus a balance between upfront detailed flow testing, and an algorithmic approach is generally the most practical. After implementing any FC algorithm, it is important to evaluate its performance periodically and modify it as needed to improve its effectiveness.

Design of Effective Panels

An effective panel is the first requirement for cost-effective FC. The panel should obviously include key backbone markers, and markers characteristic of specific diseases. However, the initial FC panel need not include every diagnostic possibility, but should focus on the most likely diseases found in that sample type. In our laboratory's experience of peripheral blood FC testing for LPD, three-quarters of malignant cases are CD5[+] LPDs, mostly CLL/monoclonal B-cell lymphocytosis, with some peripheralizing mantle cell lymphoma, or atypical CLL.[6] The remaining 25% of LPD are mostly marginal zone lymphoma with a small proportion of T-cell LPDs and a rare peripheralizing follicular lymphoma. Thus these data indicate an effective FC panel for blood LPD would focus on CD5[+] disease. Similar efforts can be used to identify the most frequent diseases in other specimens and can similarly direct panel design.[10–12]

Identify Low-Yield Specimens Amenable to Limited Flow Cytometry Testing

Specimens where there is a definite but low probability of detecting a malignancy by FC are the perfect choice for performing a limited or screening flow panel. These specimens need to be identifiable by the FC laboratory using simple parameters, such as absolute lymphocyte count (ALC) and age, or specimen type, such as all lymph node fine-needle aspirations. Because these specimens still have FC performed and the FC study answers the clinical questions, there is no necessity to contact the ordering physician about the limited test; he or she will still get a result. It is much easier to perform limited studies on low-yield specimens than to cancel testing altogether, so these limited panels are the low hanging fruit if the goal is to reduce laboratory costs.

Identify "No-Yield" Specimens and Educate Clinicians on the Lack of Role for Flow Cytometry

FC studies in some circumstances are virtually no yield, such as leukocytosis secondary to neutrophilia, "screening" flow on CSF with no compelling indication of lymphoma.[13] These cases require a time investment to explain to the referring physician why FC is inappropriate. Doing this on a case-by-case basis is often

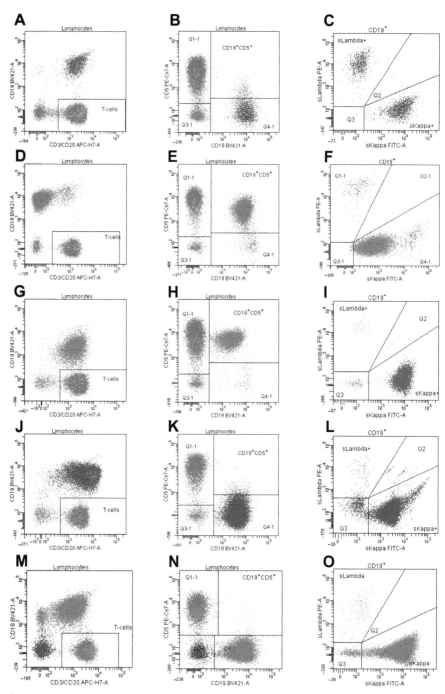

Fig. 4. FC studies of five cases with suspected LPD, where the screening algorithm was used based on ALC <5000. Each case is represented on one row, with dot plots showing CD19 versus CD3/CD20 on *left*, CD5 versus CD19 in *middle*, Lambda versus Kappa on *right*. (*A–C*) Case 1: benign lymphocytosis. The lymphocytes are mostly CD3+/CD5+/CD19− T cells (*A, B*).

impracticable and is time consuming. Therefore effective application of flow cancellation rules requires implementing strategies outside the FC laboratory. These could include education of referring physicians, development with clinicians of practice guidelines, pop up screens with questions on electronic test orders, and/or only performing tests ordered by specific physicians. Support from health care administration is fundamental to implement such policies successfully.[9,14–16] Tracking the numbers of cases canceled or with limited FC is useful because these data can be shared with health care administrators to demonstrate cost savings.

Develop Algorithms to Differentiate High- and Low-Yield Specimens and Sequential Test Strategies if a Low-Yield Sample is Positive

FC evaluation of peripheral blood for suspected LPD is one of the scenarios most amenable to an algorithmic flow approach and is described in more detail later. Patient age and ALC are key predictors for blood LPD detection.[6,17–19] Patients less than 50 years old with ALC less than 5000/µL are unlikely to have disease, whereas older patients with higher ALC probably have an LPD. Serum ferritin is also useful in predicting presence of an LPD in patients with lymphocytosis, with high ferritin (>450 µg/L) predictive of reactive lymphocytosis.[20] Because age and ALC independently predict likelihood of LPD, we have developed an algorithm that uses both pieces of data.[6]

We identify the following cases as having low likelihood of LPD: any blood with ALC less than 5000/µL, blood on patients less than 55 years old with ALC less than 7500/µL. Samples with ALC less than threshold have a single FC screening test performed (**Fig. 4**, **Table 5**). If a monoclonal B-cell disorder is detected, the reflex test performed depends on CD5 expression (**Fig. 5**, see **Table 5**). Samples with ALC over the threshold have a CD5-focused FC study performed. This testing algorithm results in a reflex rate of about 20%, which fits in with our laboratory work flow.

Modify the Algorithm Based on Laboratory Experience

Our initial flow screening tube included the T-markers CD3, CD4, and CD5. Review of follow-up data showed that further testing was being performed on some of these patients because the proportion of CD3$^+$/CD4$^+$ to CD3$^+$CD4$^-$ cells was often low, and raised concern for an undetected CD8$^+$ T-cell disorder. We therefore added CD8 to the panel, so a CD4/CD8 ratio is calculated in all cases. Such tweaking is an essential part of the laboratory operation.

The following list of keys to success and failure are a good beginning to developing targeted panels.

Keys to success of limited FC testing:

1. The limited test strategy is applicable to the laboratory's patient population.
2. The limited test strategy can be applied in a significant proportion of cases.

The CD19$^+$ B cells are polyclonal (C). (D–F) Case 2: monoclonal B-cell lymphocytosis. (D) The lymphocytes include many CD19$^+$/CD20 dim B cells (red). The B cells coexpress CD5 (E), and show weak monoclonal kappa (F). (G–I) Case 3: peripheralizing mantle cell lymphoma. The lymphocytes include B cells (red), which express CD19 and bright CD20 (G), coexpress CD5 (H), and show bright monoclonal kappa (I). (J–L) Case 4: peripheralizing marginal zone lymphoma. Many CD19/CD20 bright B cells (purple; J) are detected that lack CD5 (K) and show moderate kappa light chain (L). (M–O) Case 5: peripheralizing follicular lymphoma. CD19/CD20 moderate B cells (red; M) lack CD5 (N) and show bright kappa light chain (O).

Table 5
FC panel used for LPD detection in peripheral blood

LPD Tube #	1. BV 421	2. V500-C	3. FITC	4. PE	5. PERCP-CY5.5	6. PE-CY7	7. APC	8. APC-H7	Use
1 Screen	CD19	CD45	Kappa	Lambda	CD4	CD5	CD8	CD3/CD20	All samples for LPD
2 CD5+	CD5		CD20	CD23	CD19	CD38	CD200	CD45	Run upfront if high likelihood disease
3 CD5-	CD19	CD45	CD103	CD22	CD25	C10	CD11C	CD20	Add on if CD5- LPD identified

Tube 1 is performed on all samples, including those with low likelihood of disease based on age and ALC. Tube 2 is performed up front only on samples with ALC above threshold. Tube 3 is added if CD5$^-$ disease is detected.

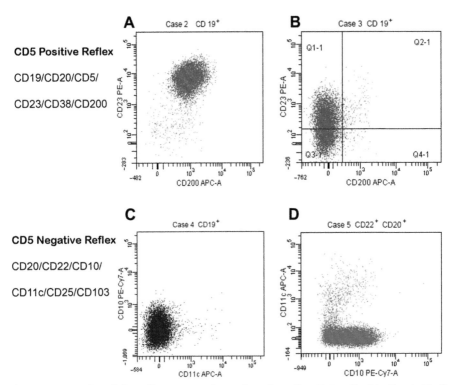

Fig. 5. FC examples of the reflex tests performed on Cases 2 to 5 described in **Fig. 4**. (*A, B*) CD23 versus CD200 expression on CD19-gated B cells for CD5+ Cases 2 and 3. (*A*) monoclonal B-cell lymphocytosis: B cells express CD23 and CD200. (*B*) Mantle cell lymphoma: B cells show dim CD23 and absent CD200. (*C, D*) Reflex flow studies on CD5⁻ Cases 4 and 5. (*C*) Marginal zone lymphoma: B cells lack CD10 and CD11c. CD10 versus CD11c. (*D*) Follicular lymphoma: neoplastic B cells express CD10 without CD11c.

3. The reflex rules are designed based on easily available and preferably numeric data, such as complete blood cell count/age.
4. The reflex rules are clearly written so the technologists can proceed to the next step of the process independently of direct pathologist oversight.
5. The FC laboratory staff is properly trained and educated in the use of the rules.
6. The reflex rules can be understood and implemented properly by the least experience FC technologist in the laboratory.
7. The reflex rules reflect an appropriate balance between limited testing and inefficiency through excess reflex testing.
8. The rules are periodically reviewed and optimized.

Keys to make the reflex testing unworkable:

1. Reflex testing requires pathologist review of initial FC screening data, or requires significant back and forth between pathologist and technical staff, wasting time and slowing the process.
2. Reflex testing rules are vague, poorly communicated, or not understandable to the least experienced FC technologist.
3. Reflex rules are complicated and involve integration of several pieces of information.

4. Reflex rules are applicable to only a small proportion of cases so do not become routine in the laboratory, and do not significantly alter work flow.
5. The rules result in an excessive proportion of cases requiring reflex testing, resulting in increased inefficiency and cost.
6. Reflex testing process is not integrated into FC laboratory workflow, resulting in slow turnaround time and impacting patient care.
7. Reflex test rules are not periodically revisited and tweaked.

SUMMARY

More cost-effective FC is possible in any clinical FC laboratory. The use of panels designed primarily to evaluate common diseases, and the development of easily followed criteria to identify cases where only a limited FC work-up is needed, are straightforward, especially as applied to peripheral blood samples. These strategies can make the laboratory more cost effective with minimal perceived impact to the user. Implementation of strategies to identify samples where FC is not indicated requires input from a broader constituency, support from health care administration, and clearly articulated goals to be successful.

REFERENCES

1. Davis BH, Holden JT, Bene MC, et al. 2006 Bethesda International Consensus recommendations on the flow cytometric immunophenotypic analysis of hemato-lymphoid neoplasia: medical indications. Cytometry B Clin Cytom 2007;72(Suppl 1):S5–13.
2. Wood BL, Arroz M, Barnett D, et al. 2006 Bethesda International Consensus recommendations on the immunophenotypic analysis of hematolymphoid neoplasia by flow cytometry: optimal reagents and reporting for the flow cytometric diagnosis of hematopoietic neoplasia. Cytometry B Clin Cytom 2007;72(Suppl 1): S14–22.
3. Reichard KK, Wood AJ. Laboratory test utilization management: general principles and applications in hematopathology. Surg Pathol Clin 2016;9:1–10.
4. David JA, Huang JZ. Diagnostic utility of flow cytometry analysis of reactive T cells in nodular lymphocyte-predominant Hodgkin lymphoma. Am J Clin Pathol 2016;145:107–15.
5. Wu D, Thomas A, Fromm JR. Reactive T cells by flow cytometry distinguish Hodgkin lymphomas from T cell/histiocyte-rich large B cell lymphoma. Cytometry B Clin Cytom 2016;90:424–32.
6. Oberley MJ, Fitzgerald S, Yang DT, et al. Value-based flow testing of chronic lymphoproliferative disorders: a quality improvement project to develop an algorithm to streamline testing and reduce costs. Am J Clin Pathol 2014;142:411–8.
7. Hoffmann DG, Kim BH. Limited flow cytometry panels on bone marrow specimens reduce costs and predict negative cytogenetics. Am J Clin Pathol 2014;141:94–101.
8. van Dongen JJM, Lhermitte L, Böttcher S, et al. EuroFlow antibody panels for standardized n-dimensional flow cytometric immunophenotyping of normal, reactive and malignant leukocytes. Leukemia 2012;26:1908–75.
9. Elnenaei MO, Campbell SG, Thoni AJ, et al. An effective utilization management strategy by dual approach of influencing physician ordering and gate keeping. Clin Biochem 2016;49:208–12.
10. Haycocks NG, Lawrence L, Cain JW, et al. Optimizing antibody panels for efficient and cost-effective flow cytometric diagnosis of acute leukemia. Cytometry B Clin Cytom 2011;80:221–9.

11. Gujral S, Polampalli SN, Badrinath Y, et al. Immunophenotyping of mature B-cell non Hodgkin lymphoma involving bone marrow and peripheral blood: critical analysis and insights gained at a tertiary care cancer hospital. Leuk Lymphoma 2009;50:1290–300.
12. Rajab A, Porwit A. Screening bone marrow samples for abnormal lymphoid populations and myelodysplasia-related features with one 10-color 14-antibody screening tube. Cytometry B Clin Cytom 2015;88:253–60.
13. Collie AMB, Hill BT, Stevens GH, et al. Flow cytometric analysis of cerebrospinal fluid has low diagnostic yield in samples without atypical morphology or prior history of hematologic malignancy. Am J Clin Pathol 2014;141:515–21.
14. Bossuyt PMM, Reitsma JB, Linnet K, et al. Beyond diagnostic accuracy: the clinical utility of diagnostic tests. Clin Chem 2012;58:1636–43.
15. Fryer AA, Smellie WSA. Managing demand for laboratory tests: a laboratory toolkit. J Clin Pathol 2013;66:62–72.
16. Kahan NR, Waitman DA, Vardy DA. Curtailing laboratory test ordering in a managed care setting through redesign of a computerized order form. Am J Manag Care 2009;15:173–6.
17. Andrews JM, Cruser DL, Myers JB, et al. Using peripheral smear review, age and absolute lymphocyte count as predictors of abnormal peripheral blood lymphocytoses diagnosed by flow cytometry. Leuk Lymphoma 2008;49:1731–7.
18. te Raa GD, Fischer K, Verweij W, et al. Use of the CD19 count in a primary care laboratory as a screening method for B-cell chronic lymphoproliferative disorders in asymptomatic patients with lymphocytosis. Clin Chem Lab Med 2011;49:115–20.
19. Tseng V, Morgan AS, Leith CP, et al. Efficient assessment of peripheral blood lymphocytosis in adults: developing new thresholds for blood smear review by pathologists. Clin Chem Lab Med 2014;52:1763–70.
20. Healey R, Naugler C, Koning L, et al. A classification tree approach for improving the utilization of flow cytometry testing of blood specimens for B-cell non-Hodgkin lymphoproliferative disorders. Leuk Lymphoma 2015;56:2619–24.

Automated Analysis of Clinical Flow Cytometry Data

A Chronic Lymphocytic Leukemia Illustration

Richard H. Scheuermann, PhD[a,*], Jack Bui, MD, PhD[b],
Huan-You Wang, MD, PhD[c], Yu Qian, PhD[a]

KEYWORDS

- Chronic lymphocytic leukemia • Minimal residual disease • Cell-based diagnostics
- Automated gating • Cluster analysis • Flow cytometry • FLOCK

KEY POINTS

- Traditional manual gating analysis of cytometry data cannot effectively address the scale and complexity of data generation from modern cytometry instrumentation.
- Bioinformatics investigators have developed a collection of computational methods for automated identification of cell populations from high-dimensional flow cytometry data; a small subset of these methods has been evaluated for their use in diagnostics applications of leukemia and lymphoma with promising results.
- By applying computational pipelines to classify and compare chronic lymphocytic leukemia (CLL) samples with healthy controls, the pilot study reported in this article illustrates the use of these methods to determine that traditional CLL definition based on CD5 and CD19 alone can be improved by also examining the expression levels of CD10 and CD79b in an automated fashion.
- Clinical validation of these computational approaches is ongoing and essential to realize the true potential of these methods for use in the clinical diagnostic laboratory.

BACKGROUND

Cells of the peripheral blood can serve as sentinels of the physiologic and pathologic state of an organism. Normal vascular recirculation and extravascular migration allow these cells to touch every part of the body. The number and phenotype of blood cells

Disclosure Statement: The authors do not have a conflict of interest to claim. This work was supported by the US National Institutes of Health - 1U01TR001801, CA157885, HHSN272201200005C, and U19AI118626 and The Hartwell Foundation-2013-1592.
[a] Department of Informatics, J. Craig Venter Institute, 4120 Capricorn Lane, La Jolla, CA 92037, USA;
[b] Department of Pathology, University of California, San Diego, Biomedical Sciences Building Room 1028, 9500 Gilman Drive, La Jolla, CA 92093-0612, USA; [c] Department of Pathology, School of Medicine, University of California, San Diego, 3855 Health Sciences Drive, La Jolla, CA 92093-0987, USA
* Corresponding author.
E-mail address: rscheuermann@jcvi.org

Clin Lab Med 37 (2017) 931–944
http://dx.doi.org/10.1016/j.cll.2017.07.011
0272-2712/17/© 2017 Elsevier Inc. All rights reserved.

labmed.theclinics.com

are also constantly influenced by the sea of cytokines, growth factors, hormones, and other small molecules they are bathed in, such that the cellular constituents of blood also reflect its molecular constituents. Thus, a detailed, accurate, and consistent representation of the qualitative and quantitative properties of blood cells can be used to understand the mechanistic underpinnings of disease and to identify potential biomarkers of disease diagnosis, prognosis, and therapeutic response.

In the 1960s, Alexander Vastem recognized that the enumeration of blood cell types (complete blood count, CBC) could be used diagnostically as evidence for certain kinds of infections and malignancies. Although the CBC has emerged as a critical laboratory assay, it cannot detect, with any detail, the phenotypes of the enumerated blood cells. Flow cytometry (FCM) represents an advancement in the analysis and characterization of blood cells, enabling researchers and clinicians to identify the surface antigen expression of blood cells using fluorochrome-conjugated antibodies, multiple lasers to provide specific excitation of fluorochromes, and several detectors to quantitate the emitted fluorescent signal. Indeed, using a simple cocktail of antibodies, each conjugated to defined fluorochromes with known emission ranges, an investigator can identify specific lymphoid and myeloid populations in peripheral blood, as well as the expression of antigenic determinants, some of which can be diagnostic or prognostic.

In 2007, Davis and colleagues[1] published recommendations from an expert panel regarding the medical indications for performing FCM-based diagnostic testing, including cytopenias, elevated leukocyte counts, atypical cells in bodily fluids, plasmacytosis or monoclonal gammopathy, and organomegaly. Based on the individual indications, specific staining panels are selected to target the likely cell suspects. For example, at the University of California, San Diego (UCSD) Center for Advanced Laboratory Medicine (CALM), 10 different tubes/panels are in routine use to aid in the diagnosis of acute and chronic leukemia. **Table 1** shows an example of 3 such tubes, the fluorescent channels used, and the antigens detected.

Although the use of these panels has demonstrated accurate and clinically actionable diagnosis and classification of hematolymphoid neoplasms, there is room for improvement, given the genetic and phenotypic diversity of blood cell diseases. For example, although flow cytometry can accurately diagnose acute promyelocytic leukemia (APL) based on multiple surface antigens, molecular subclassification of APL using cytogenetic detection of the t(15;17) translocation is diagnostic for a subtype that responds to all trans-retinoic acid. The fact that this leukemia appears to be derived from a distinct population of immature granulocytes suggests that this important subclassification could potentially be achieved using more complex staining panels alone without the need for cytogenetics. However, despite the routine use of complex (ie, >8 color) staining panels in research laboratories in recent years, high-complexity FCM panels have not been incorporated into routine use in the clinical FCM laboratory. In part, the lack of consensus of diagnostically relevant antigens and

Table 1
Markers used for diagnosis of acute and chronic leukemia

	Acute Myeloid Leukemia Panel					Chronic Lymphocytic Leukemia Panel			
	FL1	FL2	FL3	FL4		FL1	FL2	FL3	FL4
Tube 1	CD15	CD33	CD45	CD34	Tube 1	CD45	CD5	CD3	CD19
Tube 2	CD2	CD117	CD45	CD34	Tube 2	CD43	CD79a	CD5	CD19
Tube 3	HLA-DR	CD7	CD13	CD34	Tube 3	CD20	CD38	CD5	CD19

the inability to standardize analysis templates have hindered progress in clinical laboratories.

The current approach for identification of diagnostic cell populations from cytometry data is based on manual gating analysis, which is subjective, labor-intensive, and poorly reproducible, especially when dealing with higher-dimensional complex datasets. Over the last several years, our group and others have developed a suite of computational tools for the processing and analysis of cytometry data.[2,3] These include computational tools and informatics resources for: (i) data pre-processing to manipulate file formats, identify outlier events and samples, and adjust for batch effects; (ii) automated gating for supervised and unsupervised cell population identification; (iii) post-processing for cell-based biomarker identification, feature extraction, and data visualization; (iv) data standards and database resources for cytometry data dissemination. Most of these computational tools are made available as open source software with unrestrictive licensing, and most of the resources are publicly available.

In order to assess the performance of different computational approaches for cytometry data analysis and to provide guidance to end-users on their use, an international consortium - FlowCAP (Flow Cytometry Critical Assessment of Population Identification Methods, http://flowcap.flowsite.org) - was assembled to assess and compare computational methods through a series of analysis challenges. FlowCAP-I tested whether automated algorithms could reproduce expert manual gating; FlowCAP-II focused on sample classification.[4] FlowCAP-I showed that several algorithms were able to achieve similar results to expert manual analysis for 5 testing datasets from GvHD (graft-versus-host disease), DLBCL (diffuse large B-cell lymphoma), HSCT (hematopoietic stem cell transplant), WNV (symptomatic West Nile virus infection), and normal donors (NDs). As an example of their performance, multiple methods achieved F-measure scores for event-level classification accuracy of greater than 0.9 compared with expert manual gating for DLBCL in human peripheral blood mononuclear cell (PBMC) samples. In FlowCAP-II, several classification algorithms were able to effectively classify acute myeloid leukemia (AML) from non-AML samples with 100% accuracy. These computational methods have now been found to effectively identify novel cell-based biomarkers in a variety of research settings.

A few studies have now begun to evaluate the use of these methods in diagnostic settings. In 2012, Bashashati and colleagues[5] used the flowClust method to identify a subtype of diffuse large B-cell lymphoma (DLBCL), in which the lymphoma cells showed a unique high side scatter pattern reflecting internal cellular complexity. Importantly, the subset of patients carrying this DLBCL subtype showed significantly inferior overall and progression-free survival, suggesting that this lymphoma phenotype might serve as a useful biomarker to identify DLBCL patients at high risk for relapse. Zare and colleagues[6] used the SamSPECTRAL and FeaLect methods to identify features in flow cytometry data that are useful in distinguishing between mantle cell lymphoma (MCL) and small lymphocytic lymphoma (SLL), and showed that the classification accuracy increased, for MCL from 64% to 100% and for SLL from 69% to 97%, compared with standard of care manual analysis of the diagnostic flow cytometry data. Craig and colleagues[7] used the flowType and RchyOptimyx methods and found that a CD10+ CD38- B cell population showed significantly different proportions in germinal center B-cell lymphoma versus germinal center hyperplasia; however, the absolute proportion in any given patient was not considered specific enough to be used in a diagnostic setting. Dorfman and colleagues[8] used the FLOCK methods to identify discrete mast cell populations in most patients with systemic mastocytosis, with a sensitivity of 75% and a specificity of 86%. Dorfman and colleagues[9] also used FLOCK to identify discrete plasma cell populations in the bone marrow of patients with plasma cell neoplasms with a sensitivity of 97%, compared with only 81% for standard flow cytometric analysis. Finally, Levine and colleagues[10] used the PhenoGraph method, which algorithmically defines phenotypes in high-dimensional single-cell data, to stratify acute myeloid leukemia (AML) patients into subtypes with prognostic differences based on the activation of signaling pathways derived using mass cytometry data. These examples clearly indicate the promise of using computational approaches of flow cytometry data in a clinical diagnostics setting.

As the complexity of cytometry data has increased in recent years, it has been recognized by the translational research community that computational support is becoming essential for accurate single-cell phenotyping. With the advent of clinical genomics applications, the diagnostic laboratory environment will need to become familiar with the validation and use of computational pipelines in diagnostic workflows. In the case of cytometry, the integration of computational methods into the laboratory workflow would allow for the use of more complex staining panels for traditional diagnostic tests (ie, leukemia and lymphomas) where objective analysis methods could provide for more consistent disease characterization and subtype identification with therapeutic and prognostic implications. In addition, the ability to consistently manage and interpret data from complex staining panels would also allow for the validation of diagnostic tests for other diseases, including the monitoring of tumor cells for solid tumors and the diagnosis and monitoring of other immune-mediated diseases (eg, allergy, asthma, and autoimmune disease). And while diagnostic flow analysis has historically focused on the identification of neoplastic cells within the patient sample, a comprehensive elucidation of both the neoplastic and normal cellular components may also help identify candidates for cancer immunotherapy and contribute to the goals of precision medicine.

ILLUSTRATION

In order to illustrate the potential use of these computational methods in a clinical diagnostic setting, we present the results of our preliminary attempts to optimize the application of a selected set of computational methods for the automated identification of chronic lymphocytic leukemia (CLL) cells stained with a newly implemented 10-marker panel. The goal is to illustrate the process of computational pipeline optimization, to highlight the promise that these methods bring for more objective identification of CLL cells in patient samples, and to explore their potential utility for monitoring of minimal residual disease (MRD).

The computational data processing and analysis workflow we have implemented for the CLL FCM data analysis (**Fig. 1**A) consists of the following steps.

Data Preparation

Twenty FCS 3.0 files from peripheral blood samples of 20 subjects were received from UCSD clinical laboratories for CLL diagnostic evaluation. Eleven subjects received a diagnosis of CLL; 5 subjects were reported as having no evidence of CLL (no-CLL), and 4 subjects were evaluated for the presence of MRD following therapy. Protected health information (PHI) was scrubbed from the file headers and pseudo file names were used in the data analysis. Except for the corresponding subject disease status (CLL, non-CLL, MRD), no other clinical data about the

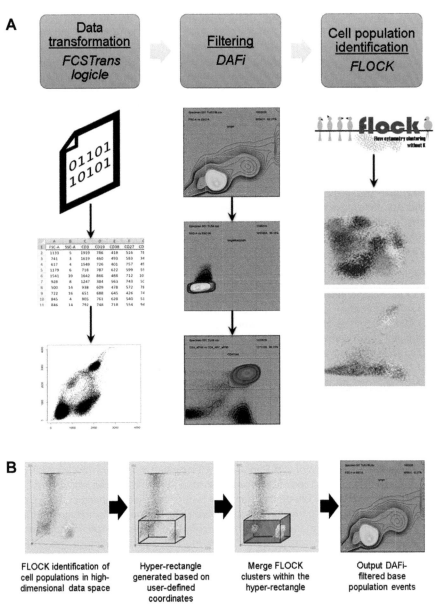

Fig. 1. Computational workflow for FCM data analysis. (*A*) The computational workflow used to analyze the CLL study data. Initial data transformation uses the FCS file format as input to the FCSTrans algorithm,[11] which applies a logicle transformation[15] to the fluorescence intensity values in order to obtain more normal distributions. The cell events are then filtered based on intensity values of selected parameters (eg, FSC and SSC to capture lymphocyte events based on size and complexity) using the DAFi-filtering method (Qian Y and Scheuermann R, 2017, unpublished data). Filtered events from all individual sample files are merged into a single file and cell populations identified using the FLOCK method[12] for unsupervised, density-based clustering. Cell events are then segregated back into sample-specific files while retaining cell population membership annotations to facilitate cross-sample comparison. (*B*) Details of DAFi filtering steps. The DAFi filtering method begins

subjects have been disclosed. The reagents used in the 10 color CLL panel were: CD45-FITC, CD22-PE, CD5-PerCP55, CD19-PECy7, CD79b-APC, CD23-APC-R700, CD81-APC-H7, CD10-BV421, CD43-BV510, and CD3-BV605. Cells were stained according to our standard protocol; acquisition was performed on a BD FACSCanto 10-color instrument, and manual analysis was done using FCS Express software (DeNovo).

Logicle Transformation

The second step in the workflow is to apply FCSTrans[11] to convert the binary FCS files, compensate them using the compensation matrices in the file headers, and transform the cellular marker expression values for optimizing the segregation of cell populations for both visualization and data analysis purposes. FCSTrans reproduces the logicle transformation procedure used in the FlowJo software (TreeStar, Incorporated) and generates consistent displays and transformed values.[11] The output of FCSTrans for each FCS file is a data matrix with each column a parameter measured in the FCM experiment and each row a cellular event.

Prefiltering

Although unsupervised data clustering methods can be applied to the whole data file for identification of cell populations, they usually generate a large number of data clusters as the number of parameters measured in an FCM experiment keeps increasing. Interpreting and annotating these data clusters is labor-intensive. Some of the data clusters were found in debris, dead cells, and doublets. Including a data prefiltering step before the cluster analysis step allows the computational pipeline to focus on the cells of interest. Depending on the data clustering method used in the pipeline, the prefiltering step also helps the identification of small cell subsets, reduces the run time of the pipeline, and allows the population summary statistics (eg, proportions) to be calculated based on the parent populations of interest.

A data prefiltering method we recently developed, called DAFi (Directed Automated Filtering and Identification of Cell Populations), is applied to identify the CLL cells from the input FCS files. The steps of DAFi are illustrated in **Fig. 1**B. In the first step of DAFi, the unsupervised FLOCK clustering method[12] is applied to partition the data into many small data clusters. Compared with unsupervised learning methods, a major feature of DAFi is that it requires a manual gating strategy from the user. For the identification of the CLL cells, the 2-dimensional coordinates in user manual gating based on FSC/SSC, CD45, CD3, CD5, and CD19, are combined into a hyper-rectangle for the computational identification of the CLL cells in the high-dimensional space, through the merging of FLOCK-identified data clusters whose centroids are located within the hyper-rectangle. Finally, the filtered data are displayed in 2-dimensional plots for visual examination. Unlike supervised methods, this approach preserves the data-driven characteristics of unsupervised learning, which identifies data clusters

---

by clustering cells into population in high-dimensional space using FLOCK. A hyper-rectangle is defined by the user to define the spatial regions that contain the cell populations of interest. The cell events of cell populations with centroids located within the hyper-rectangle of interest are then merged into a single base population for further downstream analysis using a cell population identification method, for example, FLOCK.

using all data dimensions simultaneously without preconceived bias. On the other hand, through the use of a manual gating definition and plotting high-dimensional data clusters on 2-dimensional plots, DAFi facilitates the interpretation of the data analysis results in a way that the user predefines.

Unsupervised Identification of Chronic Lymphocytic Leukemia Subsets Using FLOCK

The FLOCK-based computational pipeline[12] was applied to identify subsets in the CLL cells through unsupervised cluster analysis. In order to map the FLOCK-identified data clusters across the 20 files, the CLL data was first normalized across the files with the 0 to 1 min-max normalization method, and then merged the data together into a single file for FLOCK analysis. FLOCK returned a cluster membership file for each event in the merged data, and a custom script was then used to separate the events back into each original file together with their cluster membership. Thus, the same set of cluster IDs is used across the 20 files to indicate the mapping of these data clusters.

The FLOCK pipeline outputs summary statistics tables with each row corresponding to one experiment sample and each column a cell population identified in the sample. The contents of these tables include percentage values of cell subsets, mean fluorescence intensities (MFI) on each marker, cell phenotype profiles, and other predefined statistical analysis results. Then *P*-values based on statistical hypothesis testing can be calculated (eg, through a nonparametric Wilcoxon rank sum test) to indicate if there is a significant difference in cell population summary statistics between the subject groups.

RESULTS

The goal of this study was to determine if a computational pipeline could be developed for the identification of diagnostic cell populations in CLL patient samples using FCM data. We chose to use a new method we recently developed for directed unsupervised population identification called DAFi (Qian Y and Scheuermann R, 2017, unpublished data). The DAFi approach uses "direction" from prior knowledge about the cell populations of interest that it typically used to drive manual gating analysis. **Fig. 2** shows a typical manual gating hierarchy used in the CALM diagnostic lab to identify CLL cells from FCM data with their new 10-color panel. A plot of time versus SSC-A is used to determine if there are any instrument anomalies occurring during data acquisition; a plot of FSC-A versus FSC-H is used to gate on singlet cells with FSC-A = FSC-H. SSC-H versus CD45 is used to gate on leukocytes; FSC-A versus SSC-A is used to gate on lymphocytes, and CD5 versus CD19 is used to gate on putative CLL cells (CD5+CD19+), normal B cells (CD5-CD19+), and normal T cells (CD5+CD19-). DAFi was initially configured to produce a hyper-rectangle to recapitulate this manual gating hierarchy.

Cell events retained by these initial DAFi filters for a single CLL blood sample are shown in **Fig. 3** (*upper panels*), and for a composite of all 20 samples in the data set following unsupervised clustering using the FLOCK method in **Fig. 3** (*lower panels*). The results from individual samples show that all 3 cell populations show natural distributions with the expected marker expression levels. The composite results show that although the general expected marker expression levels are observed for all samples, there also appears to be some heterogeneity in their absolute fluorescence levels, especially in terms of CD5 expression in normal T cells (bottom middle) and both CD5 and CD19 expression in CLL cells (bottom right). The heterogeneity in CD5 expression can also be seen in plots from individual samples (**Fig. 4**), with

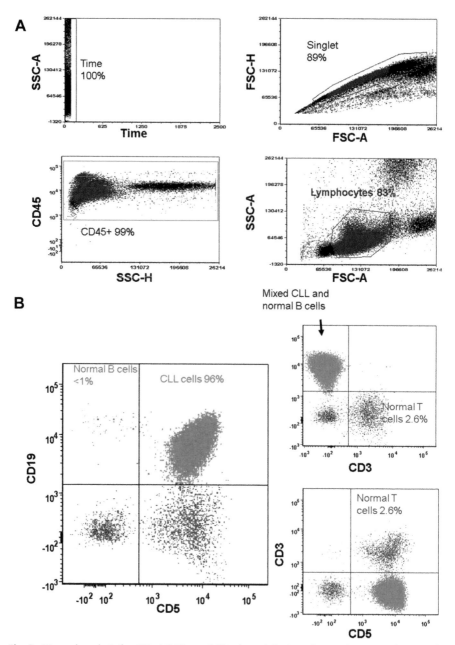

Fig. 2. Manual analysis for CLL. (*A*) Manual filtering of the lymphocyte base population. The singlet viable lymphocyte base population is captured using as FSC-H=FSC-A, CD45+, SSC-H low, SSC-A low, and FSC-A intermediate. (*B*) CLL gate. CLL cells (*red*) are classically distinguished from normal B lymphocytes (CD19+, CD3-, CD5-; *green*) and T lymphocytes (CD19-, CD3+, CD5+; *maroon*) as being uniquely CD19+, CD3- and CD5+.

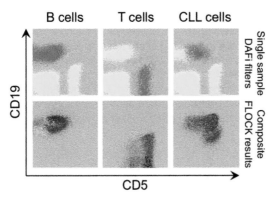

Fig. 3. DAFi filtering and FLOCK clustering of CLL FCM data. The DAFi algorithm was configured to recapitulate the manual gating strategy for capturing normal B cells (*upper left*), normal T cells (*upper middle*), and CLL cells (*upper right*) as depicted in **Fig. 2**, with the cell events retained colored in red and cell events excluded colored in yellow, from a single CLL peripheral blood sample. The cell events for each of these 3 cell types from all samples were then merged and subpopulation clusters identified using FLOCK-based unsupervised clustering, with cell events from each sample colored in a different color (*lower panels*). Considerable heterogeneity between individual samples can be observed.

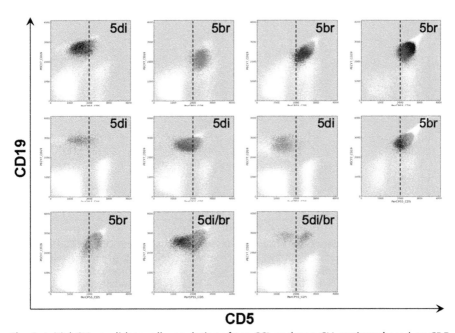

Fig. 4. Initial CLL candidate cell populations from CCL and non-CLL patients based on CD5 and CD19 expression only. DAFi filtering of CD5+CD19+ cells (putative CLL cells) from peripheral blood samples of 11 different CLL patients are shown. The putative CLL population was further subdivided into subpopulation clusters using FLOCK-based unsupervised clustering, with cell events from each putative CLL subpopulation colored in a different color. Considerable variability in absolute CD5 expression between patients can be observed, with some patients carrying putative CLL cells with relatively dim (5di) and some with relatively bright (5br) expression of CD5.

some samples showing relatively high levels of CD5 expression (bright - br), some showing intermediate levels (dim - di), and some showing a mixture of both (di/br).

In order to verify that the initial DAFi filters were specifically isolating CLL cells, we compared cells retained by the initial DAFi filters from both CLL and non-CLL patients. Unfortunately, cell retained by these initial DAFi filters were observed in 3 of the 5 non-CLL samples evaluated in the CD5 versus CD19 dot plots (**Fig. 5**A). To investigate this discrepancy further, the expression pattern of other cell surface markers that could be useful for improving the specificity of DAFi filtering was examined, and it was found

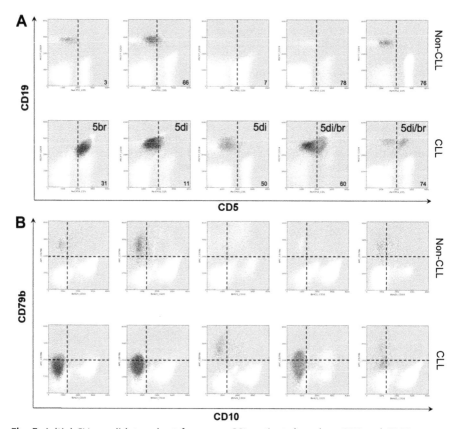

Fig. 5. Initial CLL candidate subset from non-CCL patients based on CD5 and CD19 expression only. DAFi filtering of CD5+CD19+ cells (putative CLL cells) from peripheral blood samples of 5 different patients with (CLL, *lower rows*) and without (non-CLL, *upper rows*) a definitive diagnosis of CLL from a combination of clinical, cellular, and molecular diagnostic tests are shown. The putative CLL population was further subdivided into subpopulation clusters using FLOCK-based unsupervised clustering, with cell events from each putative CLL subpopulation colored in a different color. (*A*) CD5 versus CD19 dot plots. Based on the CD5+CD19+ CLL definition, cell events captured using DAFi filtering in non-CLL patients can be observed (*upper row*). (*B*) CD10 versus CD79b dot plots. Examination of the expression of CD10 and CD79b in the CD5+CD19+ population reveals that these cells in CLL patients generally lack expression of CD10 and exhibit dim expression of CD79b (*lower row*). Whereas in non-CLL patients, the CD5+CD19+ cells express high levels of CD79b with or without CD10 expression (*upper row*). These results suggest that a revised CLL definition of CD5+CD19+CD10-CD79dim could be more specific for the identification of authentic CLL cells.

that most putative CLL cells from CLL patients were CD10- and CD79b dim, whereas the seemingly CLL cells retained by the initial DAFi filters in non-CLL patients were CD79b bright and CD10 + or -.

Based on these finding, the configuration of DAFi was adjusted to include additional filters for CD79b dim and CD10-. Although the use of these additional filtering criteria had little effect on CLL cell population identification in CLL samples (**Fig. 6**A), this

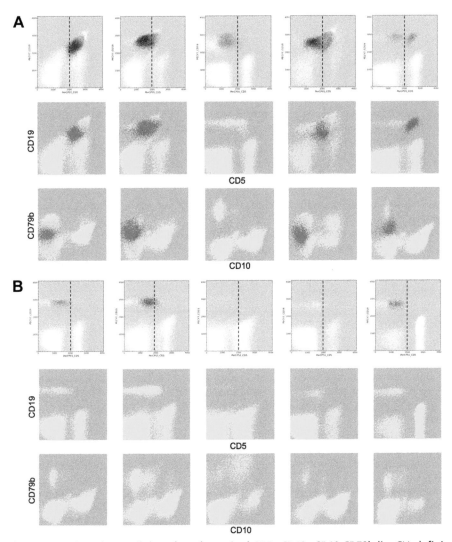

Fig. 6. Detection of CLL cells based on the revised CD5+CD19+CD10-CD79bdim CLL definition. The analysis presented in **Fig. 5** was repeated with the addition of DAFi filtering criteria to further filter based on the lack of CD10 expression and dim CD79b expression. Each of the top rows in A and B shows the results using the previous definition based on CD5+CD19+ only. The bottom 2 rows in each section show the DAFi filtering results using the revised definition, with the putative CLL cells colored in red. (*A*) Samples from 5 different CLL patients. (*B*) Samples from 5 different non-CLL patients.

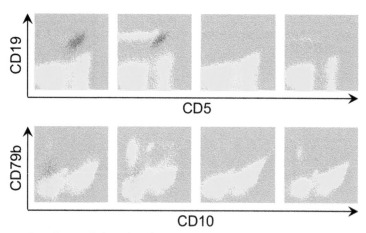

Fig. 7. Detection of CLL cells based on the revised CD5+CD19+CD10-CD79bdim definition in the setting of minimal residual disease. Peripheral blood samples from 4 different CLL patients in clinical remission following treatment were analyzed using DAFi filtering based on the revised CD5+CD19+CD10-CD79bdim CLL definition, with the CLL cells colored in red. Minimal residual disease is evident in 2 of the 4 patient peripheral blood samples.

revised definition eliminated the spurious retention of cell events in non-CLL samples (see **Fig. 6**B).

Finally, the ability of the revised DAFi filtering to detect CLL cells in the setting of MRD was examined, where distinguishing between CLL cells and normal B cells can be challenging. By including the CD10-and CD79b dim phenotypes in the revised CLL definition and DAFi filtering configuration, CLL cells could be clearly identified in 2 of the 4 MRD samples (**Fig. 7**).

DISCUSSION AND SUMMARY

In this illustration, the ability of an automated computational pipeline based on the DAFi method to identify CLL cells in multidimensional FCM data was examined. Using an initial definition based solely on the co-expression of CD5 and CD19, we found that the cell populations identified were not specific to CLL patients, but that the populations identified in CLL versus non-CLL patients differed in their expression of CD10 and CD79b. Indeed, this pattern of CD10 and CD79b expression in CLL cells has been reported previously.[7,13] By changing the cell population definition and configuration of DAFi to retain cells that are CD5+CD19+CD10-CD79bdim, cells that are specific to the CLL patient cohort could be automatically identified without manual gating.

By identifying CLL cells in multidimensional space simultaneously, DAFi filtering was robust to slight changes in marker expression. This robustness was especially important for CD5 expression, which showed considerable variability between CLL patients, ranging from bright to dim. In addition, the use of a precise multidimensional definition allowed for the sensitive identification of CLL cells in the setting of MRD.

We also observed considerable heterogeneity in CD5 expression in normal T cells (see **Fig. 3**). It should be noted that this population of normal T cells is not typically the focus of manual analysis and is considered irrelevant in the current diagnosis of CLL; however, the T cell phenotype of CLL patients could stratify responses to immune therapy and could find utility in the future. We postulate that an unbiased, automated analysis platform, as described herein, could be used to capture all of the populations in peripheral blood, thereby realizing the vision that peripheral blood samples could indeed reflect the physiology of the patient. As flow cytometry platforms become more complex and multidimensional, it may become impossible to examine and interpret all of the data manually.

The work presented here was a pilot study to demonstrate the feasibility of applying automated computational pipelines to diagnostic data using a relatively small number of samples and a subjective evaluation of the results. Based on the positive findings from this pilot, a prospective study is underway to expand the sample size and apply objective evaluation criteria to quantitatively assess the sensitivity, specificity, and predictive value of this approach for CLL diagnosis compared with standard-of-care practices. The protocol being used will allow for follow-up on any discrepancies between automated and manual analysis to determine if any additional diagnostic testing results and patient outcome information can be used to adjudicate the discrepancies. By examining the outcome of patients evaluated in the setting of MRD, one can also determine if monitoring CLL cell population levels using automated computational pipelines would have prognostic utility. In addition, in the pilot study we obtained evidence that distinct sub-types of CLL might exist based on the expression of the other markers (eg, CD22 and CD81) in the 10-color staining panel used (data not shown). However, the small sample size made it difficult to draw any definitive conclusions. The prospective study should help determine if the detection of distinct subtypes is reproducible and show different responses to therapy and prognostic outcome.

The ultimate goal of these efforts is to achieve adoption of automated computational pipelines for routine use in the clinical diagnostic laboratory. This goal presents a challenge in determining how best to validate computational pipelines for FCM data analysis for patient management use in a CLIA environment. Emerging experience with the application of computational methods for the processing and interpretation of next-generation sequencing data for diagnostic use[14] could be used to establish the necessary computational method validation plan for FCM data.

Flow cytometry analysis of patient samples has become an indispensable component of the modern diagnostic toolkit for various different hematopoietic diseases, especially leukemias, lymphomas, and myeloproliferative disorders. Advancements in cytometry instrumentation and the availability of more complex staining panel collections promise to allow for more accurate identification and monitoring of disease for improved diagnosis and prognosis of patients. However, these advances result in an increase in the complexity of data that feed into the diagnostic process. The validation and use of computational pipelines to assist in the processing and interpretation of these data will be essential to realize their true potential in the clinical laboratory.

REFERENCES

1. Davis BH, Holden JT, Bene MC, et al. 2006 Bethesda International Consensus recommendations on the flow cytometric immunophenotypic analysis of hematolymphoid neoplasia: medical indications. Cytometry B Clin Cytom 2007; 72(Suppl 1):S5–13.

2. O'Neill K, Aghaeepour N, Spidlen J, et al. Flow cytometry bioinformatics. PLoS Comput Biol 2013;9(12):e1003365.

3. Kvistborg P, Gouttefangeas C, Aghaeepour N, et al. Thinking outside the gate: single-cell assessments in multiple dimensions. Immunity 2015 Apr 21;42(4): 591–2.

4. Aghaeepour N, Finak G, Hoos H, et al, FlowCAP Consortium, DREAM Consortium. Critical assessment of automated flow cytometry data analysis techniques. Nat Methods 2013;10(3):228–38 [Erratum appears in Nat Methods 2013;10(5):445].

5. Bashashati A, Johnson NA, Khodabakhshi AH, et al. B cells with high side scatter parameter by flow cytometry correlate with inferior survival in diffuse large B-cell lymphoma. Am J Clin Pathol 2012;137(5):805–14.

6. Zare H, Bashashati A, Kridel R, et al. Automated analysis of multidimensional flow cytometry data improves diagnostic accuracy between mantle cell lymphoma and small lymphocytic lymphoma. Am J Clin Pathol 2012;137(1):75–85.

7. Craig FE, Foon KA. Flow cytometric immunophenotyping for hematologic neoplasms. Blood 2008;111(8):3941–67.

8. Dorfman DM, LaPlante CD, Pozdnyakova O, et al. FLOCK cluster analysis of mast cell event clustering by high-sensitivity flow cytometry predicts systemic mastocytosis. Am J Clin Pathol 2015;144(5):764–70.

9. Dorfman DM, LaPlante CD, Li B. FLOCK cluster analysis of plasma cell flow cytometry data predicts bone marrow involvement by plasma cell neoplasia. Leuk Res 2016;48:40–5.

10. Levine JH, Simonds EF, Bendall SC, et al. Data-driven phenotypic dissection of AML reveals progenitor-like cells that correlate with prognosis. Cell 2015;162: 184–97.

11. Qian Y, Liu Y, Campbell J, et al. FCSTrans: an open source software system for FCS file conversion and data transformation. Cytometry A 2012;81(5):353–6.

12. Qian Y, Wei C, Eun-Hyung Lee F, et al. Elucidation of seventeen human peripheral blood B-cell subsets and quantification of the tetanus response using a density-based method for the automated identification of cell populations in multidimensional flow cytometry data. Cytometry B Clin Cytom 2010;78(Suppl 1):S69–82.

13. Hulkkonen J, Vilpo L, Hurme M, et al. Surface antigen expression in chronic lymphocytic leukemia: clustering analysis, interrelationships and effects of chromosomal abnormalities. Leukemia 2002;16(2):178–85.

14. Rehm HL, Bale SJ, Bayrak-Toydemir P, et al, Working Group of the American College of Medical Genetics and Genomics Laboratory Quality Assurance Committee. ACMG clinical laboratory standards for next-generation sequencing. Genet Med 2013;15(9):733–47.

15. Parks DR, Roederer M, Moore WA. A new "Logicle" display method avoids deceptive effects of logarithmic scaling for low signals and compensated data. Cytometry A 2006;69(6):541–51.

Applications of Mass Cytometry in Clinical Medicine

The Promise and Perils of Clinical CyTOF

Gregory K. Behbehani, MD, PhD

KEYWORDS

- Mass cytometry • CyTOF • Flow cytometry • Minimal residual disease
- Acute leukemia • Aberrant marker expression

KEY POINTS

- Mass cytometry enables cytometric measurement of up to 50 parameters per single cell through the use of time-of-flight mass spectrometry and heavy-metal tagged antibodies.
- The high number of parameters facilitates analysis of highly complex cell populations and could be extremely useful for the diagnosis of malignant hematologic disorders, monitoring of minimal residual disease, and selection of treatment modalities.
- Mass cytometry could also be very useful for characterization of autoimmune disorders and monitoring of immunotherapy approaches.
- Several unique challenges associated with mass cytometry analysis need to be addressed before the technology could be used for clinical testing.
- The large amounts of data generated from mass cytometry assays are best analyzed using bioinformatic algorithms that enable a range of new approaches to the analysis of clinical samples.

INTRODUCTION

Flow cytometry has become an increasingly important diagnostic tool in the clinical laboratory for the study of malignancies, infectious diseases, and immune system function. Its utility stems from its ability to analyze single cells for their expression of virtually any protein to which an antibody, or similar reagent, can be specifically bound. This enables the identification and quantification of different cell types in complex biologic samples as well as the simultaneous assessment of a wide variety of functional properties of each cell. These many advantages have led flow cytometry to become

The author has nothing to disclose.
Division of Hematology, The Ohio State University and James Cancer Hospital, B305 Starling Loving Hall, 320 West 10th Avenue, Columbus, OH 43210, USA
E-mail address: Gregory.behbehani@osumc.edu

Clin Lab Med 37 (2017) 945–964
http://dx.doi.org/10.1016/j.cll.2017.07.010 labmed.theclinics.com
0272-2712/17/© 2017 Elsevier Inc. All rights reserved.

a critical tool for the diagnosis of hundreds of medical disorders, and it is now routinely used for making critical treatment decisions. Despite its tremendous utility, however, most current clinical flow cytometry technologies are limited to analysis of 4 to 12 simultaneous measurement parameters. The dependence on fluorescent reporter molecules also makes flow cytometry susceptible to various artifacts due to the fluorescent properties of the cells being studied and interactions between the reagents being used to study them. Correcting for these artifacts requires extensive controls and experienced operators. Fortunately, the technology of cytometry continues to advance rapidly with newer machines and newer reagents being developed to improve upon these limitations. Perhaps none of these innovations is more transformative than the recent development of mass cytometry. Although there are now numerous publications using this technology and many excellent reviews,[1–4] this review focuses on its potential use in the clinical cytometry laboratory, where it may soon arrive and become an important tool to enhance cytometry's role in clinical practice.

Mass cytometry is a cytometric technique similar to fluorescent flow cytometry that detects antibody binding to cellular antigens through the use of mass spectrometry rather than fluorescent detection.[1,5] The technology uses binding of the same antigen-specific antibodies used in conventional flow cytometry, but measures this binding by attaching isotopically purified heavy metal atoms to the antibodies instead of fluorophores. The presence of the bound antibodies is then detected through the use of inductively coupled plasma ionization and time-of-flight mass spectrometry (ICP-MS TOF) analysis of the metal ions that were attached to each antibody. The advantage of this approach stems from the ability of ICP-MS to distinguish ions of different atomic weight with less than 1% signal spillover between adjacent masses. When done properly, mass cytometry data are nearly identical to fluorescent flow cytometry data for most antigens, and currently up to 40 to 50 parameters can be simultaneously recorded per cell without significant compensation or background from autofluorescence. Theoretically, the technology could measure up to 120 simultaneous parameters. This huge increase in parameters enables a broad range of new applications, all of which have the capacity to analyze highly complex cell populations in ways that were previously extremely difficult or impossible. The goal of this review is to provide a broad overview of the mass cytometry technology and how it might be applied in clinical settings. Specifically, the author addresses the major strengths of mass cytometry analysis, some limitations that will be particularly relevant for clinical applications, and some of the most common analysis methodologies used to explore the resulting data.

MASS CYTOMETRY BASICS

Mass cytometry is essentially a fusion of flow cytometry and ICP-MS, with the sample collection and processing steps being nearly identical to a flow cytometry workflow, and the data acquisition almost entirely based on ICP-MS TOF. The basic workings of a mass cytometer have been described in numerous publications,[1,5,6] so they will only be briefly summarized here. A schematic diagram of mass cytometry analysis (from Di Palma and Bodenmiller[4]) is shown in **Fig. 1**. Cells are first collected and processed in the same manner as a regular flow cytometry experiment. In general, the same cell processing methods used to assay the antigens of interest by fluorescent flow cytometry should be used for mass cytometry analysis of those same antigens. The cells are incubated (or "stained") with antibodies just as in standard flow cytometry assays (with the exception that the antibodies are conjugated to heavy metals rather than fluorophores). In most cases, the same antibody clones and protocols

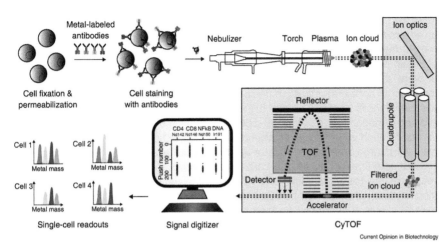

Current Opinion in Biotechnology

Fig. 1. Schematic of mass cytometry analysis. Cells are typically fixed before analysis to preserve the intracellular state being studied. Cells are then permeabilized (if needed) and stained with antibodies specific for surface and intracellular antigens of interest using antibodies conjugated to atoms of isotopically purified heavy metal. The cells with bound antibodies are then nebulized into a stream of argon gas and passed through a radiofrequency-induced argon plasma that vaporizes and ionizes the cells, antibodies, and the attached heavy metal atoms. After passing through the plasma, each cell becomes an ion cloud that enters the quadrupole filter, which removes all ion masses below approximately 75 Da. The remaining cloud of heavy metal ions then enters the TOF analysis where each cell ion cloud is segmented across several "pushes" of the TOF analysis. The electrical potential applied during each "push" imparts an acceleration to each metal ion inversely proportional to the ion's mass. As a result, the lightest ions strike the detector first with the heaviest striking last (the exact "mass windows" are tuned daily). The mass cytometer's software converts the signal data from each of the "pushes" back into cell events and then integrates the mass signals from each measurement channel for each cell event. The integrated mass signal for each channel and each cell event is then recorded as a standard FCS file. (*From* Di Palma S, Bodenmiller B. Unraveling cell populations in tumors by single-cell mass cytometry. Curr Opin Biotechnol 2015;31:124; with permission.)

used for flow cytometry can be used for staining of both surface and intracellular antigens. Unlike traditional fluorescent flow cytometry, however, cells must be incubated with a heavy metal DNA intercalator or other stain before analysis to allow identification of cell events that may lack antibody binding (as light scatter characteristics cannot be used for this purpose). Mass cytometry samples must also be analyzed in pure water (to prevent salt build-up and signal loss in the instrument), and this necessitates that samples are fixed after antibody staining to prevent cell lysis and ensure antibodies remain attached to their antigens in the absence of physiologic salt concentrations.

Once cells have been processed, they are diluted before analysis to ensure that cells are analyzed at an appropriate acquisition rate. Unlike traditional flow cytometers, the rate of liquid flow into the machine is kept constant to maintain plasma stability, and cell acquisition rate is thus controlled by adjusting the cell concentration in solution. The diluted cell suspension is pumped into a nebulizer that aerosolizes the cells into single-cell droplets. The aerosolized sample is funneled by a sheath of argon gas through a heating element to evaporate the water and then into an induced argon plasma at a temperature of about 7000°K. The plasma completely vaporizes and ionizes the cell and the attached antibodies into a cloud of single-atom ions. This cloud then enters the mass spectrometer where ions with a mass of less than ~75 Da are removed from the ion stream. This filtering step removes essentially all of the atoms that would normally be present in normal human cells, leaving only the heavy metals that were attached to the staining antibodies or reagents. The ion stream is then directed to an accelerator that creates a pulse of electrical potential every 13 μS accelerating any ions in front of it toward the ion detector. (The ion cloud generated by each cell is large enough that it takes 100–300 μS to cross the plane of the accelerator and, as a result, each cell event is segmented across 8–20 pulses.) Because the ions all have a +1 charge and the accelerator applies the same force to each of them, the acceleration and final speed attained are directly proportional to the mass of each ion. Because of this, the lightest ions cross the machine and hit the detector in the shortest period of time, whereas the heaviest take the longest. The time between when the accelerator pulses and when an ion hits the detector (measured in nanoseconds) is recorded as the "time-of-flight" and allows determination of which atoms are present in cell ion cloud. Ions of each 1-Da increment of mass typically strike the detector within a window of approximately 25 ns, and these mass windows are tuned based on a standard solution of atoms of known mass. The stream of data from these pulses is then computationally processed to determine the beginning and end of each cell ion cloud, and the total signal from each mass channel is integrated across all of the measurement pulses that detected ions from that cell. The integrated signal from each cell is then recorded in Flow Cytometry Standard (FCS) file format, which can be analyzed and processed just like an FCS file generated by a fluorescent flow cytometer.[1,6]

ADVANTAGES OF MASS CYTOMETRY

The biggest advantage of mass cytometry is the large increase in the number of simultaneous parameters that can be recorded from each cell event as compared with fluorescent flow cytometry. This is particularly useful in the analysis of highly complex or heterogeneous populations wherein the additional parameters can allow numerous cell types or functional states to be uniquely identified and characterized. A common criticism of mass cytometry is that the same experiments could be done with several overlapping flow cytometry panels, but this criticism both oversimplifies what would be involved in creating equivalent overlapping flow cytometry panels to characterize 30+ antigens and fails to recognize the many advantages afforded by having all parameters measured simultaneously. A typical mass cytometry experiment might involve utilization of 15 to 20 cell surface markers to identify 30 or more distinct immunophenotypic subsets within a complex cell mixture while simultaneously characterizing each cell with another 15 to 20 intracellular markers of cell function (eg, intracellular signaling, DNA damage, cell cycle, intracellular cytokines). This type of high-parameter experimental design affords many advantages over traditional flow cytometry approaches. First, specific relationships between every marker present in the experiment can be analyzed simultaneously without the need for complex patterns of overlapping smaller flow cytometry panels. Second, measuring all parameters simultaneously allows immunophenotypic classification to be performed through clustering techniques. Analysis through clustering enables each cell to be placed into one, and only one, classification group, ensuring both that every cell is accounted for and that it is only placed into one classification group (eg, CD4+ T cells, promyelocyte). Importantly, this approach also allows identification and enumeration of cells in the experiment that are negative for most, or even all, of the markers included in the analysis. Third, the interrelationship of the multiple markers can allow for identification of cell populations without the need for many markers classically used to identify them, for instance, natural killer (NK) cells in peripheral blood can be readily clustered into separate groups without the use of CD56 (through the use of CD3, CD7, CD45RA, and CD38), and plasma cells can be readily identified in human bone marrow without the need to stain with CD138 (based on CD45, CD38, CD19, and CD20 expression levels).

Obviously, the use of mass-tagged antibodies instead of fluorophore-conjugated antibodies also eliminates many fluorescence-associated complications and sources of error in traditional flow cytometry experiments. Chief among these is that, in properly designed antibody panels, there is no significant signal overlap between measurement channels and no need for compensation. In addition, there is no autofluorescent background, and as such, no problems related to exposure of samples to agents that are fluorescent (eg, daunorubicin) or that change the fluorescent properties of the cells being studied (such as fixation with glutaraldehyde). This lack of background fluorescence can also allow for more precise comparison of low levels of antigen expression that might otherwise be undetectable amid autofluorescent background. The mass cytometer also has only a single detector for all mass channels, eliminating the complexity of adjusting and monitoring the sensitivity of multiple detectors. Finally, current mass cytometry reagents are all created using the same DTPA chelator backbone to attach the heavy metal ions to each antibody, and these conjugates are stable after treatment with methanol or other alcohols, allowing sequential surface and intracellular staining protocols without restrictions related to the stability of the antibody conjugates used for the prepermeabilization staining step.

A final major advantage of mass cytometry is the ability to stain cells with other metal reagents that are not used as part of the ~40 antibody measurement channels. The most prominent application of this is cellular barcoding, which allows several (typically up to 20) samples to be combined into a single tube to allow for processing, antibody staining, and mass cytometry analysis to be performed simultaneously on all samples within a single tube.[7–9] Barcoding enables a dramatic reduction in the technical variation of measurements across the barcoded samples (to coefficients of variation as low as 3%) and allows for reference or control samples to be included in the same tube with the experimental samples. This can allow for very precise comparisons between different samples in the context of time-course experiments, or head-to-head comparisons of samples treated with experimental agents to controls. Barcoding also enables the same immunophenotypic gates to be applied across all samples within an experiment. This approach can be extremely useful when studying malignant or otherwise abnormal cells for which there are no routine gate boundaries. By mixing normal cells with the abnormal ones, gates can be drawn on the normal cells and then applied to all of the other abnormal ones without adjustment.[10] In addition, barcoding can reduce the time required for sample processing and analysis and can frequently reduce reagents costs as well. Along with barcoding, several other nonantibody reagents are available to characterize other cell properties, such as membrane content,[11] nucleotide incorporation into DNA,[12] cell membrane integrity (ie, live/dead staining),[13] total DNA content,[5] and even hypoxia.[14]

CHALLENGES OF CLINICAL MASS CYTOMETRY

There are also some significant challenges specific to mass cytometry that bear discussion. These challenges are particularly relevant to potential clinical applications, because these issues must be rigorously controlled in order to achieve data sufficiently consistent and reliable to allow for its use in making clinical decisions. First among these is that removal of photometric measurement precludes measurement of forward and side scatter. This can significantly complicate assessment of populations such as blasts that are typically identified by their scatter properties. The iridium-based intercalator used for identifying cell events in mass cytometry binds both DNA and nonspecifically binds to cellular protein and thus represents a correlate to cell size, allowing it to be used as an approximate substitute for forward light scatter. Currently, however, there is no good mass cytometry surrogate for side scatter, and thus it is not possible to identify an exact correlate to some commonly measured cell populations such as blasts gated on CD45 and side scatter. As a result, population identification by mass cytometry must be performed almost solely on the basis of cell immunophenotype, which fortunately can be done with extremely high resolution.

A second major issue is that mass cytometry has a significantly lower throughput than fluorescent flow cytometry. To collect high-quality data, cells can typically be run no faster than 200 to 400 cells per second, which is almost an order of magnitude slower than current fluorescent flow cytometers. This limitation stems from the fact that cell ionization is achieved by vaporizing each cell into a cloud of ions, and the borders of these clouds can easily fuse if cells are run at too high of a concentration. This throughput limitation is also related to another significant caveat of mass cytometry, which is the much higher frequency of doublet events observed in mass cytometry measurement. Much like clouds in the sky, the ion clouds formed by plasma ionization can fuse with one another when cell analysis rate is high, and it can be difficult to determine the boundaries of the original cell event clouds. Similar to flow cytometry, a singlet gate can be used to reduce the frequency of doublet events; however, only about half of total doublet events can be removed under most circumstances without leading to significant (and potentially biased) loss of real single-cell events. So far, the best strategies for doublet management are slow rates of cell acquisition and the use of barcoding techniques featuring nonredundant metal codes that allow for identification of doublet events through detection of an "illegal barcode."

Mass cytometry also suffers from 2 issues related to signal intensity. First, because of the inherit efficiency of ion transmission and the amount of metal ions that can currently be attached to an antibody, a particular antibody clone conjugated to a heavy metal and analyzed by mass cytometry typically gives a detection sensitivity similar to a fluorescein isothiocyanate–conjugated (FITC) reagent made from the same monoclonal antibody analyzed on a flow cytometer. This level of sensitivity is sufficient for the large majority of antigens of clinical interest; however, certain antigens may have a sufficiently low abundance that they can only be reliably detected with antibodies conjugated to very bright fluorophores, such as phycoerythrin or allophycocyanin. Detection of such low abundance antigens can be difficult by mass cytometry, although it is worth noting that the lack autofluorescent background does allow for detection of significantly smaller absolute signal differences than can be typically measured with fluorescence-based instruments. Fortunately, new methods to enhance the amount of metal that can be attached to each antibody are being developed that can increase this sensitivity.

The second signal intensity issue that requires attention is inherent to ICP-MS analysis, which suffers from a consistent, time-dependent decrease in sensitivity that occurs due to the accumulation of salt and oxidized molecules of sample on the cones and other surfaces of the machine. In the mass cytometer, this buildup reduces the efficiency with which ions are transmitted through the machine and leads to a decrease in the ion sensitivity and an apparent loss of signal. Over the course of many hours, this can lead to a decrease of 30% to 50% in apparent signal. Fortunately, this effect occurs very predictably and is generally uniform across the mass range. Because of this, this signal decrease can be readily measured and normalized by mixing metal-containing polystyrene standard beads with cell samples. Because these beads are evenly distributed across the cell sample, they also provide a real-time indicator of the mass cytometer's performance throughout the course of sample analysis.[15] These standards should be included in all mass cytometry experiments, and the data from these bead events are extremely useful in determining the cause of any problems in machine performance and can be used to remove any data collected during any time period when machine performance is not within specifications (eg, reduced signal intensity, increased oxidation).

The metals used to label antibodies can also create unique artifacts and errors in mass cytometry analysis. Although the excellent atomic resolution of the mass cytometer means that less than 1% of the signal of one atomic mass detection channel spillover into the adjacent channel, some "spillover" artifacts are still present in the data. Chief among these are isotopic impurities present in the lanthanide metal isotopes used to label the antibodies. To achieve the high number of mass channels available, multiple isotopic forms of each metal species are used for antibody labeling. For example, the metal Neodymium (Nd) has 7 stable isotopes with masses of 142, 143, 144, 145, 146, 148, and 150 Da, and each can be purified from the others. By separately conjugating these purified isotopes to antibodies, 7 different measurement channels can be created using Nd. However, the purification process is not perfect, particularly for isotopes of low natural abundance, so the isotopically purified metal salt solutions used to label the antibodies frequently have 1% to 4% of other isotopic species present as a contaminant. Most commonly, the contamination is from the isotopic species 1 Da heavier (although other contaminating isotopic species may also be present). For instance, the Nd143 salt used to label antibodies contains 2.2% Nd144, and this creates an apparent 2.2% spillover from the 143 channel into the 144 channel. In most panel designs, this spillover is negligible because a signal of 100 counts in the 143 channel will only result in a spillover signal of 2 counts in the 144 channel, which would typically not be above measurement background. However, just like in fluorescent flow cytometry, such spillovers can create significant data artifacts and reduce measurement sensitivity when a very highly expressed marker spills into a marker with a very low expression level. Thus, the same considerations of expected marker intensities and expected spillovers used in fluorescent antibody panel designs are relevant to mass cytometry, although to a much less significant degree. In rare cases, these spillovers require compensation, and this can be performed similar to fluorescent flow cytometry compensation, with reasonable accuracy on the newer mass cytometers. Furthermore, the isotopic impurities of each metal are known and consistent, and investigators can consider these impurities when designing mass cytometry reagent panels. A second common artifact comes from the oxidation of the metal ions by oxygen during the interval between ionization in the plasma and detection. The addition of an oxygen atom creates an apparent spillover into the channel 16 Da above. The propensity for this oxidation to occur depends on the chemical properties of each individual metal and is greatest for Lanthanum (La; for this reason, the oxidation of La is used to tune the mass cytometer so that the fraction of oxide formed is <2.5%). For these reasons, "M+1" and "M+16" spillovers are the most common artifacts in mass cytometry data, and these should be assessed in all mass cytometry experiments (particularly when the intensity of a marker is above several hundred ion counts). Fortunately, the absence of significant background in mass cytometry makes the presence of these artifacts quite obvious in biaxial plots of any given marker compared with the mass channels 1 and 16 Da above it. Thus, use of "minus one" controls are not typically needed to identify and compensate for such artifacts. In certain experimental systems, however, panels will need to be redesigned to eliminate particularly large or problematic spillovers.

Finally, mass cytometry analysis can be complicated by clogs and sample carryover in the fluidics systems of the instrument. In the newest mass cytometer design (Helios), these issues have been greatly improved, but remain an important consideration for the analysis of clinical samples. When cells aggregate within the fluidics system, either complete or partial clogs can form disrupting data analysis, requiring downtime for instrument maintenance. Partially clogging cell aggregates are most problematic, because they may shear other cells as they pass around the aggregate or clumps of these cells can come loose and pass into the nebulizer, giving rise to doublet events. It is thus important to monitor the mass cytometer carefully during data collection so that any fluidics problems are detected quickly before sample is wasted and potentially misleading data are collected.

POTENTIAL CLINICAL APPLICATIONS

Despite the additional complexities of mass cytometry analysis, the technology has tremendous potential for the analysis of clinical samples. This potential has been most notable in analysis of malignant diseases and in the characterization and monitoring of immune system function. In both contexts, the high number of parameters afforded by mass cytometry enables the organization of numerous distinct cell populations within very complex cell samples, while still allowing sufficient additional measurement parameters to characterize functional properties of the different cell populations. The data generated from such studies would be very difficult to obtain using overlapping fluorescent flow cytometry panels, and in some cases, mass cytometry represents the only technology capable of performing these types of experiments.

High-parameter analysis of malignant diseases, particularly leukemias, is an area in which mass cytometry could be particularly useful in the clinic, and initial experiments have been performed by several research groups.[10,16–19] These studies highlight a particular strength of high-parameter analysis: the ability to define rare cell types, such as leukemia stem cells, and simultaneously characterize the functional properties of these cells. The author's group used mass cytometry for the analysis of ex vivo samples from patients with acute myeloid leukemia (AML) and myelodysplastic syndrome (MDS).[10] By barcoding patient samples with normal reference control samples, each patient sample could be compared with normal bone marrow samples across a panel of 25 cell surface markers and 20 intracellular markers. This allowed grouping of cells by developmental stage and direct comparison of the malignant cells from patient samples to developmentally similar normal cells. This process enabled identification of abnormal expression levels of multiple surface markers in cells from every patient sample at all stages of myeloid development. This type of analytical approach, only possible through high-parameter analysis, has the potential to greatly increase the sensitivity of minimal residual disease (MRD) detection. In addition, the leukemia cells with abnormal surface marker expression patterns were also shown to exhibit abnormal basal intracellular signaling and altered cell cycle properties. Because malignant cells by their nature have disrupted gene expression programs, it is likely that sufficiently precise and sufficiently high-parameter analysis of surface and intracellular antigens could very reliably distinguish almost any malignant cell from normal ones at the single-cell level.

Using these principles, mass cytometry could be used to not only detect rare persistent cancer cells, but to also identify therapeutically targetable functional properties of these cells (such as up-regulated signaling pathways, increased expression of immune checkpoint inhibitors, or altered DNA damage response pathways). For example, we could identify rare immunophenotypic stem cell populations with extremely low S-phase fractions in samples from patients with AML subtypes (such as those with FLT3-ITD mutations) known to respond poorly to S-phase specific consolidation therapy.[10] Importantly, these patients with FLT3-ITD AML also exhibited increased expression of CD33 and CD123 on the quiescent progenitor cells, suggesting these antigens as therapeutic targets. Preliminary evidence from clinical trials supports the suggestion that these targets may be particularly efficacious in this AML subtype.[20] An example of this aberrant antigen detection is shown in **Fig. 2**. Spanning-tree Analysis of Density Normalized Events (SPADE) analysis (described in detail in later discussion) was used to simultaneously analyze several bone marrow samples from leukemia patients and healthy donors. The SPADE plot allows visualization of all of the immunophenotypically

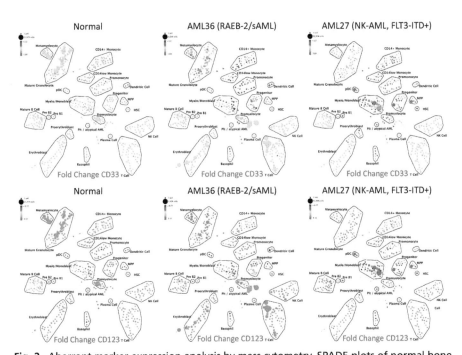

Fig. 2. Aberrant marker expression analysis by mass cytometry. SPADE plots of normal bone marrow samples compared with samples from a patient with NK, FLT3-ITD+ AML, and a patient with high-risk MDS transforming to sAML. SPADE clustering was performed on all samples (normal and AML) simultaneously to generate a single tree structure for all samples. All of the cell events from each sample were then mapped to the common tree structure. Each node of the SPADE tree is colored for the fold change in the median expression of the indicated markers relative to the average median from 14 control samples. Coloring ranges from decreased expression in blue to increased expression in red; yellow-green shades represent no change in expression relative to the average of the control samples. Aberrant increased expression of CD33 and CD123 is present across multiple stages of immunophenotypic development in the patient with FLT3-ITD + AML but not in the patient with RAEB-2 MDS/sAML where an aberrant decreased CD33 can be seen in the maturing monocytes. The size of each node is correlated to the fraction of cells mapping to the node; however, a minimum size was enforced for most nodes to allow visualization of node color. Immunophenotypic grouping of nodes was performed manually on the basis of the median marker expression level of each node, and based on analysis of the relevant biaxial plots (eg, CD38 vs CD34).

identifiable marrow populations and comparison of all of the measured parameters between each of the samples. These high-dimensional comparisons can enable the rapid identification of aberrant expression patterns.

Several other researchers have now performed similar studies leveraging mass cytometry for analysis of leukemia. Ferrell and colleagues[17] used a mass cytometry approach to identify phenotypic changes that occur in the AML blast population in serial samples taken over the course of AML treatment. The phenotypic changes noted in this analysis allowed the cells to be more readily distinguished from normal HSCs and could potentially be used for MRD analysis (although formal MRD analysis was not preformed). Fisher and colleagues[18] performed an analysis of bone marrow samples from a patient with myelofibrosis and associated secondary AML (sAML) to identify abnormal NF-κB pathway signaling in progenitor cell populations from patients with these diseases. Each of these assay approaches could eventually be harnessed to select cytotoxic, antibody-drug conjugate, or small molecule therapeutic treatment strategies. This type of functional information could eventually be used to enable adaptive treatment strategies to eliminate rare persistent leukemia cells from patients in remission before these cells can proliferate and lead to disease relapse. Such approaches could lead to mass cytometry eventually being used for aberrant marker detection, MRD monitoring, detection of aberrant differentiation patterns, and the identification of therapeutic targets against malignant cell populations in MDS, myeloproliferative neoplasms, and both acute and chronic leukemia. Importantly, with close attention to detail and careful validation, mass cytometry experiments could be performed almost as quickly as traditional flow cytometry experiments, enabling diagnostic results to be available within a clinically useful time frame.

A closely related application of mass cytometry is the assessment of response to novel therapeutic agents. Currently, most of the pharmacodynamic measurements used in clinical trials are still conducted on bulk cell samples using techniques such as western blotting or gene expression analysis. Although very useful, these types of assays cannot capture the effects of a therapeutic agent on the rare quiescent or resistant cell populations that commonly lead to the failure of therapeutic strategies. Mass cytometry assays could be used to both identify these rare cells and characterize a novel agent's effects upon them. This approach could be used to predict late therapeutic failures and potentially to develop synergistic treatment approaches that target unique functional properties of the resistant cells. The author's group has used mass cytometry approaches to monitor responses to novel therapeutic kinase inhibitors in vivo (Behbehani GK and colleagues, 2017, unpublished results), and Saenz and colleagues[21] have used mass cytometry to assess ex vivo responses in AML stem/progenitor cells to a novel BET inhibitor. Similar strategies could be applied for monitoring the pharmacodynamics of virtually any therapy being tested in patients with a hematologic malignancy.

The other major clinical arena in which mass cytometry could prove extremely useful is in monitoring of the immune system. High-parameter assessment by mass cytometry allows the simultaneous assessment of a broad range of activation markers across a wide range of immunophenotypically identifiable immune effector cells. Mass cytometry has been used to measure global characteristics of immune function and to further characterize several important immune cell subsets. Strauss-Albee and colleagues[22] mapped the diversity of NK cells across a diverse panel of donors and were able to use overlapping 39-antibody mass cytometry panels to demonstrate strong relationships between viral exposure and increases in both NK diversity and terminal differentiation. A particularly elegant and powerful method was developed by Newell and colleagues,[23] who combined MHC-tetramer staining with high-parameter surface immunophenotype assessment to characterize a phenotypically distinct T-cell subset specific to the response to rotavirus infection. In the study of rheumatologic disease, Rao and colleagues[24] used mass cytometry to identify an expanded T-cell population that appears to drive B-cell activation in rheumatoid arthritis, and O'Gorman and colleagues[25] demonstrated distinct monocyte cytokine profiles associated with systemic lupus erythematous. Finally, an intriguing study of the immune response to hip surgery was recently conducted by Gaudilliere and colleagues.[26] These researchers collected samples from patients before, and at several time points after, hip replacement surgery and performed a broad mass cytometry characterization of immune function coupled with a machine-learning algorithm for analysis of the resulting data. This analysis demonstrated that changes in the intracellular signaling of several monocyte populations correlated with long-term surgical outcomes. Importantly, the signaling changes were observed during the first 24 hours after surgery, but correlated to surgical outcomes observed weeks later, such as time to improved pain, range of motion, and fatigue. This finding was not suspected a priori and was detected as a result of performing a precise and broad characterization of immune function. These examples suggest that the simultaneous and precise characterization of multiple aspects of immune function enabled by mass cytometry could potentially be diagnostic of a wide variety of medical conditions. Identifying unique subsets of aberrant cell types characteristic of pathologic immune states could one day become part of the diagnostic criteria of numerous diseases while simultaneously allowing for the mechanistic selection of immunomodulatory therapies.

Increasingly, immune responses have also been harnessed for the treatment of malignant diseases through the blockage of immune inhibitory checkpoints. High-parameter mass cytometry is ideally suited for assessment of such therapeutic approaches because it enables the detailed characterization of malignant cells with the simultaneous assessment of how therapeutic drugs might alter their expression of immune checkpoint proteins and overall activation state. An example of mass cytometry's potential for monitoring of cancer immunotherapy was recently performed by Spitzer and colleagues[27] in a mouse model of immunotherapy. In this study, mass cytometry was used to characterize a broad range of tissues from mice receiving either a successful immunotherapy or one known to be incapable of inducing tumor rejection. This study demonstrated that a successful immunotherapy response was associated with an expanded CD4 T-cell population systemically, rather than specifically in the tumor microenvironment. This suggests that human immunotherapy responses could likely also be monitored systemically, and several early attempts have been made at doing so.[28,29] Clinically, the ability to make such assessments could enable the early detection of treatment resistance and allow for adaptive changes of therapeutic strategy through increasing the dose of an immunostimulatory therapy or changing treatments to one targeting another checkpoint pathway.

HIGH-DIMENSIONAL ANALYSIS APPROACHES

Achieving the potential goals outlined above requires methodologies to synthesize the highly complex data generated by mass cytometry experiments into detectable patterns that can be reliably identified. Although mass cytometry data can readily be analyzed using the same gating strategies used in similar fluorescent flow cytometry experiments, these approaches can be cumbersome and limiting when used for high-dimensional data. For instance, a 42-antibody mass cytometry panel would require 861 different biaxial plots to completely visualize the data generated. Fortunately, a variety of dimensionality-reduction algorithms have been developed that can organize highly complex single-cell data into more easily recognizable patterns that can be readily compared across samples. Several such approaches have gained wide acceptance within the mass cytometry community, and it is worth briefly overviewing the strengths and weaknesses of 3 of these (SPADE, viSNE, and Citrus) with respect to how they might be applied to clinical analyses. The author has selected these analysis methods because of their popularity and in part because each are available in the commonly used online platform, Cytobank,[30] although several other excellent analysis tools are available that could also be used for mass cytometry data.[31–33]

To begin, there are several general considerations that are applicable to the most commonly used mass cytometry analysis approaches. As in flow cytometry, batch effects can be quite significant in mass cytometry, and most of these data analysis methodologies work best on data sets that are highly comparable (same reagents; same panel design; same machine with same acquisition settings). The sensitivity of each technique to batch effects is somewhat variable, and one technique, Scaffold, was specifically designed to be compatible with data sets created using different analysis methods and can be used in situations where data files may not be perfectly comparable.[34] The first step of each approach is similar: all cell event files from the experiment are sampled to create a single data set that is representative of all of the cells from all of the samples in the experiment. The cells of this pooled data set are then organized into groups based on their similarity across several user-specified parameters; essentially organizing the cells "like with like" across the expression levels of the selected markers. (Typically, the parameters chosen are surface markers known to differentiate functionally distinct cell types, but all of these analysis approaches can also be used to organize cells on the basis of intracellular signaling properties, cell cycle state, or progression through a process such as apoptosis or DNA damage response.) The result of this organization is a common data structure for the entire experiment that groups together the most similar cells across the specified parameters (ie, SPADE nodes, or regions of the viSNE plot). From here, the common data pool is then separated back into individual files, and the cells of each sample populate the common data structure to form separate, sample-specific, versions of the data projection. Most of the enhanced power of these analysis approaches comes from performing the cell organizing step simultaneously on all cells from the experiment and then projecting the individual samples onto this common data structure. This process allows similar cells from different samples to be compared with one another without respect to differences in the frequencies of these populations. For example, in a study of acute leukemia, a patient might have several different immunophenotypically distinct blast populations (making up 80% of bone marrow cellularity) before chemotherapy treatment, whereas after chemotherapy treatment, only one of these blast populations may persist (at 0.8% of bone marrow cellularity). If the pretreatment and posttreatment samples are analyzed together with SPADE or viSNE (described in later discussion), this persisting blast population can be differentiated from normal cells and compared with the same blast population before therapy to determine which functional properties are different between normal blasts, the persisting blast population, and the blast populations that were eliminated by treatment.[17] This type of analysis is only possible with high-dimensional single-cell data and is greatly facilitated by the use of dimensionality-reduction algorithms.

SPADE

SPADE stands for Spanning-tree Analysis of Density Normalized Events and was the first high-dimensional analysis technique commonly used for mass cytometry data.[35,36] SPADE analysis starts by pooling a sample of events from each sample through a process of density-dependent down-sampling. This density-dependent down-sampling step compares cells to one another across the user-specified clustering parameters and preferentially removes cells for which many other similar cells are present. This creates a very important advantage of SPADE, because it allows for a much better representation of rare cell events in the final data projection than would be achieved through a random sampling of events from each sample. In the second step, this pool of down-sampled data is used to perform an agglomerative clustering. Both this clustering step and the previous down-sampling step are performed on the basis of the total distance (ie, the sum differences in all clustering parameters) between cells across the parameters specified by the user. This step essentially groups cells with their most similar neighbors with respect to the parameters used for clustering. The number of clusters formed (typically 200–300) can be specified by the user and should be empirically determined based on the complexity of the cell samples being studied. In the third analysis step, these clusters are converted into nodes and connected to one another in a branching minimum spanning tree, which connects the nodes together in a way that minimizes the total distance separating each of the nodes from their nearest neighboring nodes. After the conclusion of this step, a single common SPADE tree structure has been created from the pool of down-sampled data. In the final step, termed "up-sampling," each cell event from each of the original FCS files is added to its most closely related node from the common SPADE tree to create a unique version of the SPADE tree specific for each individual sample file.

SPADE is an excellent tool for analysis of high-dimensional mass cytometry and is well suited to analysis of clinical samples.[36] It has two particularly useful properties: First, as mentioned above, the initial density-dependent down-sampling step ensures that rare cell populations are well represented in the final data structure. This step is not present in the other common analysis approaches and makes SPADE somewhat better suited for the analysis of rare events, because these will be well represented in the final SPADE tree structure, whereas in other analysis methods, these cells may or may not form into distinct clusters and might be difficult to discern because of their rarity in final data projection. Second, SPADE is excellent for making comparisons between small cell subsets within complex samples. This strength stems from the fact that the clustering and up-sampling steps force all cells into the nodes of the common tree structure. This is similar to a binning analysis and allows the user to easily recognize samples that are unique to one or a few samples (these nodes will only be populated in some samples) and compare similar cell types (cells in the same nodes) across different samples. Cells within the same SPADE node will be highly similar to one another across the clustering dimensions and thereby allow "apple-to-apple" comparisons between similar cell populations of different samples. The SPADE software further simplifies these comparisons by allowing the nodes of each sample's tree structure to be colored by the fold-change of each marker median compared with the median in the same node of the control sample. The clustering of SPADE also has the important advantage that all cells are placed into the final data representation once and only once, which means that cells will readily cluster on the basis of both the markers they express and the markers that they lack. This property enables the identification of populations that are not positive for any of the makers in the staining panel. Clustering analysis also ensures that a given cell event is only represented in one node of the SPADE tree, preventing events from being in more than one population and increasing the utility of comparisons of the frequencies of cell events in different populations.

As above, the author's group has used these properties of SPADE to make very sensitive comparisons between patients with AML and MDS to healthy donors.[10] In their experience, this greatly increased the sensitivity of detecting aberrant surface marker expression and intracellular signaling by allowing the intensities of individual markers to be directly compared between patient and control cells of the same developmental stage. As shown in **Fig. 2**, comparing AML bone marrow samples to healthy donor bone marrow allows for the grouping of cells into developmental stages and comparison of marker expression levels across each clustered group of cells. For instance, the sample from the patient with FLT3-ITD$^+$ AML demonstrated increased CD33 and CD123 expression across all stages of monocyte development, whereas a patient with RAEB-2 MDS/sAML demonstrated decreased CD33 in the monocyte lineage and no significant changes in CD123. In the author's experience, this analysis approach can find surface marker aberrancies in almost every AML sample tested. SPADE has also been broadly used for analysis of both high-dimensional mass and flow cytometry data. Studies from other researchers have performed comparisons of intracellular signaling responses across immune cell subsets,[35] predicted clinical outcomes in HIV,[31] dissected leukemia progenitor subsets,[37,38] analyzed aberrant monocyte subsets in chronic myelomonocytic leukemia,[39] and identified T-cell populations predictive of immunomodulatory treatment responses in aplastic anemia[40] and graft-versus-host disease.[41]

There are some weaknesses of the SPADE algorithm relevant to its use in analysis of clinical data. A major drawback is that the minimum spanning tree is generated in a stochastic way, resulting in a unique tree structure every time the analysis is run. This is true even if SPADE is run multiple times on the same data set. In general, the algorithm will create similar cell clusters each time it is run, but the way in which these clusters will connect in the minimum spanning tree can vary significantly. This property can be confusing to researchers unfamiliar with SPADE, even though the overall interrelationships between cell nodes are similar each time. This property can make comparing SPADE trees from different experiments challenging. This weakness has been addressed in a modification of the SPADE approach known as Scaffold.[34] In this approach, clustering of each sample is performed to create similar nodes of cells; however, these nodes are then organized into a tree around a common tree structure already populated with manually gated (or otherwise selected) known cell populations. Scaffold has the advantage of creating a common tree structure onto which samples from different experiments (even using different technologies) can be overlaid. Although this approach can allow meaningful projection of data onto a common tree structure, comparisons between the same node from different samples can still only be made accurately if the underlying data are highly comparable and can be clustered as a single group simultaneously. In addition, forcing all cell events to be organized in accordance with the same reference populations from control samples limits observation of unique patterns of data structure (eg, an aberrant cell differentiation lineage) that do not exist in the reference populations.

viSNE

viSNE is an FCS-specific modification of the t-distributed Stochastic Neighbor Embedding approach first published by Van der Maaten and Hinton.[42] This approach has been widely used in data science and performs very well for the analysis of a broad range of data types. The t-SNE algorithm maps data points from high-dimensional space to low-dimensional space by converting the distances between them into similarities and then uses an optimization algorithm to plot these in a 2- (or 3-) dimensional map by iteratively aligning and realigning the events until the low-dimensional map most closely matches the cell distribution in high dimension. Although the underlying mathematics of the t-SNE algorithm are complex, the end result is a 2- (or 3-)

dimensional map that is most similar to a principal component analysis plot, but importantly, the plot is essentially nonparametric and not overly influenced by the absolute intensity difference in the individual markers. This property makes viSNE significantly less sensitive to batch effects and the specific panel design used. This also makes viSNE maps more consistent from run to run; however, just like SPADE, each analysis run (even of the same exact data set) yields a unique result. Another important distinction is that viSNE runs on individual cell events, and this requires that analysis runs be performed on smaller numbers of cell events (because of computational constraints). These constraints typically limits analysis to a total 1 to 2 million cells per experiment, which are typically randomly sampled from the total number of events in all files of the experiment.

Like SPADE, viSNE analysis can use the additional information present in high-dimensional data allowing cells to be positioned in the final data projection on the basis of the presence of markers as well as their absence. Because viSNE maps individual cells, by definition, cells are only represented once in the final data projection. A major strength of viSNE analyses is that the analysis is nonparametric and thus not highly influenced by high degrees of variation in marker expression level, which are commonly found in biologic systems. This makes it very useful for observing the global interrelationships between the cells of a complex population. viSNE is also extremely good at dissecting subtle changes in marker expression between individual cells (because each cell event is uniquely positioned on the viSNE map). This makes viSNE very useful for studying progressive changes that occur during a biologic response or as part of a differentiation program. Such progressive changes will leave a "trail" of cells in intermediate stages of the process, and the trajectory of these changes can be visualized in high detail using a viSNE map. Thus far, viSNE has most commonly been used for performing broad characterizations of cell systems or large subsets of a cellular system (eg, lymphoid cells or progenitor cells) to discern global changes between individuals or for the discovery of novel cell subtypes.[7,10,17,22,24,29,40,43]

viSNE has been used to analyze cell samples for MRD or MRD correlates in both AML and acute lymphoblastic leukemia (ALL). Amir and colleagues[16] used a synthetic MRD experiment to detect a unique cell population generated by adding ALL patient cells into normal bone marrow, and Ferrell and colleagues[17] used viSNE to track persistence of immunophenotypically abnormal progenitor cells during AML induction treatment. However, viSNE's limitation on the total number of events that can be analyzed requires random sampling from each test sample, which can reduce the ability to detect rare events and easily visualize them among all of the other cell events on the viSNE plot. To address this, viSNE analysis can be performed on pre-gated cell subsets to make the analysis more sensitive for analysis of rare events and more subtle intersample variation (because the total immunophenotypic space represented on the viSNE map is significantly smaller). This initial subgating essentially results in a viSNE plot that is "zoomed-in" on the immunophenotypic population of interest. This approach has been used for detection of MRD from fluorescent flow cytometry analyses of B-cell ALL (after gating on B-cells),[44] and for analysis of abnormal early stem and progenitor cell populations in patients with AML.[10] An example of using this type of viSNE approach for MRD analysis is shown in **Fig. 3**. In this analysis, mass cytometry data from 3 patients with AML who achieved a complete remission (CR) after intensive chemotherapy was first gated on $CD34^+CD38^{lo}Lin^-$ events, and then this small subset of events was analyzed by viSNE across 19 cell surface markers. Although very preliminary, this type of analysis was able to identify small cell clusters of apparently abnormal cells in the two patients who ultimately relapsed.

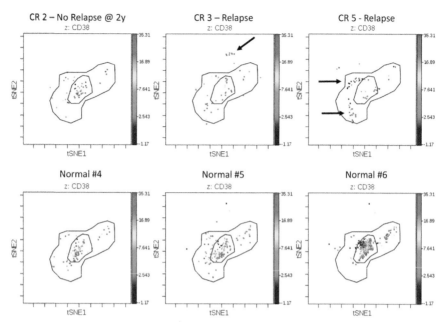

Fig. 3. viSNE analysis of CD34⁺CD38ˡᵒ subset demonstrates consistent normal immunophenotypic patterns in high-dimensional space that are altered in patients with presumed residual disease. Gated CD34⁺CD38ˡᵒ cells from each sample were analyzed by viSNE (up to 5000 sampled events per individual) using 19 (surface marker) dimensions. Two gates encompassing the vast majority of normal CD34⁺CD38ˡᵒ events are shown for reference (*blue outlines*). Altered patterns in the 2 patients in CR who ultimate relapsed are indicated by arrows. Each cell event is colored for its expression level of CD38 from blue (0 ion counts) to red (approximately 40 ion counts). Red cell events still fall within the CD34⁺CD38ˡᵒ gate and demonstrated dim CD38 expression.

The unique properties of viSNE, however, also lead to a few drawbacks. With respect to clinical analyses, the fact that a viSNE map places every cell into a unique position (relative to the other events in the experiment) makes comparing similar subpopulations of cells from different samples difficult. The user is left to determine which groups of cell events are most similar for the purposes of making comparisons, and this can significantly complicate determinations of aberrant marker expression or analysis of changes in the frequency of cells with a particular immunophenotype. This drawback can be partially mitigated by including known normal samples in each analysis, but the nonparametric nature of the tSNE algorithm makes it difficult to decide how far the boundaries of any given normal population should extend on the viSNE plot. For these reasons, viSNE is not ideally suited for clinical analyses in which abnormal cell populations need to be directly compared with one another (cell population to cell population) or to normal samples. SPADE tends to be better in this regard because all cells within each SPADE analysis populate the same tree structure, making comparable nodes fairly obvious. (Although it could be argued that the SPADE node assignments are somewhat arbitrary, they are at least determined in an unbiased manner.) viSNE's powerful ability to accurately represent the variance across the cell events within a sample also leads to a second significant drawback; even small or random variations in a data set can appear to have meaningful structure in a viSNE map. This is because the nonparametric nature of viSNE rescales the variance across all of the cells in the experiment to populate the viSNE map. As a result, if nearly uniform cell events (with small amounts of random variation) are analyzed in viSNE, a complete viSNE map will still be created that will appear to have significant differences if not carefully inspected. (SPADE can also suffer from this problem, but the connections of the minimum spanning tress and the process of manual annotation in SPADE makes the true variance much more apparent.) Thus, as with all high-dimensional data projections, it remains very important to look at the original raw data to confirm any apparently significant differences or data trends observed in a viSNE map.

Citrus

Citrus (cluster identification, characterization, and regression) is an algorithm developed by Bruggner and colleagues[45] for the purpose of automating the detection of condition-specific differences between cell populations in single-cell data sets. Citrus combines clustering of cell events with automated regression modeling across the resulting high-dimensional clusters to determine which data features are significantly different between samples from different groups (eg, treated vs untreated; good outcome vs bad outcome). Similar to both SPADE and viSNE, Citrus starts by first randomly sampling events from each sample into a single pool of data representing the entire experiment. Citrus then clusters this aggregated data pool into hierarchical clusters across user-specified clustering dimensions. The user can specify the number of clusters by specifying a minimum percentage cluster size, which can be set to relatively low percentages of the total cell events (working well down to percentages of 0.5%). Because all events will be clustered, however, clustering down to small fractions of cells generates a large number of clusters that can become computationally intensive. Each of the clusters is then merged with its nearest neighbor to form a hierarchical tree until all of the clusters merge into a single cluster, thus each cell event will be included in multiple, ever larger, clusters. Citrus then splits the combined clustered data back into individual sample components and can then calculate the characteristics of each cluster for each file. This allows calculation of the median level of each marker, and the proportion of cell events for each cluster of each samples. Citrus then uses regularized supervised learning algorithms (different algorithms may be chosen by the user) to identify cluster features that best predict the condition difference (eg, treated vs untreated; good outcome vs bad outcome). Finally, Citrus performs a cross-validation using a subset of the experimental samples that allows for estimation of the false-discovery rate. The Citrus data output then displays the cell clusters and cluster features that were most predictive of the user-specified condition of interest.

Citrus is best suited to analysis of relatively large data sets and will work best if the underlying data files are highly comparable (although if batch effects are evenly distributed across the conditions of interest, they should have less effect on the predictive model). For such datasets, Citrus can be very powerful and, unlike SPADE and viSNE that require human interpretation and annotation, Citrus can identify classifiers with almost no human intervention beyond identification of relevant clustering parameters and cluster sizes. This makes Citrus well suited for experiments designed to look for novel classifying characteristics for which the researcher may not have any a priori hypotheses. One of the first publications to use Citrus was an investigation into the immune activation state of patients before and after hip replacement surgery, discussed previously.[26]

The main drawback of Citrus is its requirement for a reasonably large number of samples in each condition being compared. Analysis of smaller numbers of samples will be prone to errors of overfitting, and the small number of samples will also reduce the effectiveness of the cross-validation methodology within Citrus designed to reduce such errors. Citrus, like viSNE, also randomly samples events from all samples, which makes detection of changes in important but rare subpopulations (eg, cancer stem cells; antigen-specific immune cells) significantly more difficult. Finally, Citrus's additional flexibility in giving the user the ability to specify the association model may be intimidating to clinicians or biologists unfamiliar with the specific association models. For these reasons, an eventual role for an algorithm like Citrus in clinical practice would likely be limited to hypothesis-generating studies or analysis of experimental agents (eg, responders vs nonresponders).

SUMMARY

The research community continues to increase the understanding of the immense heterogeneity of malignant diseases and the tremendous complexity of the human immune responses. Unfortunately, the ability to personalize clinical treatments in accordance with these complexities remains limited. Mass cytometry is uniquely well suited to organize the complex cell populations targeted by cancer therapies and immunomodulatory agents and could be used in the near future for the personalization of these therapies. Achieving these goals will require careful attention to several unique aspects of mass cytometry analysis, and a paradigm shift in how clinical cytometry data are analyzed. Although challenging, the rewards of this work could be tremendous, because clinical mass cytometry assays could combine the power of rare event analysis with the broad scope of genomic assays all within a clinically actionable timeframe, creating an extremely powerful tool for personalized medicine.

REFERENCES

1. Tanner SD, Baranov VI, Ornatsky OI, et al. An introduction to mass cytometry: fundamentals and applications. Cancer Immunol Immunother 2013;62:955–65.
2. Spitzer MH, Nolan GP. Mass cytometry: single cells, many features. Cell 2016; 165:780–91.
3. Bjornson ZB, Nolan GP, Fantl WJ. Single-cell mass cytometry for analysis of immune system functional states. Curr Opin Immunol 2013;25:484–94.
4. Di Palma S, Bodenmiller B. Unraveling cell populations in tumors by single-cell mass cytometry. Curr Opin Biotechnol 2015;31:122–9.
5. Ornatsky OI, Lou X, Nitz M, et al. Study of cell antigens and intracellular DNA by identification of element-containing labels and metallointercalators using inductively coupled plasma mass spectrometry. Anal Chem 2008;80:2539–47.
6. Ornatsky O, Baranov VI, Bandura DR, et al. Multiple cellular antigen detection by ICP-MS. J Immunol Methods 2006;308:68–76.
7. Behbehani GK, Thom C, Zunder ER, et al. Transient partial permeabilization with saponin enables cellular barcoding prior to surface marker staining. Cytometry A 2014;85:1011–9.
8. Bodenmiller B, Zunder ER, Finck R, et al. Multiplexed mass cytometry profiling of cellular states perturbed by small-molecule regulators. Nat Biotechnol 2012;30: 858–67.
9. Zunder ER, Finck R, Behbehani GK, et al. Palladium-based mass tag cell barcoding with a doublet-filtering scheme and single-cell deconvolution algorithm. Nat Protoc 2015;10:316–33.
10. Behbehani GK, Samusik N, Bjornson ZB, et al. Mass cytometric functional profiling of acute myeloid leukemia defines cell-cycle and immunophenotypic properties that correlate with known responses to therapy. Cancer Discov 2015;5:988–1003.

11. Stern AD, Rahman AH, Birtwistle MR. Cell size assays for mass cytometry. Cytometry A 2017;91:14–24.

12. Behbehani GK, Bendall SC, Clutter MR, et al. Single-cell mass cytometry adapted to measurements of the cell cycle. Cytometry A 2012;81:552–66.

13. Fienberg HG, Simonds EF, Fantl WJ, et al. A platinum-based covalent viability reagent for single-cell mass cytometry. Cytometry A 2012;81:467–75.

14. Edgar LJ, Vellanki RN, Halupa A, et al. Identification of hypoxic cells using an organotellurium tag compatible with mass cytometry. Angew Chem Int Ed Engl 2014;53:11473–7.

15. Finck R, Simonds EF, Jager A, et al. Normalization of mass cytometry data with bead standards. Cytometry A 2013;83:483–94.

16. Amir el AD, Davis KL, Tadmor MD, et al. viSNE enables visualization of high dimensional single-cell data and reveals phenotypic heterogeneity of leukemia. Nat Biotechnol 2013;31:545–52.

17. Ferrell PB Jr, Diggins KE, Polikowsky HG, et al. High-dimensional analysis of acute myeloid leukemia reveals phenotypic changes in persistent cells during induction therapy. PLoS One 2016;11:e0153207.

18. Fisher DA, Malkova O, Engle EK, et al. Mass cytometry analysis reveals hyperactive NF Kappa B signaling in myelofibrosis and secondary acute myeloid leukemia. Leukemia 2017. [Epub ahead of print].

19. Levine JH, Simonds EF, Bendall SC, et al. Data-driven phenotypic dissection of AML reveals progenitor-like cells that correlate with prognosis. Cell 2015;162:184–97.

20. Renneville A, Abdelali RB, Chevret S, et al. Clinical impact of gene mutations and lesions detected by SNP-array karyotyping in acute myeloid leukemia patients in the context of gemtuzumab ozogamicin treatment: results of the ALFA-0701 trial. Oncotarget 2014;5:916–32.

21. Saenz DT, Fiskus W, Qian Y, et al. Novel BET protein proteolysis-targeting chimera exerts superior lethal activity than bromodomain inhibitor (BETi) against post-myeloproliferative neoplasm secondary (s) AML cells. Leukemia 2017. [Epub ahead of print].

22. Strauss-Albee DM, Fukuyama J, Liang EC, et al. Human NK cell repertoire diversity reflects immune experience and correlates with viral susceptibility. Sci Transl Med 2015;7:297ra115.

23. Newell EW, Sigal N, Nair N, et al. Combinatorial tetramer staining and mass cytometry analysis facilitate T-cell epitope mapping and characterization. Nat Biotechnol 2013;31:623–9.

24. Rao DA, Gurish MF, Marshall JL, et al. Pathologically expanded peripheral T helper cell subset drives B cells in rheumatoid arthritis. Nature 2017;542:110–4.

25. O'Gorman WE, Hsieh EW, Savig ES, et al. Single-cell systems-level analysis of human Toll-like receptor activation defines a chemokine signature in patients with systemic lupus erythematosus. J Allergy Clin Immunol 2015;136:1326–36.

26. Gaudilliere B, Fragiadakis GK, Bruggner RV, et al. Clinical recovery from surgery correlates with single-cell immune signatures. Sci Transl Med 2014;6:255ra131.

27. Spitzer MH, Carmi Y, Reticker-Flynn NE, et al. Systemic immunity is required for effective cancer immunotherapy. Cell 2017;168:487–502.e15.

28. Wistuba-Hamprecht K, Martens A, Weide B, et al. Establishing high dimensional immune signatures from peripheral blood via mass cytometry in a discovery cohort of stage IV melanoma patients. J Immunol 2017;198:927.

29. Romee R, Rosario M, Berrien-Elliott MM, et al. Cytokine-induced memory-like natural killer cells exhibit enhanced responses against myeloid leukemia. Sci Transl Med 2016;8:357ra123.

30. Kotecha N, Krutzik PO, Irish JM, Web-based analysis and publication of flow cytometry experiments. Current Protocols in Cytometry. 53:10.17:10.17.1–10.17.24.

31. Aghaeepour N, Chattopadhyay P, Chikina M, et al. A benchmark for evaluation of algorithms for identification of cellular correlates of clinical outcomes. Cytometry A 2016;89:16–21.

32. Diggins KE, Greenplate AR, Leelatian N, et al. Characterizing cell subsets using marker enrichment modeling. Nat Methods 2017;14:275–8.

33. Samusik N, Good Z, Spitzer MH, et al. Automated mapping of phenotype space with single-cell data. Nat Methods 2016;13:493–6.

34. Spitzer MH, Gherardini PF, Fragiadakis GK, et al. IMMUNOLOGY. An interactive reference framework for modeling a dynamic immune system. Science 2015;349: 1259425.

35. Bendall SC, Simonds EF, Qiu P, et al. Single-cell mass cytometry of differential immune and drug responses across a human hematopoietic continuum. Science 2011;332:687–96.

36. Qiu P, Simonds EF, Bendall SC, et al. Extracting a cellular hierarchy from high-dimensional cytometry data with SPADE. Nat Biotechnol 2011;29:886–91.

37. Gibbs KD, Jager A, Crespo O, et al. Decoupling of tumor-initiating activity from stable immunophenotype in HoxA9-Meis1 driven AML. Cell Stem Cell 2012;10: 210–7.

38. Sachs Z, LaRue RS, Nguyen HT, et al. NRASG12V oncogene facilitates self-renewal in a murine model of acute myelogenous leukemia. Blood 2014;124: 3274.

39. Selimoglu-Buet D, Wagner-Ballon O, Saada V, et al. Characteristic repartition of monocyte subsets as a diagnostic signature of chronic myelomonocytic leukemia. Blood 2015;125:3618.

40. Kordasti S, Costantini B, Seidl T, et al. Deep phenotyping of Tregs identifies an immune signature for idiopathic aplastic anemia and predicts response to treatment. Blood 2016;128:1193.

41. Kim B-S, Nishikii H, Baker J, et al. Treatment with agonistic DR3 antibody results in expansion of donor Tregs and reduced graft-versus-host disease. Blood 2015; 126:546.

42. van der Maaten L, Hinton G. Visualizing data using t-SNE. J Mach Learn Res 2008;9:85.

43. Ribas A, Shin DS, Zaretsky J, et al. PD-1 blockade expands intratumoral memory T cells. Cancer Immunol Res 2016;4:194–203.

44. DiGiuseppe JA, Tadmor MD, Pe'er D. Detection of minimal residual disease in B lymphoblastic leukemia using viSNE. Cytometry B Clin Cytom 2015;88(5): 294–304.

45. Bruggner RV, Bodenmiller B, Dill DL, et al. Automated identification of stratifying signatures in cellular subpopulations. Proc Natl Acad Sci U S A 2014;111: E2770–7.

UNITED STATES POSTAL SERVICE ® Statement of Ownership, Management, and Circulation (All Periodicals Publications Except Requester Publications)

1. Publication Title	2. Publication Number	3. Filing Date
CLINICS IN LABORATORY MEDICINE	000 – 713	9/18/2017

4. Issue Frequency	5. Number of Issues Published Annually	6. Annual Subscription Price
MAR, JUN, SEP, DEC	4	$258.00

7. Complete Mailing Address of Known Office of Publication (Not printer) (Street, city, county, state, and ZIP+4®)

ELSEVIER INC.
230 Park Avenue, Suite 800
New York, NY 10169

Contact Person
STEPHEN R. BUSHING

Telephone (Include area code)
215-239-3688

8. Complete Mailing Address of Headquarters or General Business Office of Publisher (Not printer)

ELSEVIER INC.
230 Park Avenue, Suite 800
New York, NY 10169

9. Full Names and Complete Mailing Addresses of Publisher, Editor, and Managing Editor (Do not leave blank)

Publisher (Name and complete mailing address)

ADRIANNE BRIGIDO, ELSEVIER INC.
1600 JOHN F KENNEDY BLVD. SUITE 1800
PHILADELPHIA, PA 19103-2899

Editor (Name and complete mailing address)

STACY EASTMAN, ELSEVIER INC.
1600 JOHN F KENNEDY BLVD. SUITE 1800
PHILADELPHIA, PA 19103-2899

Managing Editor (Name and complete mailing address)

PATRICK MANLEY, ELSEVIER INC.
1600 JOHN F KENNEDY BLVD. SUITE 1800
PHILADELPHIA, PA 19103-2899

10. Owner (Do not leave blank. If the publication is owned by a corporation, give the name and address of the corporation immediately followed by the names and addresses of all stockholders owning or holding 1 percent or more of the total amount of stock. If not owned by a corporation, give the names and addresses of the individual owners. If owned by a partnership or other unincorporated firm, give its name and address as well as those of each individual owner. If the publication is published by a nonprofit organization, give its name and address.)

Full Name	Complete Mailing Address
WHOLLY OWNED SUBSIDIARY OF REED/ELSEVIER, US HOLDINGS	1600 JOHN F KENNEDY BLVD. SUITE 1800 PHILADELPHIA, PA 19103-2899

11. Known Bondholders, Mortgagees, and Other Security Holders Owning or Holding 1 Percent or More of Total Amount of Bonds, Mortgages, or Other Securities. If none, check box ▶ ☐ None

Full Name	Complete Mailing Address
N/A	

12. Tax Status (For completion by nonprofit organizations authorized to mail at nonprofit rates) (Check one)
The purpose, function, and nonprofit status of this organization and the exempt status for federal income tax purposes:
☒ Has Not Changed During Preceding 12 Months
☐ Has Changed During Preceding 12 Months (Publisher must submit explanation of change with this statement)

13. Publication Title	14. Issue Date for Circulation Data Below
CLINICS IN LABORATORY MEDICINE	JUNE 2017

15. Extent and Nature of Circulation			Average No. Copies Each Issue During Preceding 12 Months	No. Copies of Single Issue Published Nearest to Filing Date
a. Total Number of Copies (Net press run)			189	131
b. Paid Circulation (By Mail and Outside the Mail)	(1)	Mailed Outside-County Paid Subscriptions Stated on PS Form 3541 (Include paid distribution above nominal rate, advertiser's proof copies, and exchange copies)	56	48
	(2)	Mailed In-County Paid Subscriptions Stated on PS Form 3541 (Include paid distribution above nominal rate, advertiser's proof copies, and exchange copies)	0	0
	(3)	Paid Distribution Outside the Mails Including Sales Through Dealers and Carriers, Street Vendors, Counter Sales, and Other Paid Distribution Outside USPS®	36	27
	(4)	Paid Distribution by Other Classes of Mail Through the USPS (e.g. First-Class Mail®)	0	0
c. Total Paid Distribution (Sum of 15b (1), (2), (3), and (4))		▶	92	75
d. Free or Nominal Rate Distribution (By Mail and Outside the Mail)	(1)	Free or Nominal Rate Outside-County Copies included on PS Form 3541	51	56
	(2)	Free or Nominal Rate In-County Copies Included on PS Form 3541	0	0
	(3)	Free or Nominal Rate Copies Mailed at Other Classes Through the USPS (e.g. First-Class Mail)	0	0
	(4)	Free or Nominal Rate Distribution Outside the Mail (Carriers or other means)	0	0
e. Total Free or Nominal Rate Distribution (Sum of 15d (1), (2), (3) and (4))		▶	51	56
f. Total Distribution (Sum of 15c and 15e)		▶	143	131
g. Copies not Distributed (See Instructions to Publishers #4 (page 83))		▶	46	0
h. Total (Sum of 15f and g)		▶	189	131
i. Percent Paid (15c divided by 15f times 100)		▶	64.34%	57.25%

* If you are claiming electronic copies, go to line 16 on page 3. If you are not claiming electronic copies, skip to line 17 on page 3.

16. Electronic Copy Circulation		Average No. Copies Each Issue During Preceding 12 Months	No. Copies of Single Issue Published Nearest to Filing Date
a. Paid Electronic Copies	▲	0	0
b. Total Paid Print Copies (Line 15c) + Paid Electronic Copies (Line 16a)	▲	92	75
c. Total Print Distribution (Line 15f) + Paid Electronic Copies (Line 16a)	▲	143	131
d. Percent Paid (Both Print & Electronic Copies) (16b divided by 16c × 100)	▲	64.34%	57.25%

☒ I certify that 50% of all my distributed copies (electronic and print) are paid above a nominal price.

17. Publication of Statement of Ownership
☒ If the publication is a general publication, publication of this statement is required. Will be printed
in the DECEMBER 2017 issue of this publication.   ☐ Publication not required.

18. Signature and Title of Editor, Publisher, Business Manager, or Owner

STEPHEN R. BUSHING - INVENTORY DISTRIBUTION CONTROL MANAGER

Date 9/18/2017

I certify that all information furnished on this form is true and complete. I understand that anyone who furnishes false or misleading information on this form or who omits material or information requested on the form may be subject to criminal sanctions (including fines and imprisonment) and/or civil sanctions (including civil penalties).

PS Form 3526, July 2014 (Page 3 of 4)   PRIVACY NOTICE: See our privacy policy on www.usps.com

PS Form 3526, July 2014 [Page 1 of 4 (see instructions page 4)]   PSN 7530-01-000-9931   PRIVACY NOTICE: See our privacy policy on www.usps.com

Moving?

Make sure your subscription moves with you!

To notify us of your new address, find your **Clinics Account Number** (located on your mailing label above your name), and contact customer service at:

Email: journalscustomerservice-usa@elsevier.com

800-654-2452 (subscribers in the U.S. & Canada)
314-447-8871 (subscribers outside of the U.S. & Canada)

Fax number: 314-447-8029

Elsevier Health Sciences Division
Subscription Customer Service
3251 Riverport Lane
Maryland Heights, MO 63043

*To ensure uninterrupted delivery of your subscription, please notify us at least 4 weeks in advance of move.

Printed and bound by CPI Group (UK) Ltd, Croydon, CR0 4YY

03/10/2024

01040395-0009